Ethics in Medical Coding

MEDICAL NECESSITY DOCUMENTATION BUNDLING COMPLIANCE OVERCODING UNDERCODING FRAUD WASTE ICD-10
TION COMORBIDITIES INTRACTABLE SEQUELAE PAYMENT DIFFERENTIAL MACROECONOMICS RIGHTS THEORY MOD
ONOMIES OF SCALE SITUATIONAL ETHICS ENTITLEMENT MENTALITY LATERALITY MORBIDITY TRANSPOSITION U
NT ACUTE CONDITION INDIVIDUAL ETHICS PRICE CONTROLS COMMENSURATE METAETHICS UNDERCODING ORGA
ETAL ETHICS MORTALITY CLEAN CLAIM DE FACTO ARBITERS SEQUELAE LATE EFFECT CAPITATED OVERCODIN
NTOLOGICAL ETHICS FRAUD COMPLIANCE PROGRAM REVENUE TELEOLOGICAL ETHICS OPHTHALMIC APPLIED ET
DITIES PAY-FOR-PERFORMANCE OCCUPATIONAL ETHICS HIPAA PROACTIVE APPROACH SUPERBILLS COPAYMENT B
AFFIRMATIVE UNETHICAL ACT VIRTUE ETHICS ACCOMMODATIVE APPROACH NORMATIVE ETHICS COINSURANCE I
APPROACH TEMPLATE EHR MEDICAL NECESSITY DOCUMENTATION BUNDLING COMPLIANCE OVERCODING UNDERC
TLEMENT CONDITION BUNDLING DIFFERENTIAL COMORBIDITIES INTRACTABLE SEQUELAE PAYMENT DIFFERENTIA
LATE EFFECT OVERCODING SEQUELAE INTRACTABLE ECONOMIES OF SCALE SITUATIONAL ETHICS ENTITLEMENT
ANSPOSITION UNBUNDLING JUSTICE THEORY EMERGENT ACUTE CONDITION INDIVIDUAL ETHICS PRICE CONTROL
CODING ORGANIZATIONAL ETHICS SUBORDINATES SOCIETAL ETHICS MORTALITY CLEAN CLAIM DE FACTO ARBI
D OVERCODING GLOBAL PROCEDURE NEOPLASMS DEONTOLOGICAL ETHICS FRAUD COMPLIANCE PROGRAM REVE
MIC APPLIED ETHICS DIFFERENTIAL DIAGNOSIS COMORBIDITIES PAY-FOR-PERFORMANCE OCCUPATIONAL ETHICS
BILLS COPAYMENT BUNDLING CODIFICATION CREDENTIAL AFFIRMATIVE UNETHICAL ACT VIRTUE ETHICS ACCOM
ICS COINSURANCE DUE DILLIGENCE OBSTRUCTIONIST APPROACH TEMPLATE EHR MEDICAL NECESSITY DOCUME
VERCODING UNDERCODING FRAUD WASTE ICD-10 ACUTE CONDITION BUNDLING CODIFICATION COMORBIDITIES I
ENTIAL MACROECONOMICS RIGHTS THEORY MODIFIERS EXTRAPOLATION INTRACTABLE MOTALITY WASTE FRAUD
ENT MENTALITY LATERALITY MORBIDITY TRANSPOSITION UNBUNDLING JUSTICE THEORY EMERGENT ACUTE CO
NTROLS COMMENSURATE METAETHICS UNDERCODING ORGANIZATIONAL ETHICS SUBORDINATES SOCIETAL ETHICS
ARBITERS SEQUELAE LATE EFFECT CAPITATED OVERCODING GLOBAL PROCEDURE NEOPLASMS DEONTOLOGICAL
TELEOLOGICAL ETHICS OPHTHALMIC DIFFERENTIAL DIAGNOSIS COMORBIDITIES PAY-FOR-PERFORMANCE OCCUPA
ROACH SUPERBILLS COPAYMENT BUNDLING CODIFICATION CREDENTIAL AFFIRMATIVE VIRTUE ETHICS ACCOMMO
CS COINSURANCE DUE DILLIGENCE OBSTRUCTIONIST APPROACH EHR MEDICAL NECESSITY DOCUMENTATION BU
AUD WASTE ICD-10 ACUTE CONDITION BUNDLING CODIFICATION COMORBIDITIES INTRACTABLE SEQUELAE PAYM
RIGHTS THEORY MODIFIERS EXTRAPOLATION INTRACTABLE ECONOMIES OF SCALE SITUATIONAL ETHICS ENTI
ETAL ETHICS MORTALITY CLEAN CLAIM DE FACTO ARBITERS SEQUELAE LATE EFFECT CAPITATED OVERCODIN
NTOLOGICAL ETHICS FRAUD COMPLIANCE PROGRAM REVENUE TELEOLOGICAL ETHICS OPHTHALMIC APPLIED ET
DITIES PAY-FOR-PERFORMANCE OCCUPATIONAL ETHICS HIPAA PROACTIVE APPROACH SUPERBILLS COPAYMENT B
FFIRMATIVE UNETHICAL ACT VIRTUE ETHICS ACCOMMODATIVE APPROACH NORMATIVE ETHICS DUE DILLIGENCE
ATE EHR MEDICAL NECESSITY DOCUMENTATION BUNDLING COMPLIANCE OVERCODING UNDERCODING FRAUD W
DLING CODIFICATION COMORBIDITIES DIFFERENTIAL MACROECONOMICS RIGHTS THEORY MODIFIERS EXTRAPOLA

Ethics in Medical Coding
Theory and Practice

Bradley Hart, MBA, MS, CMPE, CPC, COBGC

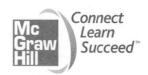

Mc Graw Hill

Connect
Learn
Succeed™

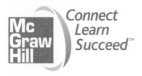

ETHICS IN MEDICAL CODING: THEORY AND PRACTICE

Published by McGraw-Hill, a business unit of The McGraw-Hill Companies, Inc., 1221 Avenue of the Americas, New York, NY, 10020. Copyright © 2013 by The McGraw-Hill Companies, Inc. All rights reserved. Printed in the United States of America. No part of this publication may be reproduced or distributed in any form or by any means, or stored in a database or retrieval system, without the prior written consent of The McGraw-Hill Companies, Inc., including, but not limited to, in any network or other electronic storage or transmission, or broadcast for distance learning.

Some ancillaries, including electronic and print components, may not be available to customers outside the United States.

This book is printed on acid-free paper.

1 2 3 4 5 6 7 8 9 0 QDB/QDB 1 0 9 8 7 6 5 4 3 2

ISBN 978-0-07-337493-2
MHID 0-07-337493-8

Vice president/Director of marketing: *Alice Harra*
Editorial director: *Michael S. Ledbetter*
Senior sponsoring editor: *Natalie J. Ruffatto*
Director, digital products: *Crystal Szewczyk*
Managing development editor: *Michelle L. Flomenhoft*
Development editor: *Raisa Priebe Kreek*
Executive marketing manager: *Roxan Kinsey*
Director, Editing/Design/Production: *Jess Ann Kosic*
Project manager: *Jean R. Starr*

Buyer II: *Sherry L. Kane*
Senior designer: *Anna Kinigakis*
Senior photo research coordinator: *John C. Leland*
Manager, digital production: *Janean A. Utley*
Media project manager: *Brent dela Cruz*
Media project manager: *Cathy L. Tepper*
Cover design: *Cody Wallis*
Interior design: *Kay Lieberherr*
Typeface: *10.5/13 Palatino*
Compositor: *MPS Limited, a Macmillan Company*
Printer: *Quad/Graphics*

Credits: *The credits section for this book begins on page 450 and is considered an extension of the copyright page.*

Library of Congress Cataloging-in-Publication Data

Hart, Bradley.
    Ethics in medical coding : theory and practice / Bradley Hart.
        p. ; cm.
    Includes bibliographical references and index.
    ISBN-13: 978-0-07-337493-2 (alk. paper)
    ISBN-10: 0-07-337493-8 (alk. paper)
    I. Title.
    [DNLM: 1. Clinical Coding--ethics--United States. 2. Attitude of Health Personnel—United States. 3. Clinical Coding--methods--United States. 4. Clinical Coding--standards--United States. 5. Guideline Adherence--ethics--United States. W 80]
    174.29073--dc23
                                                                2011040643

www.mhhe.com

Brief Contents

Chapter 1

Defining Coding: The Accurate Reporting of Medical Services 1

PART I THE FUNDAMENTALS OF ETHICS 29

Chapter 2

Ethics and the Importance of Ethical Systems 30

Chapter 3

Why Ethical Dilemmas Occur 70

About the Author

Brad Hart, MBA, MS, CMPE, CPC, COBGC, earned a BA in Bible and pastoral ministry from Central Bible College, a master's of science degree in health care administration from Des Moines University–Osteopathic Medical Center, and a master's of business administration degree from the University of Iowa. Committed to lifelong learning, he has maintained involvement in education and teaching by serving as a faculty member for the American Congress of Obstetricians and Gynecologists' Coding Workshops and as an adjunct faculty member in the MHA program at Des Moines University–Osteopathic Medical Center. He frequently speaks at national and regional conferences on topics related to health care administration, with an emphasis on the revenue cycle and billing and coding.

Hart brings an intense focus on practical application in his teaching through his more than 20 years' experience in health care administration, billing, and coding. Starting as an administrative assistant at an HMO, he became a reimbursement analyst at an academic health center clinic system and was promoted to director of the patient billing services department. Over the next 13 years, he was the administrator of several OB/GYN and OB/GYN subspecialty clinics, including one of the leading fertility clinics in the country. During this time, he started Reproductive Medicine Administrative Consulting, Inc. (RMACI), which provides billing, coding, and financial consulting services to clinics around the country.

He has achieved recognition as a Certified Medical Practice Executive (CMPE) by the American College of Medical Practice Executives (ACMPE), the certification body of the Medical Group Management Association (MGMA). Additionally, he is a Certified Professional Coder (CPC) through the American Academy of Professional Coders (AAPC) with subspecialty credentials as a Certified Obstetrics and Gynecology Coder (COBGC).

Hart lives in West Orange, New Jersey, with his wife and is blessed to have two daughters. He is actively involved in his church and enjoys reading and continuous learning.

No matter where you work, everyday tasks, challenges, and conflicts can make it hard to make the right choices and behave ethically. In the field of health care, where patients, physicians, and payers intersect, ethical decisions can be even more complex. Medical coders and billers, who coordinate the relationships between all of these parties, play a crucial role in managing the financial, legal, and personal pressures within the health care system. Choosing the most appropriate code to report a service, or submitting a claim less quickly to ensure its accuracy first, are some of the many tough decisions awaiting coders and billers in today's world of health care.

But behaving ethically doesn't have to be a negative decision, and you don't have to make that decision alone. *Ethics in Medical Coding* gives you the tools to make ethical choices by demonstrating that these choices can actually contribute to a more positive, compliant, and profitable medical practice overall. *Ethics* walks you through the potential challenges of correctly coding for diagnoses and services and shows how ethical coding leads to a positive revenue cycle by reducing claim denials and processing time. *Ethics in Medical Coding* also explores technologies and trends in health care, from EHRs to ICD-10, equipping you to make ethical and legally compliant choices in a changing health care field. Throughout the book, case studies and questions illustrate the subtleties of ethical behavior, preparing you to make ethical decisions in any aspect of health care administration.

Here's What Instructors and Students Can Expect from *Ethics in Medical Coding*

- A book by Brad Hart, MBA, MS, CMPE, CPC, COBGC, an experienced medical practice professional, coder, and instructor.
- Dedicated chapters about new trends and challenges in health care ethics, including ICD-10-CM,

EHRs recent legislation, and compliance programs.
- A practical, case-based approach to understanding and applying ethical choices.
- Presentation of ethics in context—how coding and billing intersect to produce ethical dilemmas.
- Tools for making ethical choices in all health care settings.
- Comprehensive explanation of how coders can navigate the difficult choices posed by both procedural and diagnostic coding.

Here's How Instructors Have Described *Ethics in Medical Coding*

"This book is fabulous. It presents coding ethical challenges in a practical, easy to understand fashion, with real-life examples."

Nancy Parent, MBA, CPC, Seacoast Career Schools

"Expresses the importance of compliance by great examples. . . . Hart captures all the topics needed for students to understand ethics in coding."

Angela Hennessy, MS, Corning Community College

"The writing style was unique and refreshing. I have read numerous books on coding and other books on ethics, but this is the first book that unites the two to this depth."

Marybeth Pieri-Smith, RHIA, CCS-P, CPC, CMA, Davenport University

"This book will be an excellent addition to any coding program. Ethics is a necessity especially in light of the economy and upcoming changes in medical documentation and billing. Helping students to understand and prioritize ethical behavior prior to being in the workforce is a must. Great book!"

Jerri Rowe, MA, CPC, MedVance Institute

Organization of *Ethics in Medical Coding*

Ethics in Medical Coding consists of an introductory chapter followed by three parts:

Part	Coverage
Defining Coding: The Accurate Reporting of Medical Services	Chapter 1 defines the process of medical coding and shows how accurate code assignment involves ethical action, just as a journalist must act ethically in reporting a story.
Part 1: The Fundamentals of Ethics	Part 1 lays the groundwork for ethical coding by emphasizing the importance of ethics in the workplace and explaining the many ethical systems used in workplaces.
Part 2: Ethics in Coding	Part 2 traces the ethical implications and decisions related to procedural and diagnostic coding, including a focus on coding for E/M services and coding in ICD-10. Part 2 goes on to discuss the ethical implications of coding for the revenue cycle, as well as exploring how professional certification supports ethical coding. New issues in coding that affect ethics are also described in detail.
Part 3: Applying Ethical Principles	Part 3 equips students seeking coding certifications by providing strategies for avoiding ethical problems, as well as for resolving ethical problems when they occur.

Chapter-by-Chapter Highlights of *Ethics in Medical Coding*

- **Chapter 1** defines medical coding and explores the kinds of ethical challenges seen in the coding process.
- **Chapter 2** introduces the concept of ethics, discusses existing ethical systems, and emphasizes the importance of ethics in the workplace and beyond.
- **Chapter 3** explores the reasons why ethical dilemmas occur in professional situations, with a focus on the kinds of dilemmas that most often occur in medical coding and billing.
- **Chapter 4** explains the implications of health care financing and insurance on ethical coding.
- **Chapter 5** describes the potential ethical hazards in coding for E/M services and offers ways to remedy these issues.
- **Chapter 6** discusses ethical challenges when coding for surgical and procedural services.
- **Chapter 7** explores the ethical landscape of how to assign diagnosis codes accurately and honestly when documentation is unclear or when the third-party payment system introduces pressure.
- **Chapter 8** explains the impact of ICD-10 on the coding process and identifies ethical challenges that the transition may cause.
- **Chapter 9** dives deeper into the intersection between coding and billing, exploring how ethical, accurate coding is essential to a healthy revenue cycle and to the long-term prospects of medical practices.
- **Chapter 10** explains how professional certification supports coders in acting ethically.
- **Chapter 11** discusses new trends and issues in coding ethics, from legislation to technology.
- **Chapter 12** offers methods for avoiding ethical problems by establishing and maintaining ethical practices in the workplace.
- **Chapter 13** proposes strategies for solving ethical problems when they do occur.

To the Instructor

McGraw-Hill knows how much effort it takes to prepare for a new course. Through focus groups, symposia, reviews, and conversations with instructors like you, we have gathered information about what materials you need to facilitate successful courses. We are committed to providing you with high-quality, accurate instructor support.

Instructor Resources

You can rely on the following materials to help you and your students work through the exercises in the book:

- Instructor Edition of the Online Learning Center (OLC) at **www.mhhe.com/codingethics**. Your McGraw-Hill sales representative can provide you with access and show you how to "go green" with our online instructor support. The OLC contains a number of resources to assist you in planning and teaching your course:

Resource	Description
Instructor's Manual (organized by Learning Outcomes)	Lesson plans and sample syllabi to assist you in incorporating ethics into your course
	Answer keys for end-of-section and end-of-chapter questions
PowerPoints (organized by Learning Outcomes)	Key Terms
	Key Concepts
	Teaching Notes
Electronic Testbank	Available as Word documents or within EZ Test Online (computerized)
	Questions are tagged with:
	• Learning Outcome
	• Level of Difficulty
	• Level of Bloom's Taxonomy
	• Feedback
Tools to Plan Course	Correlations of the Learning Outcomes to Accrediting Bodies such as CAHIIM, ABHES, and CAAHEP
	Sample Syllabi and Lesson Plans
	Asset Map—clickable PDF with links to all key supplements, broken down by Learning Outcomes

Need Help with the Book? Contact McGraw-Hill Higher Education's Customer Experience Team

Visit our Customer Experience Team Support website at www.mhhe.com/support. Browse our FAQs (Frequently Asked Questions) and product documentation, and/or contact a Customer Experience Team representative. The Customer Experience Team is available Sunday through Friday.

CodeitRightOnline™: Your Online Coding Tool

So that your students can gain experience with the use of an online coding tool, they will have access for a 14-day period to CodeitRightOnline, produced by Contexo Media, a division of Access Intelligence. CodeItRightOnline is available online at **www.codeitrightonline.com**.

Features

Features offered with a subscription to CodeItRightOnline include:

- CodeitRightOnline Search—The ability to find a CPT, HCPCS Level II, or ICD-9-CM code either using the Index or Tabular search sections, by code terminology, description, keyword, or code number to locate the correct code.

- Coding Crosswalks—Essential coding links from CPT codes to ICD-9-CM to HCPCS Level II codes and to Anesthesia codes.

- Articles from CMS, OIG, carriers, intermediaries, payers, and other government websites along with newsletter articles from AMA, AHA, Decision Health, Coding Institute, and others.

- ICD-10-CM/PCS Code Sets—Helps you prepare for 2013 mandatory implementation with ICD-10-CM/PCS full code sets and descriptions.

- NCCI Edits Validator™—Validates codes to help you remain in compliance with the correct coding guidelines established by the Centers for Medicare and Medicaid Services (CMS).

- Build-A-Code™—Allows students to build codes from the ground up, helping them understand how ICD-10 codes are constructed.

- Interactive tools that help reinforce the student's knowledge of anatomy.

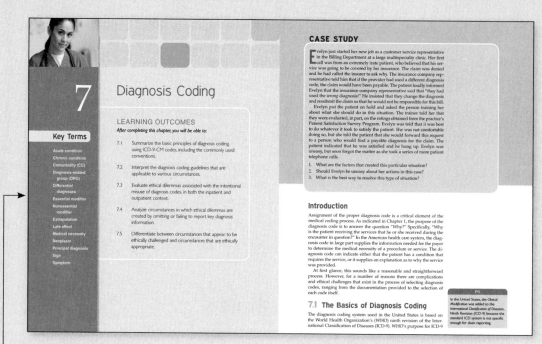

Chapter Opener

The **chapter opener** sets the stage for what will be learned in the chapter.
Learning Outcomes are written to reflect the revised version of Bloom's Taxonomy and to establish the key points the student should focus on in the chapter. In addition, major chapter heads are structured to reflect the Learning Outcomes and are numbered accordingly.
Key Terms are first introduced in the chapter opener so the student can see them all in one place.
A chapter-opening **case study** highlights the ethical decisions that will be further discussed throughout the chapter.

Learning Aids

Key Terms are bolded and defined in the margin so that students will become familiar with the language of coding. These are reinforced in the **Glossary** at the end of the book.

Commodities
Articles of trade or commerce; something useful that can be turned to commercial or other advantage.

CODING TIP

It's important to phrase questions appropriately so that patients aren't allowed to passively answer questions incorrectly.

FYI

Medical coding did not exist until much later in the development of the U.S. health care system. There were no health insurance companies until the 1930s.

WARNING

Just because preoperative services are provided more than one day in advance of a surgical procedure does not mean that the services are automatically separately billable.

COMPLIANCE TIP

Concerns about compliance became an issue when additional parties were introduced to the health care system. When medical services were originally a direct transaction between patient and provider, reporting was not necessary. The primary purpose of compliance programs is to ensure that reporting is consistent with the services actually delivered.

BILLING TIP

Each medical practice should ensure that the length of its billing cycle is appropriate. Billing cycles that are too long or too short can be equally ineffective and potentially wasteful.

Tips

Coding Tips and **FYI** features highlight helpful information for students.
Warning features point out areas where coders and billers should pay special attention to avoid ethical problems.
Compliance Tips emphasize the link between ethical choices and compliance with regulations.
Billing Tips demonstrate the link between coding, billing, and ethics.

Guided Tour

Exercises

Thinking It Through questions within the chapter prompt students to recall and think critically about each topic.

Thinking It Through 9.1

1. Coding is a critical part of the entire revenue cycle, but it is not the only part. Rank the five stages of the revenue cycle in order, from most important to least important. Explain the basis for your opinion.

2. Based on your personal experience with the medical industry, where have you seen the most significant problems in the revenue cycle of the practices from which you have received services? What caused you to form this opinion?

3. Failure to have an effective revenue cycle can have an obvious financial impact. What other possible effects could an ineffective revenue cycle have on nonfinancial elements of the practice?

4. Before we examine the ethics of the revenue cycle, what do you think is the most significant opportunity for ethical issues within the cycle? Why?

End-of-Chapter Resources

The **Chapter Summary** is in a tabular, step-by-step format with page references to help with review of the materials.

The **Chapter Review** contains the following questions, all tagged by Learning Outcomes: multiple-choice, short answer, and Applying Your Knowledge (applying what was learned in chapter-opening case study) to test students' critical thinking skills. Internet Research activities train students to use online resources for further education in coding and ethics.

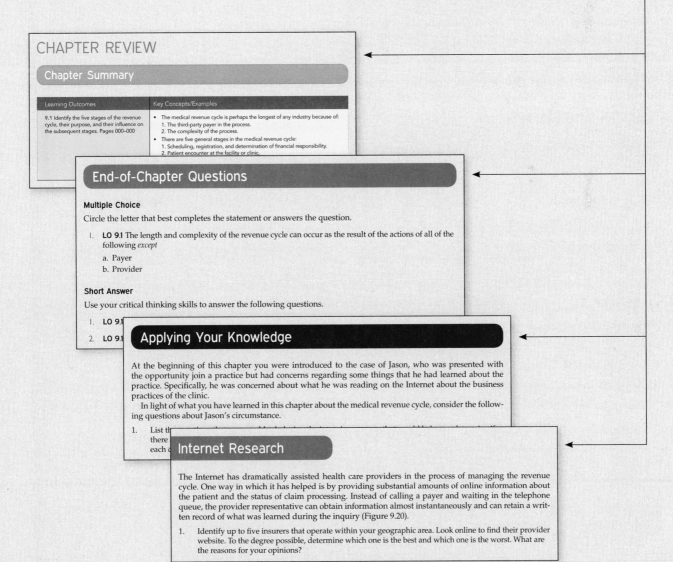

CHAPTER REVIEW

Chapter Summary

Learning Outcomes	Key Concepts/Examples
9.1 Identify the five stages of the revenue cycle, their purpose, and their influence on the subsequent stages. Pages 000–000	• The medical revenue cycle is perhaps the longest of any industry because of: 1. The third-party payer in the process. 2. The complexity of the process. • There are five general stages in the medical revenue cycle: 1. Scheduling, registration, and determination of financial responsibility. 2. Patient encounter at the facility or clinic.

End-of-Chapter Questions

Multiple Choice

Circle the letter that best completes the statement or answers the question.

1. **LO 9.1** The length and complexity of the revenue cycle can occur as the result of the actions of all of the following *except*
   a. Payer
   b. Provider

Short Answer

Use your critical thinking skills to answer the following questions.

1. LO 9.1
2. LO 9.1

Applying Your Knowledge

At the beginning of this chapter you were introduced to the case of Jason, who was presented with the opportunity join a practice but had concerns regarding some things that he had learned about the practice. Specifically, he was concerned about what he was reading on the Internet about the business practices of the clinic.

In light of what you have learned in this chapter about the medical revenue cycle, consider the following questions about Jason's circumstance.

1. List th
   there
   each

Internet Research

The Internet has dramatically assisted health care providers in the process of managing the revenue cycle. One way in which it has helped is by providing substantial amounts of online information about the patient and the status of claim processing. Instead of calling a payer and waiting in the telephone queue, the provider representative can obtain information almost instantaneously and can retain a written record of what was learned during the inquiry (Figure 9.20).

1. Identify up to five insurers that operate within your geographic area. Look online to find their provider website. To the degree possible, determine which one is the best and which one is the worst. What are the reasons for your opinions?

Acknowledgments

Suggestions have been received from faculty and students throughout the country. We rely on this vital feedback with all of our books. Each person who has offered comments and suggestions has our thanks.

The efforts of many people are needed to develop and improve a product. Among these people are the reviewers and consultants who point out areas of concern, cite areas of strength, and make recommendations for change. In this regard, the following instructors provided feedback that was enormously helpful in preparing *Ethics in Medical Coding*.

Workshops

In 2010 and 2011, McGraw-Hill conducted 13 health professions workshops, providing an opportunity for more than 700 faculty members to gain continuing education credits as well as to provide feedback on our products.

Book Reviews

Many instructors participated in manuscript reviews throughout the development of the book.

Gina M. Augustine, MLS, RT, RHIT, CPC, CPC-H, CPhT
Fortis College

Gerry A. Brasin, CMA (AAMA), CPC
Premier Education Group

Lisa G. Bynoe, MBA
Argosy University

Mary M. Cantwell, RHIT, CPC, CPC-I, CPC-H, CPC-P
Metro Community College

Rhoda Cooper, CPC, RMC, NCICS
Piedmont Virginia Community College

Gerard G. Cronin, BS, DC
Salem Community College

Ruth E. Dearborn, CCS, CCS-P
University of Alaska Southeast

Laurie Dennis, CBCS
Florida Career College

Amy Ensign, CMA (AAMA), RMA (AMT)
Baker College of Clinton Township

Madeline Flanagan, MA, CPC
Branford Hall Career Institute

Paula Hagstrom, MM, RHIA
Ferris State University

Greg Hartnett, BS, CPC, HIA, MHP
Sanford-Brown Institute

Angela G. Hennessy, MS
Corning Community College

Jennifer Lame, MPH, RHIT
Southwest Wisconsin Technical College

JanMarie C. Malik, MBA, RHIA
Shasta Community College

Barbara Marchelletta, CMA (AAMA), CPC, CPT
Beal College

Phillip A. Mayo, CPC
Premier Education Group

Lane Miller, MBA/HCM
Medical Careers Institute

Vivian Mills, RHIT, CPAR, CPC
Virginia College

Kathleen O'Gorman, BS, CPC
Tunxis Community College

Nancy R. Parent, CPC, MBA
Seacoast Career Schools

Tatyana G. Pashnyak, COI
Bainbridge College

Marybeth Pieri-Smith, MBA, RHIA, CCS-P, CPC, CMA
Davenport University

Ponsella Poindexter, AA, AHI, CMAS
Fortis College

Kimberly Rash
Gateway Community and Technical College

Christine D. Ringer, BS
Pittsburgh Technical Institute

Diane Roche Benson, CMA (AAMA), BSHCA, MSA, CFP, CPC, CMRS, NSC-SCFAT, ASE, CDE, AHA BCLS, PALS, ACLS, CCT, NCI-I
Johnston County Community College
University of Phoenix
Wake Technical Community College

Jerri Rowe, MA, CPC
MedVance Institute

Chris Schram, DBA, CCS-P
Corinthian College

Gene Simon, RHIA, RMD
Florida Career College

Anna M. Slaski, JD
Brookline College

Patricia A. Stich, MA, CCS-P
Waubonsee Community College

John Varas, MSCIS, CCS, CPC
Florida Career College

Jennifer Williams, RHIA, RMA
Neosho County Community College

Jane F. Yakicic, CMA, CCS-P
Cambria-Rowe Business College

Carole Zeglin, MS, BS, MT, RMA
Westmoreland County Community College

Accuracy Panel

A panel of instructors completed a technical edit and review of all content in the book page proofs to verify its accuracy, along with the supplements.

Laurie Dennis, CBCS
Florida Career College

Barbara L Donnally, CPC
University of Rio Grande

Kelly A. Dudden, CPC, CPMA
Cayuga Community College

Madeline Flanagan, MA, CPC
Branford Hall Career Institute

Mary Beth Finn, M.Ed., CST, CSS, MCP
Herzing University

Nancy R. Parent, CPC, MBA
Seacoast Career Schools

Jane F. Yakicic, CMA, CCS-P
Cambria-Rowe Business College

Susan Zolvinski, BS, MBA
Brown Mackie College-Michigan City

Acknowledgments from the Author

I want to take this opportunity to thank the editorial team at McGraw-Hill. First, to Natalie Ruffatto and Michelle Flomenhoft—thank you for embracing my vision and taking a chance in giving an opportunity to a rookie. Next, to Raisa Kreek, whose consistent, enthusiastic encouragement and patient guidance kept me focused on the task—I am deeply grateful.

I would also like to thank project manager Jean Starr and copyeditor Sharon O'Donnell, who took my words and thoughts and made them better. Senior designer Anna Kinigakis created a terrific design, which was implemented through the production process by Jean Starr, along with Sherry Kane, senior buyer; John Leland, photo research coordinator; and Cathy Tepper, media project manager.

Thank you to all of the instructors and professors who kindly gave of their time to review my first drafts and provide suggestions for improvement and enhancement of the material. The students are unquestionably beneficiaries of your input.

Finally, to my wife Mary Lou—who understands my passion for coding and teaching and endlessly supported my efforts to write this text—thank you for believing in me more than I believe in myself. And thanks to my daughters Katelyn and Emily, who gave up some time with Dad to let him do something that he wanted to do in order to make a difference.

Brad Hart, MBA, MS, CMPE, CPC, COBGC

A COMMITMENT TO ACCURACY

You have a right to expect an accurate textbook, and McGraw-Hill invests considerable time and effort to make sure that we deliver one. Listed below are the many steps we take to make sure this happens.

OUR ACCURACY VERIFICATION PROCESS

First Round—Development Reviews

STEP 1: Numerous **health professions instructors** review the draft manuscript and report on any errors that they may find. The **author** makes these corrections in his final manuscript.

Second Round—Page Proofs

STEP 2: Once the manuscript has been typeset, the **author** checks his manuscript against the page proofs to ensure that all illustrations, graphs, examples, and exercises have been correctly laid out on the pages, and that all codes have been updated correctly.

STEP 3: An outside panel of **peer instructors** completes a review of content in the page proofs to verify its accuracy. The **author** adds these corrections to his review of the page proofs.

STEP 4: A **proofreader** adds a triple layer of accuracy assurance in pages by looking for errors; then a confirming, corrected round of page proofs is produced.

Third Round—Confirming Page Proofs

STEP 5: The **author** reviews the confirming round of page proofs to make certain that any previous corrections were properly made and to look for any errors he might have missed on the first round.

STEP 6: The **project manager,** who has overseen the book from the beginning, performs **a final check of proofread pages to confirming proof** to make sure that no new errors have been introduced during the production process.

Final Round—Printer's Proofs

STEP 7: The **project manager** performs a **final check** of the book during the printing process, providing a final accuracy review. In concert with the main text, all supplements undergo a proofreading and technical editing stage to ensure their accuracy.

RESULTS

What results is a textbook that is as accurate and error-free as is humanly possible. Our authors and publishing staff are confident that the many layers of quality assurance have produced books that are leaders in the industry for their integrity and correctness. *Please view the Acknowledgments section for more details on the many people involved in this process.*

1st Round
Author's Manuscript

Multiple Rounds of Review by Health Professions Instructors

2nd Round
Typeset Pages

Accuracy Checks by
- Author
- Peer Instructors
- 1st Proofreader

3rd Round
Typeset Pages

Accuracy Checks by
- Author
- 2nd Proofreader

Final Round
Printing

Accuracy Checks by
Final Proofreader

Supplements
- Proofreading
- Accuracy Checks

Defining Coding: The Accurate Reporting of Medical Services

LEARNING OUTCOMES

After completing this chapter, you will be able to:

1.1 Formulate and communicate a basic definition of medical coding.

1.2 Differentiate between the various code sets used to report medical services.

1.3 Describe the forms used by health care entities to report medical services.

1.4 Explain the direct correlation between the six key elements of journalism and the task of medical coding.

Key Terms

Adjudicate
Ambulatory surgery
    center
Cognitive
Commensurate
Complicit
Credential
Exploratory
Fraud
Global period
Incident to
Iteration
Morbidity
Mortality
Non-participating
Obsolete
Ophthalmic
Outpatient surgery
    center
Participating
Payment differential
Resource Based
    Relative Value
    Scale (RBRVS)
Standardized
Transposition
Venue
Verification

CASE STUDY

Medical coding can be thought of as a way to gather and report information accurately. In this respect, it bears many similarities to journalism. Just as in journalism, there are specific ethical guidelines that apply to the performance of medical coding. In addition, both journalists and coders are required to interpret the situations they face in light of these ethical guidelines.

Jayson Blair was a rising star with a significant interest in journalism. As a high school student in Clifton, Virginia, he asked to interview the new school principal for the student newspaper just minutes after she was introduced to the faculty. He majored in journalism at the University of Maryland, becoming editor-in-chief of the student newspaper for the 1996–1997 school year. At that time there was some controversy related to his tenure when 30 staff members wrote a letter to the board of directors of the newspaper, citing four serious errors as a reporter and editor—going as far as to call his integrity into question. In one specific incident, Blair wrote a story about the death of a student who allegedly died due to a cocaine overdose when, in fact, the student died of a heart ailment. The board took no action against Blair.

In the summer of 1997, he obtained a prestigious internship at the *Boston Globe.* In the summer of 1998, Blair secured an extended internship at the *New York Times.* He told the *Times* that he had to complete some coursework to graduate, which the *Times* agreed to defer. During his 10 weeks at the *Times,* he wrote 19 news articles and assisted other reporters. Generally, he was positively regarded, although some staff members were concerned about his perceived overemphasis on socializing.

Blair returned to the *New York Times* in June 1999 when he was hired as a reporter in the Police Bureau, reporting on the crimes of the day. The *Times* assumed that he had graduated from the University of Maryland. In reality, he needed to complete more than a year's coursework to obtain a degree ("Times Reporter Who Resigned," 2003).

Jayson Blair showed that he could produce articles very quickly and he worked long hours. In November of 1999, he was promoted to an intermediate reporter, which was the next step toward being a full-time staff reporter. Several editors working with Blair expressed concern to one another and directly to him that his work was, at times, sloppy. He promised to improve his accuracy while, at the same time, engaging in behavior that was reckless, such as charging expenses from a local bar to the *Times,* taking company cars for extended periods, and distributing confidential internal memos.

However, his popularity grew within the newspaper. He made a special effort to get to know the newsroom support staff and compliment other writers on specific elements of their stories. One editor stated that he had "remarkable charisma." As a result, in January 2001 he was made a full-time reporter. However, this did not change the charges of inaccuracy and poor performance. In fact, his performance became worse.

Following the attacks on September 11, 2001, Blair claimed that he lost a cousin in the attack on the Pentagon and used that as a reason for him not to participate in a series of articles on the victims of the attack.

It was later discovered that he had no relationship with the man or his family. In the chaotic atmosphere of the times, including fear of future attacks, anthrax scares, and so on Blair's behavior became more erratic and his errors more frequent, although this was attributed to the stress that many were feeling.

Blair's undoing was his assignment to cover the Washington, DC, sniper situation in October 2002. A native of the area, he wrote compelling stories about the victims of the sniper, including detailed interviews with the victims' families. He filed reports indicating that he was on the scene in the Washington area, but in fact he never left New York. He interviewed the family members—on the telephone, not in person. He created careful descriptions of details of the family homes by observing news reports by other interviewers—he never actually set foot in their homes. To make matters worse, other reporters began to complain that he was plagiarizing their work by taking large sections of their work and claiming it as his own. However, the families that were interviewed were thrilled with his reporting, and told the *Times* in letters to the editor.

1. If you were Blair's supervisor, would his behavior have concerned you? Why or why not?
2. What elements of Blair's reporting practices seem problematic? Why were they problematic? Why were they not detected sooner?
3. Would you have hired Blair if you worked for the *New York Times*? Why or why not?
4. Do you see any connections between the job responsibilities of a journalist and a coder, based on what you read in this story? If so, what are they?

Introduction

This text will emphasize two primary themes throughout—ethics and medical coding (Figure 1.1). It will place the greatest focus on the intersection of these two important concepts. How do ethical considerations affect coding? How do the elements of coding create ethical dilemmas? Before these questions can be answered, the fundamentals of each concept must be examined, beginning with a working definition of each term. To clarify and encourage additional thoughts about

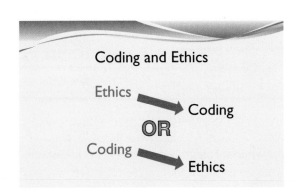

FIGURE 1.1
Coding and ethics: Which has the bigger influence? Do ethical considerations affect coding, or do coding rules, guidelines, and practices create ethical dilemmas? Or does it go both ways?

the definition of coding, throughout this chapter we will compare the profession of coding to the profession of journalism.

1.1 The Definition of *Medical Coding*

The majority of Americans are familiar with medical coding because they frequently see advertisements seeking coders to fill job opportunities. Often, these ads imply that learning to code is easy and money can be made from home. Internet search engines produce literally millions of results when the words "medical coding jobs" are entered (Figure 1.2). To a degree, it is true that coding is a unique job in that it can be successfully done outside the traditional office setting, making it an attractive option. In fact, a major women's magazine described medical coding as "one of eight legitimate ways someone can work from home" (Braff, 2009).

Although the perception of the public is that coding is easy to learn, it is not necessarily easy to define. What is medical coding?

PRACTICAL AND FUNDAMENTAL DEFINITIONS

There are many different definitions of *medical coding*. Some of them include:

Standardized
Universally used, understood, and accepted in the same fashion.

- "Medical coding is basically the process of applying formal, **standardized** medical codes to patient medical records" (*Medical Insurance Coding*, 2009).

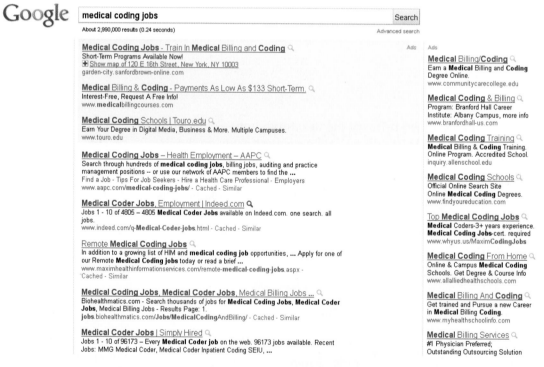

FIGURE 1.2

Internet search engines produce millions of results when a search is performed on the words "medical coding jobs."

- "Diagnostic and procedural information is translated by medical coders into easy numerical codes that can be electronically processed for payment by third party payers, [such as] insurance companies and Medicare, for example" (Dunn, 2008).
- "Millions of people get sick every day. The kinds of illnesses they suffer from range from mild to severe. Classifying these conditions and, in some cases, subsequent deaths is done with medical coding and billing. In order for a process of this magnitude to be successful, it has to be universally accepted" (Moss, 2009).
- "The placement of HCPCS codes—e.g., 99221 for an initial inpatient admission—on bills submitted to Medicare and other 3rd-party payers, identifying and defining the complexity of physician or other health care provider services" ("Coding," 2002).

Each of these definitions is technically correct. Some are more complete than others, but they all accurately describe one or more elements of the process. However, they ultimately do not capture the fundamental essence of the goals and activities of medical coding. In its simplest form, medical coding is about telling a story. In that respect, coding is very much like journalism. Journalism involves telling a story—but there are very specific guidelines and ethical considerations related to the process. Similar guidelines and considerations exist for coders.

To be effective, a journalist must follow certain nonnegotiable rules and principles, which are the same as the fundamental principles associated with medical coding and billing. These principles are shown in Table 1.1.

Coders, in essence, must adhere to the same principles. Their audience is different than a journalist's and the coder's tools are significantly different than those of the journalist. However, they ultimately do the same thing—tell a story in the context of key principles that must not be compromised.

CODING TIP

Many decisions related to coding are made easier when you look at coding as a means of telling the patient's story. "How can I best and most accurately describe this patient's situation?"

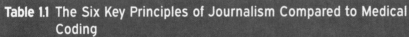

Table 1.1 The Six Key Principles of Journalism Compared to Medical Coding

Journalism	Medical Coding
First obligation is to the truth	Must be accurate and truthful at all times.
First loyalty is to citizens	Loyalty is to the truth and all parties involved in the transactions, including payers, providers, and patients.
Essence is the discipline of **verification**	Accuracy is not possible unless systems of verification are in place to ensure that what is reported reflects the service delivered.
Practitioners must maintain independence from those they cover	Coders must not code based on circumstances or individuals involved—they must be blind to the participants in the transaction.
The news must be comprehensive and proportional	Coders must reflect the services provided, ensuring that everything that should be coded/billed is reported and that the condition reported is appropriately stated.
Practitioners should be allowed to exercise their personal conscience	Coders should not be forced to engage in conduct that they find unethical or in violation of their personal moral code.

Verification
Evidence that establishes or confirms the validity or truth of something.

Source: Data on journalism from Pew Research Center's Project for Excellence in Journalism, 2006.

1. Of the various definitions of *medical coding* quoted on pages 4–5 which one do you believe best describes the role of the coder? Explain why you selected that particular definition.

2. Do you agree with the assertion that the six principles of journalism are directly linked to the role of coding? Why or why not? Which principle of journalism has the closest linkage to coding? The least? Support your answers.

3. Have you previously considered the similarities between journalism and coding? Are there other factors that link them together that were not presented? If so, what are they?

1.2 The Coder's Tools

Unlike the journalist, the coder has a very narrowly defined set of tools that are used to tell the story. Depending on the environment in which he or she is working, the tools are slightly different but the objective is still the same—to tell an accurate story to report data, obtain reimbursement, or both.

The Health Insurance Portability and Accountability Act of 1996 (HIPAA) requires that all health care providers use three code sets to report services. The Healthcare Common Procedure Coding System (HCPCS), which reports procedures performed, includes Current Procedure Terminology (CPT) and HCPCS Level II codes (Figure 1.3). The *International Classification of Diseases,* Ninth Edition, *Clinical Modification* (ICD-9-CM) provides the codes used to report patient diagnoses, although the 10th edition (ICD-10) is the designated diagnosis code set for all services provided on or after October 1, 2013.

CURRENT PROCEDURAL TERMINOLOGY, FOURTH EDITION (CPT-4)

CPT, which was introduced in 1966, is the only medical coding system owned by a private entity—the American Medical Association (AMA). It arose in connection with the Medicare program and supplied a tool by which physicians could conveniently report the procedures or

FIGURE 1.3

The chart illustrates the various components of HCPCS and their relationship to one another. Level III HCPCS codes were eliminated from use in 2000.

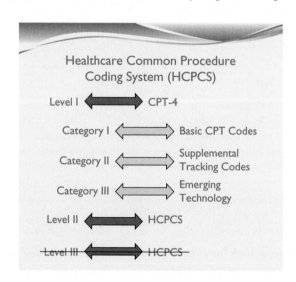

Healthcare Common Procedure Coding System (HCPCS)

Level I ⟷ CPT-4

Category I ⟷ Basic CPT Codes

Category II ⟷ Supplemental Tracking Codes

Category III ⟷ Emerging Technology

Level II ⟷ HCPCS

Level III ⟷ HCPCS

services provided to patients. Initially, the codes consisted of four digits and primarily described surgical procedures. The codes available to describe radiology, laboratory, and medicine services were extremely limited.

In 1970, a second edition (CPT-2) was published. The number of code digits increased to five and the range of services for which codes were created dramatically increased. The AMA published the third edition in the mid-1970s and published the current version, CPT-4, in 1977. New codes are created, existing codes are modified, and **obsolete** codes are deleted every year. Yet the fundamental structure and conventions of the system remain essentially unchanged to this day.

CPT codes are used by physician offices, **ambulatory** or **outpatient surgery centers** and, in some cases, hospitals to report the services provided to the patient. All of these entities must ensure that they remain aware of updates to the codes, which are issued on an annual basis and are placed into effect on January 1 of each year.

Category I.
There are three categories of CPT codes. Category I is, by far, the most commonly used and the one most thought of when CPT is discussed. Category I codes begin with CPT code 00100 and end with 99607, although they are not presented in numeric order in most CPT books. The Evaluation and Management (E/M) codes (CPT codes 99201–99607) appear first in the book because they are the most commonly used codes and are used across all specialties by all providers. These codes generally report **cognitive** and educational services, as opposed to procedural services.

Category II.
Category II CPT codes are a relatively new addition to the CPT manual. These codes have five digits—four numeric digits and one final alpha digit (the letter *F*). These codes do not report reimbursable services. Instead, they report various elements of services normally reported with E/M codes, like 99386 or 99214. Category II codes allow the provider—usually physicians—to obtain additional payment from payers who seek to compensate providers whose care meets certain defined criteria. For example, Category II CPT code 3077F is used to report that a patient with diabetes had an elevated blood pressure reading, an important marker to measure for a patient of this type. Ordinarily, taking the blood pressure of a diabetic with hypertension would be a component part of a code such as 99213 and would be reported only in the medical record. The physician does not directly receive extra payment for submitting 3077F, but the submission of the code indicates to Medicare through the billing record that quality service is being provided. If the quality standards are met, the provider receives a percentage bonus at the end of the year as a reward. The code system also supplies modifiers to report that a particular service ordinarily provided was not provided for a specific reason, such as 1000F-2P, which means a patient who smokes refused to participate in an assessment of his or her tobacco use. The patient's failure to cooperate does not result in a penalty to the physician.

Category III.
Category III CPT codes are also a relatively new addition to the CPT manual. The purpose of Category III codes is to give providers the opportunity to report new medical services for which a

Obsolete
No longer in general use, out-of-date.

Ambulatory surgery center
Often, a freestanding health care setting that provides relatively minor nonemergency surgical services.

Outpatient surgery center
Health care setting, often affiliated with a hospital or located in conjunction with a hospital facility that provides relatively minor surgical services.

Cognitive
Related to memory, judgment, and reasoning.

CODING TIP

The use of Category II CPT codes is optional and is not *directly* related to reimbursement. Additional reimbursement is obtained by using these codes to demonstrate "quality standards" that are supported by the documentation of the codes.

Category I CPT code has not yet been assigned. Category III codes are created using a different, lower standard than the Category I codes. The standards for creation of a Category I code are very high and it takes a code a long time to go through the process. However, medical advances are achieved faster than codes can be created. One of the criteria for establishing a Category I code is that it must be demonstrated that the procedure represented by the code is becoming the "standard of care." Providers, without Category III codes, did not have a way to report the new service and, therefore, could not prove that a procedure was commonly performed. Category III codes solve that problem by giving them a means to report new medical procedures. A Category III code must either be determined by the CPT panel to qualify as a Category I code within five years, or the code is removed from the book.

Category III codes are intended to be used to report reimbursable services. However, many payers will not cover services reported with a Category III code because policies often exclude payment for "experimental" services. Many services reported with a Category III code may fall into this category.

HEALTHCARE COMMON PROCEDURE CODING SYSTEM (HCPCS)

HCPCS (usually pronounced "hick-picks") codes were first created in 1978 and can be used by virtually every health care entity in the United States to report certain medical services, supplies, and equipment provided by the entity. Traditional HCPCS codes have five characters—an initial alpha character, followed by four numeric digits. The initial alpha character defines the category of service, while the remaining characters specify the individual service. For example, all *J* codes report injectible drugs and/or medications, while *E* codes are used to report durable medical equipment. All ambulance providers report their services using *A* codes.

The codes that describe the services, supplies, and medical equipment mentioned in the preceding paragraph are considered Level II HCPCS codes because the traditional CPT codes (CPT-4) are characterized as Level I HCPCS codes. This transition occurred in 1983 when the Health Care Financing Administration (HCFA) incorporated CPT codes into its HCPCS coding system. Therefore, all CPT-4 codes are HCPCS codes, but not all HCPCS codes are CPT-4 codes (see Figure 1.3).

HCPCS codes are managed by the Centers for Medicare and Medicaid Services (CMS) of the Department of Health and Human Services (HHS). CMS is the successor organization to HCFA. The Level I and II designations are organized in this fashion to indicate that a Level II code should not be used when a suitable Level I code exists to report the service. When an appropriate Level I code (CPT codes—which is the primary code set, published by the AMA) does not exist, the Level II code can and should be used.

To provide codes on a timely basis, HCPCS codes are published quarterly on the HHS website (Figure 1.4).

Prior to 2000, Level III HCPCS codes also existed. These were codes used by local insurers and payers—often state Medicaid programs—to

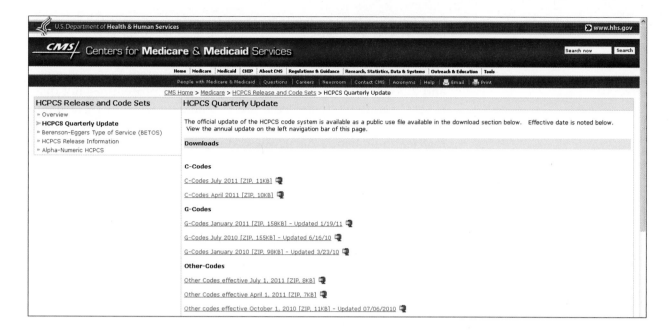

report special services for which there was no Level I or II code. Level III codes were eliminated in conjunction with the implementation of the "code set" element of HIPAA. HIPAA defined the code sets that were permissible for providers to use in reporting their services. HCPCS Level I (CPT-4) and HCPCS Level II were the only code sets authorized to report procedures, supplies, and other services to limit and streamline the unmanageable number of codes created by payers that previously existed.

INTERNATIONAL CLASSIFICATION OF DISEASES (ICD)

The *International Classification of Diseases*, Ninth Edition, *Clinical Modification* (ICD-9-CM) is the tool used by providers of all types and settings to report the diagnosis or diagnoses associated with the services provided, as well as sometimes defining the services and procedures delivered in the hospital setting. ICD-9, although used extensively in the U.S. health care system, did not originate in the United States. The ICD system is actually a product of the World Health Organization (WHO). Its purpose is to classify and facilitate the reporting of the causes of **morbidity** and **mortality** around the world, for the purpose of public health issues.

The U.S. health care system has taken the basic classification of diseases and added the Clinical Modification (the *CM* in ICD-9-CM), which allows a much greater degree of specificity than exists in the WHO system. WHO considers broad categories of disease, such as 250—Diabetes Mellitus—while third-party payers in the United States need more specificity, such as 250.53—Diabetes Mellitus, Type 1 with **ophthalmic** manifestations. This greater degree of specificity helps define the severity of the patient's condition and helps justify the level and quantity of service that the physician bills.

The ICD-9 system is published in three volumes. Volume 1 is the Tabular Index, in which the codes are listed in numeric order, ranging from 001.0 to E999.1. Volume 2 is the Alphabetic Index, where, as in the

---

FIGURE 1.4

On a quarterly basis, the Centers for Medicare and Medicaid Services (CMS) publishes updates to the HCPCS codes. These codes are found at **www.cms.hhs.gov**. For example, in 2009, during the outbreak of the H1N1 flu, CMS issued a HCPCS code (G9142—H1N1 flu vaccine) for providers to use before a CPT-4 code for that service (90663) could be published in January 2010.

FYI

The Clinical Modification (fourth and fifth digits) is what makes ICD-9 usable for reporting medical services and determining appropriate claim payment levels. ICD-9, as published by the World Health Organization, is not nearly specific enough for claim payment purposes.

Morbidity
The statistical reporting of the incidence of disease.

Mortality
The statistical reporting of the incidence of death.

Ophthalmic
Related to the eye.

traditional index of a book, key words and terms are listed in alphabetical order. Interestingly, most publishers print the ICD-9 codes with Volumes 1 and 2 in the same book—with Volume 2 first.

The codes in Volume 3 are significantly different than Volumes 1 and 2 because these codes report services and procedures, not diagnoses. In addition, these codes are available for use only by hospitals to report services delivered in the inpatient setting (National Center for Health Statistics, 2005). The codes each have either three or four digits and are organized by body system. While the diagnosis codes in Volumes 1 and 2 are used almost universally in the U.S. health care system, Volume 3 codes are used to a lesser degree, depending on the preference of the payer to whom the services are being reported. The codes in the ICD-9-CM book are published and made effective on October 1 of each year.

ICD-10-CM. The implementation of ICD-10-CM on October 1, 2013, will change the professional lives of nearly every medical coder in the United States. An entirely new code set needs to be learned, computer systems need to be changed to accommodate these different codes, and the same levels of productivity need to be maintained, which will be an enormous challenge.

ICD-10 has been adopted by nearly every country in the world. Leading countries, such as the United Kingdom, implemented ICD-10 in 1995, with France, Australia, Germany, and Canada following close behind. One of the major reasons for implementing ICD-10 is that it provides better data for detecting fraud and abuse (Centers for Medicare and Medicaid Services, 2008). Coders who are inclined to be less than fully truthful in reporting diagnosis codes will find it more challenging to do so with ICD-10.

On the other hand, ICD-10 may produce ethical dilemmas because of the fact that it is new. Coders and payers may not be fully familiar with proper coding or use of the codes, and their lack of knowledge may lead to misuse. Providers and coders may (knowingly or unknowingly) receive more payment than they are entitled to because of gaps or shortfalls in coding knowledge at some stage in the process. Similarly, providers may experience payment shortfalls if they are not diligent in obtaining adequate training on the use of ICD-10 codes.

Thinking It Through 1.2

1. Examine the three specific code sets discussed in this section (CPT, ICD-9, and HCPCS Level II). They are each owned/managed by different organizations. Is this good or bad, or does it matter? Why or why not?

2. CPT code changes are effective on January 1 of each year and ICD-9-CM code changes are effective on October 1 of each year. Why do you think there is a variance in the effective dates? What influence does the variance have on health care providers?

3. ICD-10 will make a significant change to coding in the U.S. health care system. Based on the information provided and a brief Internet search, what do you believe will be the most significant effect of this change?

1.3 Methods of Reporting Codes

Journalists have many communication tools at their disposal as well as a growing number of ways to distribute their work. While they still have the print and broadcast media to disseminate the news, they now also have Internet-based tools such as webcasts, blogs, and formal on-line news organizations. Coders, on the other hand, have relatively few tools and limited **venues** in which to report their "stories"—the CMS-1500 and the CMS-1450 claim forms.

Venue
The scene of an action or event.

CMS-1500 CLAIM FORM

Historically known as the HCFA-1500 claim form, since it was the HCFA that first oversaw the development of uniform claim tools, the HCFA-1500 was the standard reporting form for all services delivered by nonfacility providers such as physicians, chiropractors, physical therapists, and so on. All services had to be submitted on this paper form to standardize the submission of claims. The first commonly used **iteration** of the HCFA-1500 was the 12/90 (December 1990) version, which was fully implemented in January 1992. The HCFA-1500 form became the CMS-1500 claim form when HCFA was renamed the Centers for Medicare and Medicaid Services (CMS) in June 2001.

Iteration
The repeating of a procedure, often to achieve the desired result more closely.

The first major modification to the CMS-1500 claim form occurred when the use of the 08/05 version was implemented (Figure 1.5, p. 12). Providers could begin using the new form on October 1, 2006, and the new form was required by most payers on or after April 1, 2007, although Medicare delayed full implementation until July 2, 2007 ("Frequently Asked Questions," 2007).

A few payers prefer that facilities use the CMS-1500 form to report services. This, however, is an exception. It is never acceptable when facilities submit claims to government payers such as Medicare, which requires the CMS-1450 form. The National Uniform Claim Committee, a partnership among a diverse group of payers, providers, public health organizations, the AMA, and CMS, developed and now maintains the CMS-1500 claim form ("National Uniform Claim Committee," 2009).

CMS-1450 CLAIM FORM

As in the case of the CMS-1500, the CMS-1450 was originally known as the HCFA-1450 (Figure 1.6, p. 13). Its history is clearly defined because of the intensive involvement of the American Hospital Association (AHA). The AHA had interest in this form because it is the designated form used when reporting facility services, such as hospitals. The National Uniform Billing Committee (NUBC) participated with HCFA in creating the original form, commonly known as the UB-82 (Uniform Bill, 1982), although it was the mid-1980s before the form gained wide acceptance.

The UB-82 became obsolete with the introduction and mandated usage of the UB-92 in October 1993. The purpose was to take the best features of the UB-82 and add various elements and data fields that payers requested. The UB-92 remained in common use until the UB-04 replaced it in early 2007. The primary reason for creating the UB-04 was to allow the reporting of NPI information—as was the case with the 08/05 version of the CMS-1500. Ongoing monitoring and modifications of the rules for usage are overseen by the NUBC.

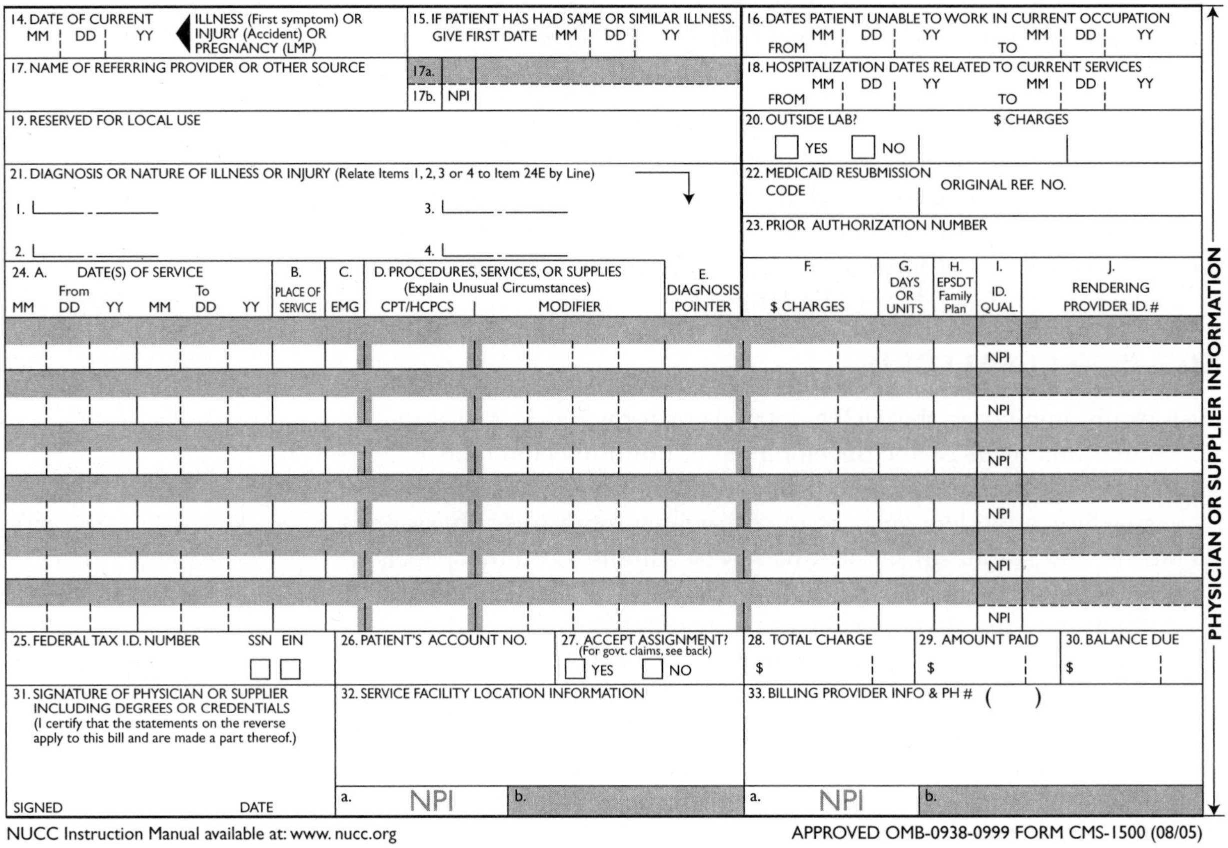

14. DATE OF CURRENT   ◄ ILLNESS (First symptom) OR   15. IF PATIENT HAS HAD SAME OR SIMILAR ILLNESS.   16. DATES PATIENT UNABLE TO WORK IN CURRENT OCCUPATION
MM DD YY   INJURY (Accident) OR   GIVE FIRST DATE   MM DD YY   MM DD YY   MM DD YY
    PREGNANCY (LMP)   FROM   TO

17. NAME OF REFERRING PROVIDER OR OTHER SOURCE   17a.   18. HOSPITALIZATION DATES RELATED TO CURRENT SERVICES
    MM DD YY   MM DD YY
    17b. NPI   FROM   TO

19. RESERVED FOR LOCAL USE   20. OUTSIDE LAB? $ CHARGES
    ☐ YES   ☐ NO

21. DIAGNOSIS OR NATURE OF ILLNESS OR INJURY (Relate Items 1, 2, 3 or 4 to Item 24E by Line)   22. MEDICAID RESUBMISSION
    CODE   ORIGINAL REF. NO.
1. L___ . ___   3. L___ . ___

    23. PRIOR AUTHORIZATION NUMBER
2. L___ . ___   4. L___ . ___

24. A. DATE(S) OF SERVICE						B.	C.	D. PROCEDURES, SERVICES, OR SUPPLIES		E.	F.	G.	H.	I.	J.
From			To			PLACE OF	EMG	(Explain Unusual Circumstances)		DIAGNOSIS		DAYS OR	EPSDT Family	ID.	RENDERING
MM	DD	YY	MM	DD	YY	SERVICE		CPT/HCPCS	MODIFIER	POINTER	$ CHARGES	UNITS	Plan	QUAL.	PROVIDER ID. #
1															NPI
2															NPI
3															NPI
4															NPI
5															NPI
6															NPI

PHYSICIAN OR SUPPLIER INFORMATION

25. FEDERAL TAX I.D. NUMBER   SSN EIN   26. PATIENT'S ACCOUNT NO.   27. ACCEPT ASSIGNMENT? (For govt. claims, see back)   28. TOTAL CHARGE   29. AMOUNT PAID   30. BALANCE DUE
    ☐ ☐   ☐ YES ☐ NO $ $ $

31. SIGNATURE OF PHYSICIAN OR SUPPLIER INCLUDING DEGREES OR CREDENTIALS (I certify that the statements on the reverse apply to this bill and are made a part thereof.)   32. SERVICE FACILITY LOCATION INFORMATION   33. BILLING PROVIDER INFO & PH # (   )

SIGNED   DATE   a. NPI   b.   a. NPI   b.

FIGURE 1.5

The bottom half of the CMS-1500 claim form (08/05 version). This section is used to report patient procedures and diagnoses. The primary reason for the change in claim form was the implementation of the National Provider Identifier (NPI), a major part of the HIPAA legislation. The new form provided space for the NPI numbers of the treating provider, the referring provider, and the facility where the service was delivered.

ELECTRONIC CLAIMS

The overwhelming majority of claims from all types of providers are submitted to payers via electronic means. Over the years, a wide variety of formats were used to communicate claim information electronically. These various formats created problems between providers and payers because there was no common language to facilitate communication between them. In recent years, organizations such as the Workgroup for Electronic Data Interchange (WEDI) have come together to advocate and promote single electronic formats, such as 5010, so that claims can flow easily from providers to payers and be processed efficiently.

The details of communicating claims information electronically are highly complex and, therefore, will not be reviewed at length in this context. However, it is accurate to state that the fundamental information communicated on paper claim forms (CMS-1500 and CMS-1450) is also the fundamental information communicated electronically. Therefore, when discussing claim data submission, the paper forms will be used for illustration purposes to enable the visualization of the information being discussed.

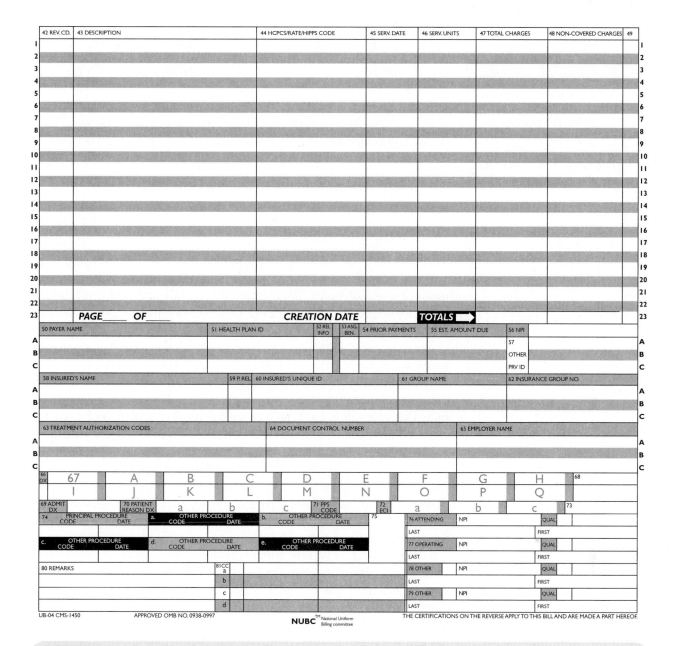

FIGURE 1.6

The bottom half of the CMS-1450 claim form (best known as the UB-04). It is used primarily by facilities to report services that they deliver.

Thinking It Through 1.3

1. Do you believe that the claim forms used today collect too much data, too little data, or just the right amount? Support your position.

2. Should the insurance claim forms be updated more frequently than they have been updated historically? Defend your position.

3. Does the electronic method of claim submission allow for more accurate coding? Does it enable more ethical coding? Justify your position.

1.4 The Fundamentals of Coding

On the surface, it may seem that journalism and coding do not have much in common. In reality, they perform the same tasks—only with different tools. The parallel objectives are illustrated in Table 1.2.

Both journalism and coding have specific ethical issues and concerns. The remainder of this text addresses the foundational issues of ethics and their specific application in coding. However, before beginning that study, it is necessary to examine briefly the elements of how coders perform their role.

THE "WHO" IN CODING

The Patient. The "who" reported by the coder would seem to be a very straightforward matter—it is the person who was in the exam room or the emergency department or the hospital room. While that certainly is true, the proper identification of that person can sometimes be the source of improper claim reporting.

Three primary elements are used to identify a patient: the patient's name, the patient's date of birth, and the patient's insurance identification number (Figure 1.7). If any one of these three elements is incorrect, the claim can be denied because the patient cannot be properly identified. This seemingly basic task is not the most common denial reason, but it is easily the most avoidable cause of delayed claim payments.

With regard to the patient's identification number, misidentifying the patient is not as difficult as you might think. The **transposition** of a single number can make the patient unidentifiable to the payers' computer systems. In the case of family coverage, each member of the family may have a different identification number. If the wrong number is used with the wrong family member, the claim will be denied because it is inaccurately reported. Conversely, some family policies may have a number of covered people—all with the same identification number. If an incorrect birth date is used, the system may not be able to identify the patient as a person covered under the policy and the claim could be denied.

Although it is less common because of the electronic submission of claims, a claim may be denied because the patient's name does not match the name in the payer's system. For example, a patient may present to the office as Rebecca Rogers, when her insurance identification

Transposition
The improper interchange of two or more numbers within a sequence.

Table 1.2 Similarities Between Goals of Coders and Journalists

	Journalists	Coders
Who	What parties were involved in the events of the story?	What parties received services?
What	What events occurred that are relevant to the story?	What services or supplies were provided to the patient?
When	When did the events occur?	When did the services occur?
Where	Where did the events occur?	Where did the services occur?
Why	Why did the events occur?	Why were the services provided?
How	How did the events occur (what were the circumstances)?	How were the services performed (specific techniques, etc.)?

1500

HEALTH INSURANCE CLAIM FORM

APPROVED BY NATIONAL UNIFORM CLAIM COMMITTEE 08/05

☐☐☐ PICA

1. MEDICARE ☐ (Medicare #)	MEDICAID ☐ (Medicaid #)	TRICARE CHAMPUS ☐ (Sponsor's SSN)	CHAMPVA ☐ (Member ID #)	GROUP HEALTH PLAN ☐ (SSN or ID)	FECA BLK LUNG ☐ (SSN)	OTHER ☐ (ID)	1a. INSURED'S I.D. NUMBER (For Program in Item 1)

2. PATIENT'S NAME (Last Name, First Name, Middle Initial)	3. PATIENT'S BIRTH DATE MM ┊ DD ┊ YY SEX M☐ F☐	4. INSURED'S NAME (Last Name, First Name, Middle Initial)

5. PATIENT'S ADDRESS (No., Street)	6. PATIENT RELATIONSHIP TO INSURED Self☐ Spouse☐ Child☐ Other☐	7. INSURED'S ADDRESS (No., Street)

CITY	STATE	8. PATIENT STATUS Single☐ Married☐ Other☐	CITY	STATE

ZIP CODE	TELEPHONE (Include Area Code) ( )	Employed☐ Full-Time Student☐ Part-Time Student☐	ZIP CODE	TELEPHONE (Include Area Code) ( )

9. OTHER INSURED'S NAME (Last Name, First Name, Middle Initial)	10. IS PATIENT'S CONDITION RELATED TO:	11. INSURED'S POLICY GROUP OR FECA NUMBER

a. OTHER INSURED'S POLICY OR GROUP NUMBER	a. EMPLOYMENT? (Current or Previous) ☐ YES ☐ NO	a. INSURED'S DATE OF BIRTH MM ┊ DD ┊ YY SEX M☐ F☐

b. OTHER INSURED'S DATE OF BIRTH MM ┊ DD ┊ YY SEX M☐ F☐	b. AUTO ACCIDENT? PLACE (State) ☐ YES ☐ NO	b. EMPLOYER'S NAME OR SCHOOL NAME

c. EMPLOYER'S NAME OR SCHOOL NAME	c. OTHER ACCIDENT? ☐ YES ☐ NO	c. INSURANCE PLAN NAME OR PROGRAM NAME

d. INSURANCE PLAN NAME OR PROGRAM NAME	10d. RESERVED FOR LOCAL USE	d. IS THERE ANOTHER HEALTH BENEFIT PLAN? ☐ YES ☐ NO If yes, return to and complete item 9 a–d.

READ BACK OF FORM BEFORE COMPLETING & SIGNING THIS FORM.
12. PATIENT'S OR AUTHORIZED PERSON'S SIGNATURE I authorize the release of any medical or other information necessary to process this claim. I also request payment of government benefits either to myself or to the party who accepts assignment below.

SIGNED _____   DATE _____

13. INSURED'S OR AUTHORIZED PERSON'S SIGNATURE I authorize payment of medical benefits to the undersigned physician or supplier for services described below.

SIGNED _____

CARRIER — *PATIENT AND INSURED INFORMATION*

PICA ☐☐☐

FIGURE 1.7

On the CMS-1500 claim form (08/05), the most important fields used to identify patients are 1a (Insured's I.D. Number), 2 (Patient's Name), and 3 (Patient's Birthdate).

card says "Rebecca Jones." Ms. Rogers explains that she recently married, but she did not have time to notify her insurer of the change. If the provider submits the claim as "Rebecca Rogers," the claim may be denied as a noncovered party on the insurance policy. Therefore, the provider office must ensure that it submits claims under the name that appears on the patient's identification card. It should counsel the patient to notify his or her insurer as soon as possible to obtain an updated, correct insurance card.

The provider also must ensure that it is submitting the claim for the correct person. Identity fraud is increasing in our society, and health care providers are not immune to the practice. In some cases, services were delivered to patients who presented stolen health insurance cards. In other cases, the insured party was **complicit** with the patient in the fraudulent use of the insurance card. For example, an uninsured relative may claim to be an insured family member so that he or she can receive medical services that are paid by the insured family member's insurance company.

Other elements on the claim forms further identify the patient, such as the patient's relationship to the insured (self, spouse, child) and the patient's status (single, married, other; employed, full-time student, part-time student). Incorrect reporting of this information may result in claim denial because certain policy provisions may prohibit claim payment if the patient's status does not meet certain criteria. Conversely, stating that the patient is a full-time student when, in fact, the provider knows he or she is not, is not only incorrect but also potentially causes

> **FYI**
>
> Health care fraud has become a serious issue. Providers must ensure that the information submitted to payers is correct.

Complicit
Cooperative in a project or process that is inappropriate or illegal.

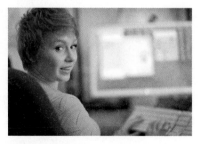

When submitting a claim, the provider's coder must ensure that the claim is being submitted for the correct person.

the provider to participate in health care **fraud.** As the journalist has a duty to report accurately the identities of those about whom he or she writes, the coder must report accurately the identities of the persons to whom service is provided.

In journalism, when an error is made in identifying a person, the problem is resolved by printing a correction as soon as the error becomes known. For the health care provider, the error can be resolved by resubmitting a corrected claim, although this has significant ramifications as it relates to cash flow because claim payment is, at best, delayed. If a journalist makes too many errors, his or her credibility and reputation are damaged. Similarly, erroneously submitted claims can damage a provider's credibility in the eyes of the patient. When the error is as simple as incorrectly identifying the patient, the patient may question the provider's competence in other areas, including clinical competence.

The Provider.   A second element of "who" is the proper identification of a number of potential providers, including the actual service provider (reported in Box 31 of the CMS-1500 claim form), the identification number or numbers of the service provider in Box 24J, the name of the referring physician (if applicable) in Box 17, and the referring physician identification number or numbers in Boxes 17a and 17b (Figure 1.8). On the CMS-1450 form (UB-04), the provider "who's" are reported in Box 82 for the attending physician's name and identification number and Box 83 to report "other" physician names and ID numbers.

Other provider identification, including the billing provider and the provider identification number or numbers, are placed in Box 33 of the CMS-1500 claim form for physician services. Both the CMS-1450 and CMS-1500 have a critical identification field in Box 5 and Box 25, respectively, that reports the Federal Tax Identification Number (TIN) for the entity billing the service. Many payers qualify a provider's status as "**participating**" or "**non-participating**" based on the TIN reported in this field.

> **BILLING TIP**
>
> Make sure that you study the regulations concerning billing "incident to" services for nurse practitioners, physician assistants, and other similar non-physician providers. If care is not taken, unethical and/or illegal billing might take place.

Particularly concerning physician-based services, it is critical to report accurately the service provider according to the payer's rules. For example, some physicians employ nurse practitioners (NPs) or physician assistants (PAs) in their practice. Some payers view these providers as extensions of the physician and require that the service be billed under the name of the physician, often under the principle of "**incident to.**" Other payers separately **credential** these non-physician

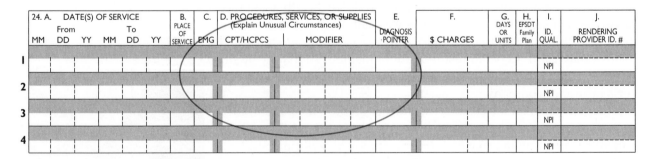

FIGURE 1.8

A small portion of the CMS-1500 claim form (08/05 version). The circled portion indicates the location in which CPT and HCPCS codes are used to report physician services (Box 24D).

providers and require that their name and identification number appear on the claim. For some payers, such as Medicare, there is a **payment differential** between physician services and the services of a NP or PA. Accurate reporting of the provider, in accordance with the requirements of the payer, is a vital task for the person billing the claim.

Payment differential
Difference between reimbursement rates for non-physician providers and physicians.

THE "WHAT" IN CODING

When the journalist communicates the "what" of a story, he or she is communicating the fundamental essence of the events that occurred or will occur. The focus is on facts and details of the story. The journalist must communicate about the action so that the reader has an accurate concept of the situation being described and can derive adequate understanding about the circumstances. Some examples of "what" include:

- A meaningful sequencing (usually chronological) of relevant events.
- A description of interaction between the parties involved.
- A listing of possible scenarios and/or outcomes that may result from the events.

For the coder, "what" is a description of the services provided (the events) to the patient on a given day or series of days. In medical coding, this is accomplished using the *Current Procedural Terminology,* Fourth Edition (CPT-4), and the Healthcare Common Procedure Coding System (HCPCS). These codes are reported by both physician and facility providers in different locations on their respective claim forms. The *International Classification of Diseases,* Ninth Edition, *Clinical Modification,* Volume 3 (ICD-9-CM, Vol. 3) is used to a lesser degree by facilities (Figure 1.9). The services that can be described with these codes include:

- Specific procedural services (e.g., appendectomy, hysterectomy, radiological exam, etc.).
- Supplies, medical equipment, or medications.
- Cognitive management services, including education, counseling, and diagnosis.

Just as the journalist reports the most relevant and compelling details, so the coder reports those services that are appropriately billable, according to the generally accepted coding rules or the specific rules of the individual payer. Legitimate journalists do not report events that never happened and that are not considered newsworthy. Similarly, coders report only the services supplied and do not bill insignificant services or services considered a component part of a larger procedure or service.

THE "WHEN" IN CODING

The timing of events in a news story is very important in providing context and relevant information that affects the reader's understanding of the events. The journalist cannot report that an event has happened before it actually happens. Conversely, the reporter who writes for the first time about an important, breaking news story three weeks after it happens is not doing his or her job appropriately.

Coders are in the same situation. Accurate reporting of the date of service is important for a number of reasons (Figure 1.10). First, any

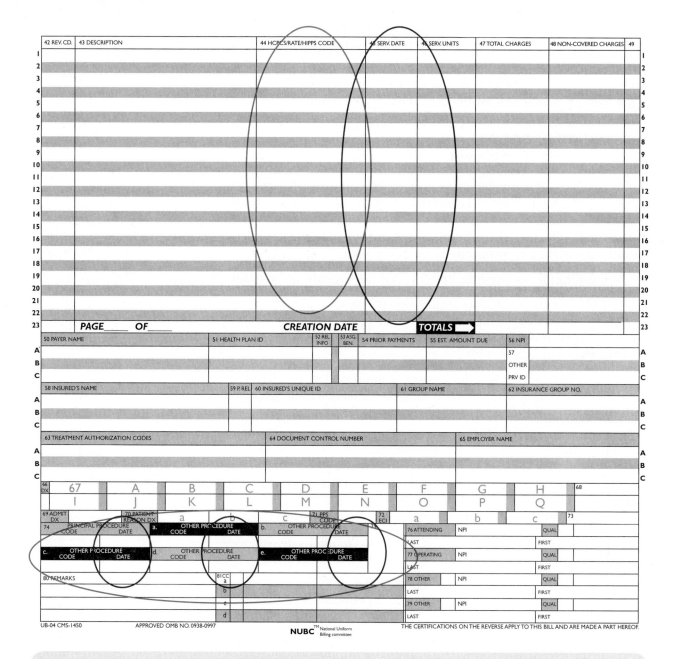

FIGURE 1.9

The bottom half of the CMS-1450 claim form (UB-04). The area circled in red at the top indicates where facilities report the CPT and HCPCS codes that describe the services provided (Box 44). The area circled in red near the bottom (Boxes 74a–e) is sometimes used to report ICD-9-CM, Vol. 3 procedure codes, as required by the third-party payer. The date the service is provided can be reported in one of several areas. Box 45 (circled in blue near the top) is the primary location, although the lower areas circled in blue (Boxes 74a–e) also can report the date of service for ICD-9-CM Vol. 3 procedures.

billing record should exactly match the patient's medical record. If the chart says that the patient received treatment on February 12 and a claim is submitted with a date of service of February 13, the claim is fundamentally flawed and incorrect. Second, on many occasions, certain services cannot be billed in proximity to another service. For example, if a Medicare patient has a hysterectomy (CPT code 58150) on March 20 and then sees the same physician for an E/M service on June 21, the

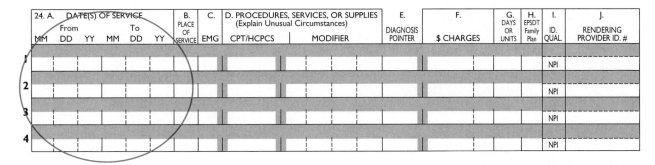

24. A.	DATE(S) OF SERVICE					B. PLACE OF SERVICE	C. EMG	D. PROCEDURES, SERVICES, OR SUPPLIES (Explain Unusual Circumstances)		E. DIAGNOSIS POINTER	F. $ CHARGES	G. DAYS OR UNITS	H. EPSDT Family Plan	I. ID. QUAL.	J. RENDERING PROVIDER ID. #
	From			To				CPT/HCPCS	MODIFIER						
	MM	DD	YY	MM	DD	YY									
1														NPI	
2														NPI	
3														NPI	
4														NPI	

FIGURE 1.10

Box 24A is used to report the dates of service for individual CPT or HCPCS codes on the CMS-1500 claim form.

claim should be paid. However, if the June 21 service is erroneously reported as having occurred on June 11, the claim would be denied by Medicare because it happened within the 90-day **global period** assigned to CPT code 58150. The correct date of service is essential to the proper payment of this hypothetical claim.

Finally, the correct reporting of the date of service is critical because of the issue of insurance claim payment. Since employers frequently make changes in insurance coverage for their employees, a patient may have different coverage from one day to the next with little or no warning. Therefore, the correct date of service is required to have the claim for that service adjudicated properly by the correct company. A more difficult situation related to the reported date of service is the situation in which the patient loses his or her coverage and asks the provider to bill the service for a date prior to their coverage termination. A coder changing the date of service at the patient's request is no different than a reporter changing substantive details regarding the time of an event reported in a story at the request of the story's subject. These actions violate the standards of both professions.

Global period
The given period of time before or after a major procedure in which another service is assumed to be associated with that procedure.

BILLING TIP

The date of service is very important as it relates to services provided near the same time as a major surgical procedure. Many claims can be denied if services are billed near the time of a surgery, but an appropriate modifier is not added.

THE "WHERE" IN CODING

The location of a service delivered by a provider must be properly reported to ensure correct payment and claim **adjudication.** This is particularly relevant for physician services because those services can be delivered in a variety of settings. The physician may perform services in an office setting, an outpatient setting (not owned by the physician), an ambulatory surgery center, an inpatient hospital setting, a home setting, and many others. The location of an event is primarily reported using a combination of two items—the place of service (POS) and, in some cases, the CPT codes. Particularly in the case of E/M codes, certain codes can be used only in certain health care settings. For example, CPT codes 99201 through 99215 can be billed only when the service is provided on an outpatient basis. CPT codes 99221 to 99223 can be billed only for the initial visit for a patient who is an inpatient in a hospital. If the CPT code reported is not consistent with the place of service reported in Box 24B of the CMS-1500 claim form, the claim will likely be denied (Figure 1.11).

The POS is also highly relevant as it pertains to reimbursement levels. Because of the structure of the **Resource Based Relative Value Scale (RBRVS),** higher payment levels are assigned when services are delivered in a physician office setting because the physician is providing all of the ancillary services (e.g., office overhead, nursing and office staff, medical equipment and supplies, etc.). If the physician provides

Adjudicate
Settle or determine.

Resource Based Relative Value Scale (RBRVS)
A reimbursement system in which each CPT code is assigned a work value, a practice expense value, and a malpractice value.

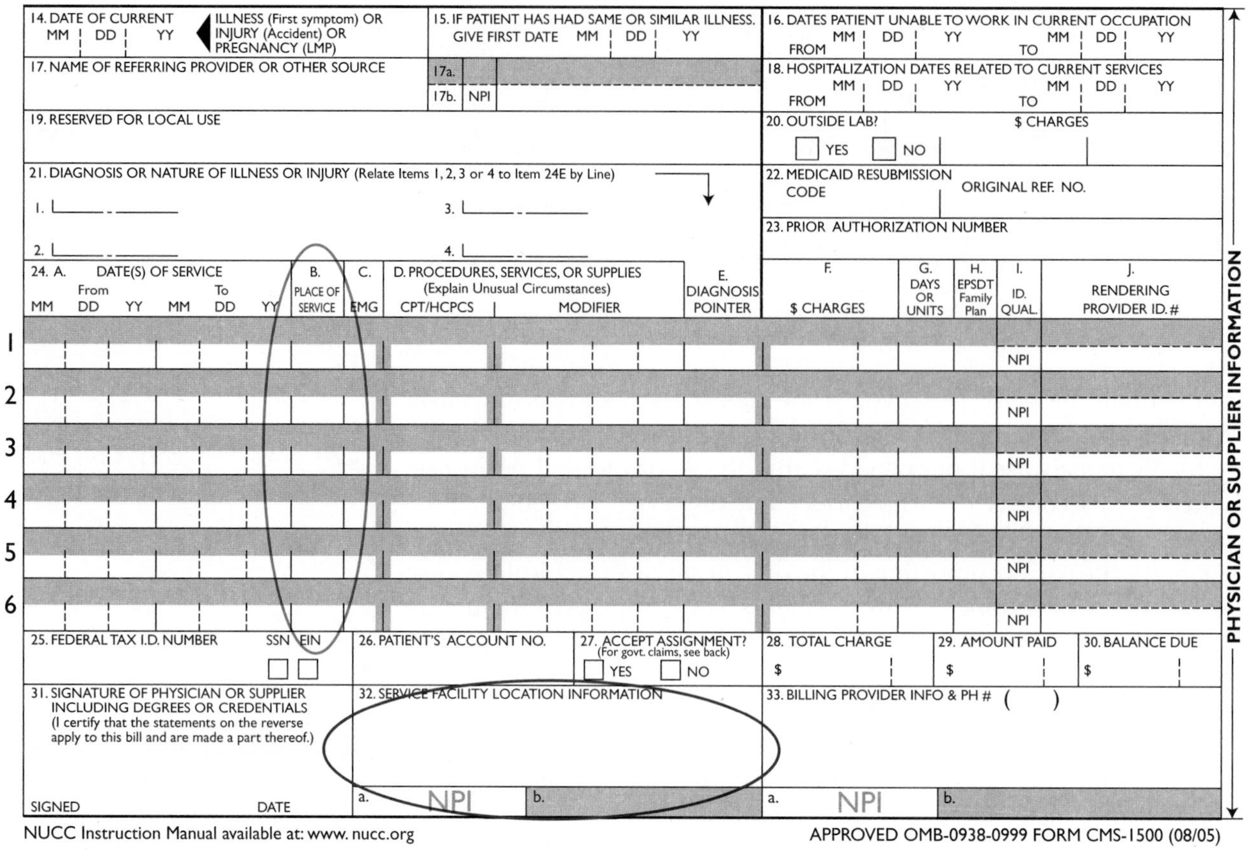
14. DATE OF CURRENT: ILLNESS (First symptom) OR INJURY (Accident) OR PREGNANCY (LMP) MM DD YY
15. IF PATIENT HAS HAD SAME OR SIMILAR ILLNESS. GIVE FIRST DATE MM DD YY
16. DATES PATIENT UNABLE TO WORK IN CURRENT OCCUPATION MM DD YY FROM TO
17. NAME OF REFERRING PROVIDER OR OTHER SOURCE
17a.
17b. NPI
18. HOSPITALIZATION DATES RELATED TO CURRENT SERVICES MM DD YY FROM TO
19. RESERVED FOR LOCAL USE
20. OUTSIDE LAB? YES NO $ CHARGES
21. DIAGNOSIS OR NATURE OF ILLNESS OR INJURY (Relate Items 1, 2, 3 or 4 to Item 24E by Line)
1. 2. 3. 4.
22. MEDICAID RESUBMISSION CODE ORIGINAL REF. NO.
23. PRIOR AUTHORIZATION NUMBER
24. A. DATE(S) OF SERVICE From To MM DD YY MM DD YY
B. PLACE OF SERVICE
C. EMG
D. PROCEDURES, SERVICES, OR SUPPLIES (Explain Unusual Circumstances) CPT/HCPCS MODIFIER
E. DIAGNOSIS POINTER
F. $ CHARGES
G. DAYS OR UNITS
H. EPSDT Family Plan
I. ID. QUAL.
J. RENDERING PROVIDER ID. #
1 NPI
2 NPI
3 NPI
4 NPI
5 NPI
6 NPI
PHYSICIAN OR SUPPLIER INFORMATION
25. FEDERAL TAX I.D. NUMBER SSN EIN
26. PATIENT'S ACCOUNT NO.
27. ACCEPT ASSIGNMENT? (For govt. claims, see back) YES NO
28. TOTAL CHARGE $
29. AMOUNT PAID $
30. BALANCE DUE $
31. SIGNATURE OF PHYSICIAN OR SUPPLIER INCLUDING DEGREES OR CREDENTIALS (I certify that the statements on the reverse apply to this bill and are made a part thereof.)
SIGNED DATE
32. SERVICE FACILITY LOCATION INFORMATION
a. NPI b.
33. BILLING PROVIDER INFO & PH # ( )
a. NPI b.
NUCC Instruction Manual available at: www. nucc.org
APPROVED OMB-0938-0999 FORM CMS-1500 (08/05)

FIGURE 1.11
By combining the information in Box 24B and Box 32, providers are able to use the CMS-1500 claim form to report the place of service (Where). Box 24B lists the codes for the places of service, such as office, ambulatory surgery center, or inpatient hospital. Box 32 provides the opportunity to report the name and address and identification numbers (Box 32a and 32b) of the specific facility where the service took place.

Commensurate
Appropriate or proportionate.

BILLING TIP

Place of service can make a huge difference in reimbursement. Physicians can either be seriously overpaid or underpaid if the incorrect place of service is used.

the service in a non-office setting but reports the claim as occurring in the office, then he or she may receive greater reimbursement than entitled to. The theory behind RBRVS is that payment for services is **commensurate** with the expenses incurred in delivering those services.

In recent years, Box 32 of the CMS-1500 claim form has become an important tool in reporting the POS for medical care delivered. When service does not occur in the physician's office, it is necessary to report the name, address, and identification numbers of the facility in which the service did occur. This helps reconfirm that the POS reported is compatible with the actual place of service and, for some payers helps confirm that the service was provided in a participating facility, which may change benefit levels for the patient.

The improper reporting of the POS (either intentionally or unintentionally) is a leading cause of improper claim payment because it mischaracterizes the nature and intensity of the service provided. As Jayson Blair, in the case study at the beginning of this chapter, mischaracterized his physical location in his bylines to add credibility to his reporting, the coder must properly categorize the place of service to accurately characterize, or weight, the service for the purpose of appropriate payment.

THE "WHY" IN CODING

Journalists face a major challenge in reporting "Why" an event occurred without reflecting bias, because the reason for an event may not be obvious. Different parties looking at the same event may arrive at two different conclusions about the reasons the event occurred or the motivations of the parties involved. A reporter responsible for news coverage is recognized as a top performer when the reader is unable to discern the reporter's personal opinion regarding the matter.

The coder must also report why a patient encounter occurred, but he or she faces a slightly different challenge related to the detail and depth of knowledge available at the time of making the report. Coders are charged with being as specific as possible, given the information they have available. However, they must not assign an illness, injury, or disease to a patient when there is not a definitive diagnosis.

The primary tool for the coder to report why an event occurred is the ICD-9-CM code. The diagnosis code reported with ICD-9-CM indicates the reason for an encounter, the condition for which the patient is being treated, and other contributory information related to the patient's condition.

An enormous challenge for coders is the proper assignment of codes to a particular procedure. Figure 1.12 shows how diagnosis codes are reported on the CMS-1500 claim form.

At several points throughout this text, the ethical implications of reporting correct diagnoses is a major topic and is discussed at significant length. Coders and physicians will often receive requests from patients and other parties to change a diagnosis to make it "payable" under the third-party payers' rules. It is the coder's task to report accurately the purpose of the treatment and to provide relevant diagnosis information that supplies context to the situation.

THE "HOW" OF CODING

The final element of the story told by both journalists and coders is "How." This includes specific information about the sequence of events, the manner in which an event occurred, or how a series of events led to an eventual outcome. In the field of journalism, masterfully explaining the "how" can differentiate an outstanding writer from an average writer. Whereas creativity and innovation in writing may be a highly valued trait for the journalist, it is skill and knowledge in both procedure and diagnosis coding that distinguishes the outstanding coder in clarifying the message of "how."

There are two components of "how" that must be communicated through coding. First, there is how a particular procedure was performed. Second, there is how an injury or illness occurred or developed.

"How"—Procedures. In CPT-4, thousands of codes exist to describe services provided to patients. Some of these codes describe the same basic procedure, with variations related to the methodology of *how* the procedure was performed. For example, an orthopedic surgeon may determine that a patient has a fractured radius (forearm). One treatment option (closed treatment of radial shaft fracture, without manipulation) is reported using CPT code 25500. Another treatment option is closed treatment of radial shaft fracture, with manipulation,

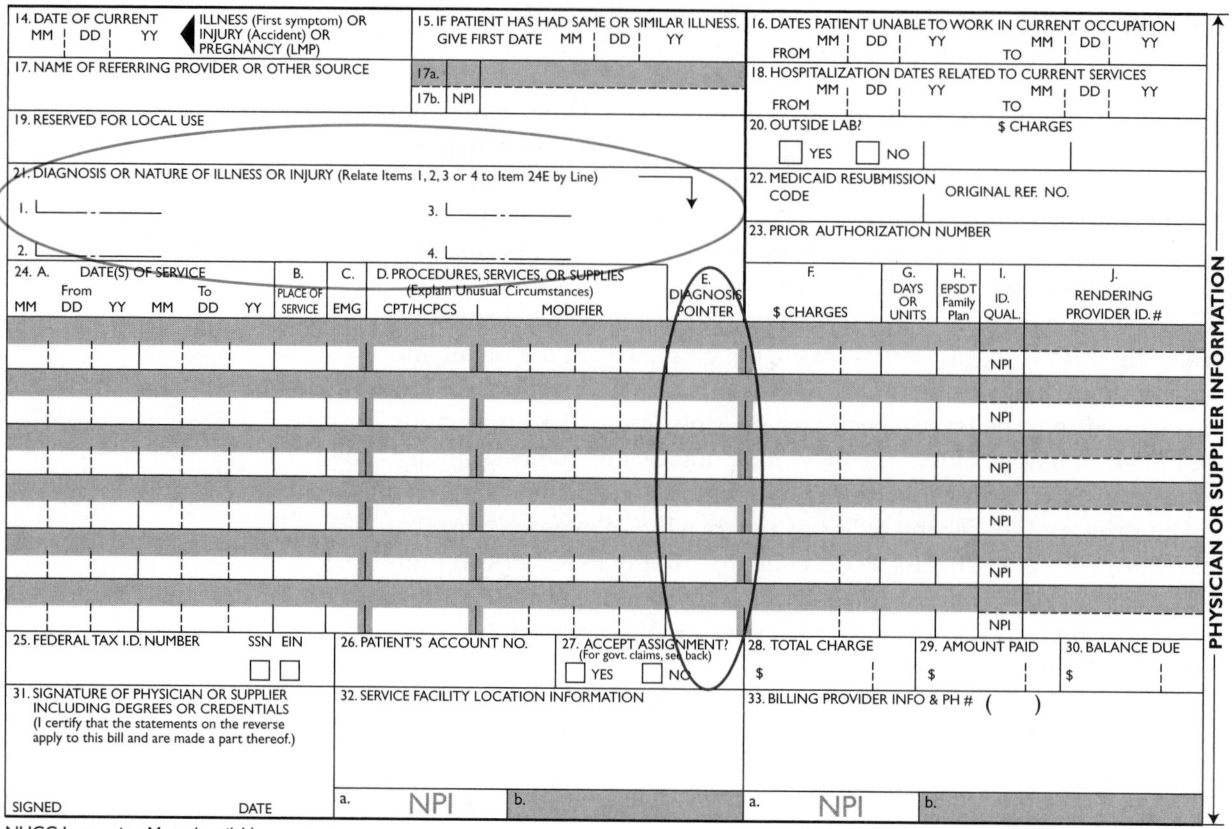

FIGURE 1.12

Box 21 provides a list of diagnosis codes associated with a given encounter, while Box 24E assigns those diagnoses to the individual services delivered during that encounter. Up to four diagnosis codes are listed in Box 21, while the associated number for the relevant diagnosis (1 through 4) for each individual procedure is placed in Box 24E. One common error is the false assumption that every diagnosis identified during an encounter is related to each individual service provided during that encounter.

reported with CPT code 25505. A third treatment option is reported using CPT code 25515, which is open treatment of radial shaft fracture, including internal fixation when performed.

In each case, the patient had a radial shaft fracture that was treated by the physician. The only difference between the codes was the method by which the physician delivered the service. Accurate description of the method is important because there can be significant differences in

Which Diagnosis Should Be Coded?

Julia, a 24-year-old female with no previous pregnancies, twisted her ankle while jogging. She went to her family physician, Dr. Washington, who examined her ankle and diagnosed an ankle sprain. He recommended conservative treatment and advised her to rest the ankle and to call him if it did not improve in the next couple of days. As Dr. Washington was getting ready to leave the room,

Julia mentioned that she was a week late for her period. Dr. Washington obtained some history about the situation and learned that Julia was sexually active and had not regularly used birth control. Dr. Washington ordered a blood pregnancy test, which produced a positive result (Figure 1.13).

21. DIAGNOSIS OR NATURE OF ILLNESS OR INJURY (Relate Items 1, 2, 3 or 4 to Item 24E by line)		22. MEDICAID RESUBMISSION	
1. 845.00 Sprain/strain ankle, unspecified site		CODE	ORIGINAL REF. NO.
2. V72.42 Pregnancy test, positive result		23. PRIOR AUTHORIZATION NUMBER	
3.			

24. A. DATE(S) OF SERVICE From / To						B. POS	D. PROCEDURES, SERVICES/SUPPLIES (Explain Unusual Circumstances) CPT/HCPCS / MODIFIER		E. DX POINTER	F. RVUs	G. DAYS OR UNITS	I. ID. QUAL	J. RENDERING PROVIDER ID. #
MM	DD	YY	MM	DD	YY								
						11	9921x		12		1	NPI	
						11	84702		2		1	NPI	

FIGURE 1.13

In this sample CMS-1500 form, diagnosis codes and diagnosis pointers accurately report why each service was provided. It would be completely incorrect to attach the first diagnosis (845.00) to a pregnancy test, since the pregnancy test was in no way related to the ankle sprain. (9921x represents the CPT code for some level of E/M service for an established patient; 84702 represents the CPT code for a beta hCG [blood pregnancy] test.)

difficulty, intensity, and time needed to perform the various procedures. This becomes critical when the service is reported to a third-party payer to obtain reimbursement. If the treatment is reported as "open" (referring to when an incision must be made or where the bone protrudes from the skin) when in fact it was a "closed" treatment (or a closed fracture, where the skin is not broken and no incision is necessary to treat it), the service will be mischaracterized and the physician will be overpaid. In addition, selecting the wrong code can also overstate the severity of the patient's condition. Conversely, a service may be underpaid if a closed procedure is reported when an open procedure was performed.

Another significant variation in terms of methodology is related to surgical approaches—laparotomy (traditional open surgery) versus laparoscopy—a less invasive surgery using specially designed tools that is performed through two or three very small incisions. The CPT code book specifically defines some procedures as being laparoscopic while others are open procedures. For example, an **exploratory** laparotomy is reported using CPT code 49000, while an exploratory laparoscopy is reported using CPT code 49320. In addition to the fact that the services may be reimbursed differently, the reimbursement for future services can be affected by the code reported. As part of the global procedure concept, Medicare includes all services delivered to the patient by the surgeon for 90 days following a laparotomy. On the other hand, Medicare includes services for only 10 days following a diagnostic laparoscopy. The physician who is tempted to report a more intensive surgical procedure to obtain additional reimbursement may actually receive less total reimbursement because of his or her inability to bill for follow-up services. Therefore, correct reporting of the methodology (the "how") of a procedure will facilitate correct reimbursement and may result in greater reimbursement than if the reporting were manipulated to maximize payment for the surgery.

"How"—Injury/Disease Cause or Process.

Certain diagnosis codes are used to indicate how a particular illness, injury, or disease state came to exist. Sometimes these diagnosis codes are part of the standard ICD-9-CM code set. More frequently, codes in the V section

CODING TIP

"Close enough" is not satisfactory in medical coding. The correct CPT code must be used to ensure proper documentation in the patient's record and proper payment from the third-party payer.

Exploratory
A surgical procedure performed to diagnose a condition or otherwise visualize an internal organ.

and E section of the ICD-9-CM code book are used to indicate the circumstances behind a condition or the specific details of the cause of the illness or injury. For example, the code V10.3—Personal history of malignant neoplasm of the breast, would be a diagnosis code used to explain why frequent mammograms are being performed to monitor the patient's condition. If a patient sustained an injury as the result of a tornado, the physician should report diagnosis code E908.1—Injury caused by tornado, in addition to supplying a code to describe the injury.

ICD-9-CM codes 740 through 759 are used to report congenital anomalies, which can be important in determining how a third-party payer may cover services related to the treatment of that condition. For example, diagnosis code 743.62 is used to report the congenital deformity of the eyelid. This may be important to the third-party payer that may not pay for elective surgery to modify the eyelids, but may pay for a correction to restore an organ that does not function properly. In this case, the code indicates that the patient had this condition at birth and was not seeking the procedure solely to improve his or her appearance.

Diagnosis codes can also be used to differentiate the ways in which patients may experience a condition. For example, diagnosis code 752.3 is used to report the congenital absence of the uterus. On the other hand, diagnosis code V88.02 is used to report the acquired absence of the uterus (with remaining cervical stump). In both cases, the patient does not have a uterus. However, these codes allow the coder to explain concisely *how* the patient came to not have a uterus.

The last codes listed in the ICD-9-CM, Volume 1, are the E codes. These codes allow the coder to report the external causes of injury and poisoning. In other words, these codes specifically explain how a patient was injured or poisoned. If a patient was injured in a high school football game, the coder would use diagnosis code E007.0 to reflect that the injury occurred during that event. If a patient incurred an injury while playing in a recreational touch football league, diagnosis code E007.1 would indicate the activity in which the patient was engaged. If the patient sprained his back while bowling, the coder would use diagnosis code E006.3 to indicate that the patient was bowling at the time the injury occurred.

These explanations of how an injury occurred can be very useful to third-party payers in adjudicating a claim. In some accident cases—particularly automobile accidents (e.g., E813.0)—responsibility for payment of the claim may be assigned to the auto insurer, as opposed to the health insurer. The proper use of E codes can be important in ensuring correct payment. However, an E code can never be a primary diagnosis code because it explains how a condition came to exist. The condition being treated must always be the primary diagnosis.

Thinking It Through 1.4

1. Which of the six fundamental elements of coding do you believe is incorrect most often? Why? Do you believe this is the result of intentional or unintentional action?

2. Do you think the use of RBRVS as a reimbursement tool has made it less or more important that precision occur with regard to "how"? Explain.

CHAPTER REVIEW

Chapter Summary

Learning Outcomes	Key Concepts/Examples
1.1 Formulate and communicate a basic definition of medical coding. Pages 4–6	• Many different definitions of medical billing and coding exist. Our fundamental definition of *coding* will be "to tell a story." • In many respects, coding is like journalism in that they both tell stories. Journalism has several strict rules concerning the way in which the story is told, which are also transferrable to coding: 1. First obligation is to the truth. 2. First loyalty is to citizens. 3. Essence is the discipline of verification. 4. Practitioners must maintain independence from those they cover. 5. The news must be comprehensive and proportional. 6. Practitioners should be allowed to exercise their personal conscience.

1.2 Differentiate between the different code sets used to report medical services. Pages 6–10	• The current code set for use in the U.S. health care system to report services, procedures, and materials is the Healthcare Common Procedure Coding System (HCPCS). The elements of it are:
	1. Level I—CPT-4 codes.
	  a. Category I—Basic CPT codes.
	  b. Category II—Supplemental Tracking codes.
	  c. Category III—Emerging Technology.
	2. Level II—HCPCS codes.
	
	• The approved code set for use in the United States to report diagnosis codes is the *International Classification of Diseases,* Ninth Edition, *Clinical Modification* (ICD-9-CM). It is presented in three volumes:
	1. Volume 1, Tabular list.
	2. Volume 2, Alphabetic list.
	3. Volume 3, Services and procedure codes for use by hospital for inpatient services.
	
	• On October 1, 2013, ICD-9 will be replaced by ICD-10.

1.3 Describe the forms used by various entities to report medical services. Pages 11–13	• A limited number of claim forms are used to report medical services. They are: 1. CMS-1500—Nonfacility providers, although they are used by facilities in certain limited cases. 2. CMS-1450—Facility providers.

1.4 Explain the direct correlation between the six key elements of journalism and the task of medical coding. Pages 14–24	• Journalism and coding both have six fundamental elements.
	1. Who: The patient and the provider.
	2. What: The service, procedure, or supply.
	3. When: The date of service.
	4. Where: The location of service.
	5. Why: The diagnosis code.
	6. How:
	  • The procedure method.
	  • The injury/disease cause or process.

End-of-Chapter Questions

Multiple Choice

Circle the letter that best completes the statement or answers the question.

1. **LO 1.1** Diagnosis and procedure codes are used by
   a. Government health programs
   b. Private health insurance companies

    c. Workers' compensation carriers

    d. All of the above

2. **LO 1.1** Which of the following is *not* similar when comparing journalists and coders?

    a. Their audience

    b. Their basic ethical principles

    c. Their tools

    d. Both a and c

3. **LO 1.2** Current Procedural Terminology (CPT) was first developed in

    a. 1958

    b. 1966

    c. 1975

    d. 1983

4. **LO 1.2** In which of the following environments are CPT codes *not* used?

    a. Physician offices

    b. Outpatient hospital settings

    c. Ambulatory surgery centers

    d. They are used in all of the above settings

5. **LO 1.2** Which type of CPT code is *not* used to report reimbursable services?

    a. Level I

    b. Level II

    c. Level III

    d. They all are used to report reimbursable services

6. **LO 1.2** Who or what was responsible for the discontinuation of Level III HCPCS codes?

    a. HIPAA

    b. CMS

    c. HCFA

    d. The Omnibus Budget Act of 1995

7. **LO 1.2** ICD-9 codes are used to report services and procedures in what setting?

    a. Physician office

    b. Outpatient setting

    c. Inpatient setting

    d. None of the above

8. **LO 1.3** The primary reason for the latest update to the CMS-1500 and CMS-1450 claims forms is to

    a. Provide space for the National Provider Identifier (NPI)

    b. Allow for the reporting of additional patient demographic information

    c. Provide space for more diagnosis codes

    d. All of the above

9. **LO 1.3** The current version of the CMS-1450 claim form is synonymous with the

    a. UB-82

    b. UB-92

    c. UB-04

    d. HCFA-1450

10. **LO 1.3** On the various claim forms, NPI numbers can be reported for

    a. The service provider

    b. The referring provider

    c. The attending provider

    d. All of the above

11. **LO 1.4** A coder can report the "How" of a service by using
    a. CPT-4 codes
    b. ICD-9-CM codes
    c. Both a and b
    d. Neither a nor b

12. **LO 1.4** The coder has a responsibility to
    a. Be concise
    b. Be complete
    c. Be truthful
    d. All of the above

Short Answer

Use your critical thinking skills to answer the following questions.

1. **LO 1.1** In Figure 1.1, the author asserts that coding rules, guidelines, and practices may sometimes create additional ethical dilemmas beyond those normally experienced in business. Do you agree? Why or why not?

2. **LO 1.1** Briefly describe the ways in which coding is like journalism.

3. **LO 1.2** CPT codes are the only code set owned by a private entity—the American Medical Association (AMA). Is this good or bad? Defend your position.

4. **LO 1.2** All CPT codes are HCPCS codes, but not all HCPCS codes are CPT codes. Explain how this is possible.

5. **LO 1.2** Explain why the Clinical Modification is necessary to enable providers in the United States to use ICD-9 to report diagnoses.

6. **LO 1.3** Why do you believe that separate claim forms are needed for physicians and hospitals/facilities?

7. **LO 1.4** What are the similarities between coders and journalists when reporting details (the "what")?

8. **LO 1.4** Why is the correct reporting of the date of service important to third-party payers?

9. **LO 1.4** What is the justification for not allowing E codes in the ICD-9-CM book to be used as a primary diagnosis?

10. **LO 1.4** Do you agree with this textbook's comparison between journalism and medical coding? Why or why not? Is there another profession that you believe has greater parallels with coding than journalism?

Applying Your Knowledge

At the beginning of this chapter, you were introduced to the case of Jayson Blair, a journalist with the *New York Times*. Once Blair's activities were identified as problematic by *Times* editors, they began to investigate further. They learned from the family of Jessica Lynch, a soldier who had famously been captured and rescued in Iraq, that Blair described the scene around their home in West Virginia in terms that were not remotely accurate. A review of receipts for meals allegedly purchased in the Washington, DC, area revealed that the receipts were actually for restaurants in Brooklyn and the greater New York metropolitan area. In the six months surrounding the sniper attacks, Blair filed reports from 20 cities in six states. However, he did not submit an expense report for a single flight, hotel room, or rental car.

Editors at the *Times* confronted Blair about his activities and reporting. He adamantly denied wrongdoing, produced pages of handwritten notes, and described in exacting detail various locations from which he claimed to have reported. It required further investigation to determine that his notes were fabricated after the fact and that his knowledge of location detail was gained by studying the digital photo archives of *Times* photographers.

The aftermath of Blair's activities was significant. While the *New York Times* obviously continues to exist, significant damage was done in relationship to the public's reliance on news reporters—could the *Times's* reporting really be trusted? The Blair incident played a role in changing the way that the public views the reporting of the news.

1.   In what ways can Blair's impact on the field of journalism parallel the effect of a "rogue" coder's impact on the field of medical coding?

2.   Why do you believe Blair was able to be successful as a journalist for so long without being detected? Would such activity be possible in the world of medical billing and coding? Why or why not?

Internet Research

The Internet provides a wealth of resources for medical coders that, until the last few years, simply did not exist. In addition to the information that is available online, communities of coders now exist that help individuals in answering difficult coding questions and addressing ethical dilemmas.

The Internet is a particularly useful tool in addressing ethics issues because of the relative anonymity that it provides, as well as the fact that it facilitates communication among coders around the United States and around the world. A coder may not feel comfortable admitting to a local colleague that he or she does not know how to code in a particular situation, but the coder may not hesitate to put the question online. The Internet's specific advantages for coders include:

*   Access to experts who are not available locally.

*   Exposure to other methodologies used in other parts of the country—introduction to best practices elsewhere.

*   Advice from disinterested third parties who do not have political or personal stakes in the decision-making process.

*   Shielding the identity of the coder and/or the practice that is struggling with a particular coding issue.

The web-based coding input can take a number of different forms. Input is available from informal chatrooms created by coders, listservs sponsored by coding and medical management organizations, websites sponsored by professional organizations or for-profit companies dedicated to coding education, and personal communication among colleagues around the country.

As the Internet has changed the world in the dissemination of information, so has the Internet changed the world of coding and coding ethics.

1.   Before reading this chapter, how would you have described the relationship between coders and the Internet?

2.   Can you think of other ways that having Internet access would be beneficial to a coder?

3.   Using the Internet search engine of your choice, enter "036.3 diagnosis" and indicate what condition this code reports.

PART ONE

The Fundamentals of Ethics

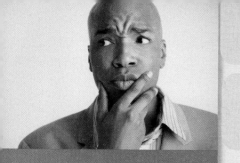

2

Ethics and the Importance of Ethical Systems

LEARNING OUTCOMES

After completing this chapter, you will be able to:

2.1   Define the term *ethics* and differentiate between the various definitions assigned to the term.

2.2   Identify and discuss the various methods available to establish ethical norms.

2.3   Elaborate on the importance of ethics on personal, business, and societal levels.

2.4   Distinguish between the factors that influence personal ethics and the factors that influence business ethics.

2.5   Explain the relationship between law and ethics.

2.6   Evaluate the range of ethical approaches in which individuals and companies can conduct themselves.

2.7   Describe the system of ethics that best serves the practice of medical billing and coding.

CASE STUDY

Sandra Hobson had been a medical biller and coder for 25 years. She started at the ground level as a billing clerk in training in a small physician office, which had two doctors. She impressed her supervisor as a diligent employee with a far-above-average work ethic. Through her career, she received consistently high reviews, received numerous merit pay increases, and was eventually promoted to the head of billing for the clinic, which had grown to eight doctors and three nurse practitioners. During this period, Sandra attended classes in medical office management at her local community college and obtained certification from a national coding organization.

Sandra was very active in her community. In her office, everyone respected her because she treated all of the employees with whom she worked with great respect. Sometimes she had to do some unpopular things as a supervisor, including terminating employees who were not performing adequately and enforcing work rules when employee behavior negatively affected productivity levels. Nevertheless, those in the practice universally saw Sandra as an outstanding biller/coder and an excellent supervisor.

The physicians in the practice elected to join their practice with a larger existing multispecialty group to improve their negotiating position with third-party payers and to achieve cost savings through **economies of scale.** Sandra worked hard to facilitate the transition and fought to protect the jobs of all the employees in her billing office. The administration of the existing multispecialty practice noticed Sandra's excellent work and reputation and named her as the associate director of billing, and she and her loyal staff all moved to the merged practice office.

After three years, the director of billing retired and Sandra was promoted to director. She was excited about the opportunity and felt that she was fortunate to have reached this level at this stage of her career. That excitement lasted until her first meeting with the practice chief financial officer (CFO). The CFO told Sandra that her first assignment was to facilitate the transition of the billing service from within the practice to an outsourced billing facility based in Bangalore, India. The practice would retain a handful of employees at the local central billing office to work with patients on a face-to-face basis. However, 90% of the employees in Sandra's department would be laid off, including all those who came with her from the previous practice. The CFO told Sandra that the realities of health care economics made the move necessary and that this was the single biggest cost savings available. Technological advances would make the outsourcing appear seamless to the patients. He assured Sandra that she would retain her position and that she would be responsible for overseeing the performance of the offshore billing company, as well as the local billing staff. He specifically instructed her not to tell anyone about this until negotiations were finalized and the plans for transition were completely in place.

Sandra returned to her office, shut the door, and stared out the window. This was not something that she expected. She did not

Economies of scale
The principle that products and services can be provided on a more cost-efficient basis when produced in larger batches.

know quite what to think, but the first things that came to her mind were:

- What about all of the employees who would be laid off? Some of them were single mothers—how would they support their families?
- Two of her employees had told her within the past week that they were going to close on the purchase of a new home within the next month. Now they were not going to have a job and they would have no income, but she could not tell them.
- Would the service truly be seamless to the patients, or would customer service suffer?
- The nature of her job would change substantially—long-distance supervision versus personal relationships and hands-on supervision. Is this something she really wanted to do?

Introduction

Coding and ethics are similar in that they both involve making hundreds of decisions (Figure 2.1). Coders have to choose and assign procedure codes from one of the thousands of Current Procedural Terminology (CPT) codes or Healthcare Common Procedure Coding System (HCPCS) codes. They have to choose and assign diagnosis codes from one of the thousands of *International Classification of Diseases, Ninth Edition, Clinical Modification* (ICD-9-CM) codes in that code set. Similarly, individuals have to make hundreds of ethical decisions every day—"How will I conduct myself in this situation?"; "What will I say to this person whom I don't like very much?"; "When will I respond to this request for assistance?"; "How much will I pay for this particular product?"

Sometimes the individual decision-making processes of coding and ethics collide and the ethical challenges that every person faces become a critical part of the coding process. However, before a detailed analysis of the application of ethical principles in coding can occur, a

FYI

Ethics is about making decisions. The medical coder has to make hundreds of decisions each day, making ethics an unavoidable issue for coders.

FIGURE 2.1
Coding and ethics both require answers to many questions. It is not possible to be an effective coder (and appropriately answer the associated questions) without also knowing the answers to the questions associated with making ethical decisions.

CODING AND ETHICS

- Coding Decisions
  - What procedure code?
  - What diagnosis code?
  - Is this procedure part of another?
  - Is this service separately billable?

- Ethical Decisions
  - How will I behave?
  - Do I tell the truth?
  - What do I do to make everyone happy?
  - This person treated me badly—how do I respond?
  - Do I have an obligation to report this matter?

complete understanding of "ethics" must first exist. The first step in the process is clarifying varying definitions and views of the concept.

2.1 Definitions and Views of *Ethics*

How a person defines and interprets the word *ethics* is shaped by past personal experience, family and peer influence, formal and informal training in ethics, and a wide variety of variables that are significantly different from person to person. However, ethics is generally recognized either as a system of moral values or principles of conduct for individuals or groups.

The definition with which a person most closely aligns his or her understanding of the concept of "ethics" significantly affects the way in which the person conducts himself or herself and applies ethical concepts. Ethics can be viewed in three different ways:

- As a field of study.
- As a set of rules and guidelines.
- As a set of personal beliefs and associated behavioral principles.

ETHICS AS A FIELD OF STUDY

One way in which ethics is considered is as a field of study. This particular field of study attempts to examine how people try to live their lives according to a standard of "right" and "wrong." The study of ethics is primarily a philosophical exercise that many, if not most, do not consciously consider on a regular basis. However, it is critically important to study this discipline to understand better the basis on which people make ethical choices.

The field of ethics is divided into three specific categories: *metaethics, normative ethics,* and *applied ethics* (Figure 2.2). They are briefly defined as follows:

- **Metaethics**—This discipline investigates where ethical principles come from and what they mean. Are they generated as part of an

Metaethics
A discipline that investigates where ethical principles come from and what they mean.

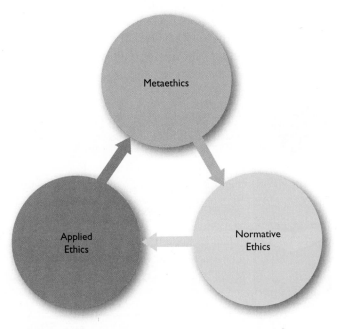

FIGURE 2.2
Metaethics (the study of the origin of ethics) informs the discussion of normative ethics (determining principles of right and wrong), which facilitates the use of applied ethics (making choices in specific daily circumstances). Often, an incident of struggling with applied ethics will drive the parties involved back to the consideration of metaethical concepts.

internal personal consideration or are they cultural or religion based? Metaethics focuses on issues of universal truths, the existence of a supreme being, the role of reason in the behavioral choices that we make, and the meaning of ethical terms themselves (Fieser, 2003).

- **Normative ethics**—Normative ethics is more practical than metaethics. It attempts to take the issues identified in metaethics and establish "normative" standards that regulate right and wrong conduct. This addresses issues such as habits to which people should aspire, the obligations that individuals have toward others, and the consequences of one person's behavior and choices on other people.

- **Applied ethics**—This discipline involves the application of ethical principles to real-world situations, often with a specific emphasis on controversial issues such as abortion, animal rights, environmental concerns, capital punishment, the justness of war, and so on. However, applied ethics is a consideration in every possible business situation, including the operation of medical practices and the day-to-day performance of medical coding duties.

At times, the lines between these fields of study are blurred. Many people believe medical coding is connected primarily to applied ethics. For example, is it right or wrong to be untruthful in submitting a claim to an insurance company if it benefits the patient (a specific application of ethical principles)? However, normative ethics must be involved because those applications cannot be discussed effectively unless the issues of truthfulness and obligations to others are fully understood. Prior to a complete discussion of normative ethics, metaethical issues such as the following must be asked and answered: "What is truth?" "On what basis is truth determined?" and "What is the logic behind the truth claim?" (Figure 2-3).

ETHICS AS A SET OF RULES AND GUIDELINES

Beyond it being a field of study, many people define *ethics* as a set of rules and guidelines by which individuals should live their lives. The difficulty with defining ethics solely as a set of rules and guidelines is that it does not adequately address the issue of the definition. What rules and/or guidelines should we follow? Who decides which rules

Normative ethics
An attempt to establish "normal" ethical standards for behavior, based on metaethical principles.

Applied ethics
The application of ethical principles to real-world situations.

FYI

We can't be ethical consistently unless we have thoroughly considered the foundation of our ethical standards. How did we decide what was acceptable behavior and what was not acceptable behavior? Why is behaving acceptably important?

FIGURE 2.3

This chart illustrates how each type of ethics is built on the previous step—applied ethics is derived from normative ethics, which originates in metaethics.

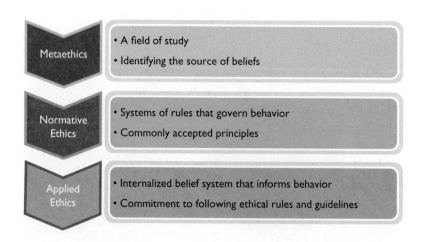

Metaethics
- A field of study
- Identifying the source of beliefs

Normative Ethics
- Systems of rules that govern behavior
- Commonly accepted principles

Applied Ethics
- Internalized belief system that informs behavior
- Commitment to following ethical rules and guidelines

Ethics and Diagnosis Codes

A 24-year-old patient, who is receiving global obstetric care from Dr. Jones, calls the office during her 13th week, reporting symptoms of a urinary tract infection (UTI). Dr. Jones's nurse asks her to come in later that same day for evaluation of her symptoms and any necessary treatment. Dr. Jones confirms a UTI.

Because this visit was not part of the global OB package (UTI is not part of a "routine" pregnancy), the service is separately billable. Dr. Jones's coder bills 9921x, with a primary diagnosis of 599.0 (urinary tract infection, unspecified) and a secondary diagnosis of V22.2 (Pregnancy, incidental). The claim is filed to the payer and it is denied as part of the global package.

Dr. Jones's coder contacts the payer and is advised that the claim was denied because it had a diagnosis of "pregnancy" attached to it. The payer representative says that if V22.2 was not attached to the claim, it would have been paid. The coder advises her manager of this information and the manager tells the coder to resubmit the claim without the pregnancy diagnosis. The coder is not comfortable with this advice because she believes it is not ethical. The manager says that the practice is entitled to this money because it was not directly related to the pregnancy—even the payer representative said so.

This case presents two points of view regarding the ethical principles. The coder says that all relevant diagnosis codes should be used to report the services—a principle with which most coders would agree. The manager desires to receive payment associated with a benefit to which the patient is entitled to keep her job and all of their workers employed—she wants them to be able to support their families. Both are sincere in their belief concerning their position and both feel that they are adhering to high standards. The fact that there is disagreement indicates that looking at ethics only as a set of rules does not solve anything when there is disagreement between the parties.

and guidelines are followed when there is a conflict between the rules? Does everyone agree on the principles that are accepted? Do all people assign the same level of value to a particular rule?

Because of the variety of family backgrounds, individual experiences, religions, and cultures, it is easy to see how there could be difficulty in arriving at a standard set of ethics accepted by all. There can be legitimate disagreement between people who are both attempting to adhere to a high set of moral standards. Which one is right and which one is wrong?

Moreover, if ethics are only a set of rules, most people will at some point encounter a circumstance in which it is not to their advantage to follow those rules. Rules are effective when the fear of the consequences of breaking the rules is greater than the benefit of breaking the rules. When the cost versus benefit analysis indicates that the risk of being caught breaking the rules is less than the perceived benefit of violating the rules, many people will take the risk and violate ethical principles. The value of those ethical principles is diminished greatly as a result.

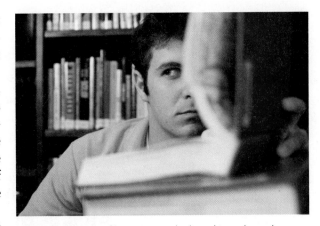

What if the risk of being caught breaking the rules is less than the perceived benefit of violating those rules? Violation of ethical principles will likely result.

ETHICS AS A SET OF PERSONAL BELIEFS AND ASSOCIATED BEHAVIORAL PRINCIPLES

A third important definition for *ethics* is associated with deeply held personal beliefs that result in behavior consistent with those beliefs. Some applications or interpretations of this definition include:

- Ethics is beliefs used to analyze and interpret situations to make decisions regarding behavior.
- Ethics is predetermined planning regarding potential actions in foreseeable situations.
- "Ethics is about how we meet the challenge of doing the right thing when that will cost more than we want to pay" (Maxwell, 2003).

DEFINING *ETHICS*

Each of these definitions references the application of ethical principles to subsequent behavior. The importance of ethics in this approach is not the rules (ethical system) so much as the behaviors that belief in and adherence to the rules produces. This is truly the center of applied ethics, which is based in real-world situations and real-world conflict. In a very practical sense, persons' ethics are defined by their behavior (actions), rather than their stated beliefs (words). However, the actions are unlikely to be consistent with the words if the person does not have a strong and clear understanding of the source of the ethical beliefs and have a serious commitment to following commonly accepted ethical rules and guidelines.

Thinking It Through 2.1

1. Describe how the way you define *ethics* affects your behavior.
2. Which type of ethics (metaethics, normative ethics, or applied ethics) is the most important? Why?
3. What is your opinion of the case study in which the secondary diagnosis (Pregnancy, incidental) is not reported? What would you do in this situation and why?

2.2 Methods of Determining Ethical Norms

Before we approach a detailed discussion of applied ethics in the field of medical coding later in this text, it is necessary to understand the available methods by which ethical norms (or generally recognized standards) are established. Different approaches in developing ethical norms will result in different outcomes in behavior. This will provide insight as to how two people concerned about ethics can arrive at two different interpretations concerning the same ethical dilemma. As reflected in Figure 2.4, we accomplish this by studying the area of normative ethics. There are four general categories of normative ethics, as illustrated.

VIRTUE ETHICS

Virtue ethics is based on the idea that a person's life should be committed to the achievement of an ideal or ideals—virtues. The philosopher

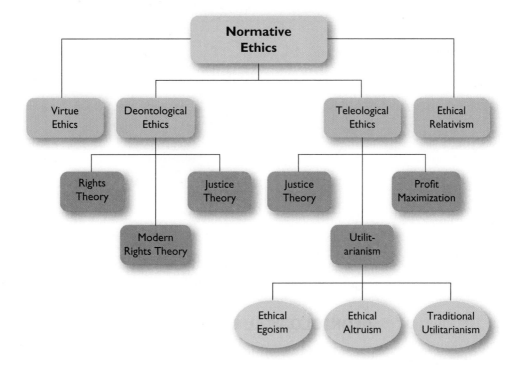

Aristotle originally introduced the concept of virtue ethics. He believed that the individual life and society, as a whole, were able to achieve optimal functionality when conducted in the pursuit of a key characteristic or behavior that was virtuous.

Virtue ethics is valuable in that the system promotes the aspiration to a higher standard—a continuous effort to improve the performance of the individual and, thereby, society as a whole. The primary difficulty with virtue ethics is that achieving the ideal level of a particular virtue may be hard to identify. For example, one commonly desired virtue is courage. An individual can have too little courage, which most people would agree is not good. On the other hand, a person can have too much courage—to the degree that he or she makes foolish decisions. Therefore, an ideal level of courage exists—but what is it? Who defines it? The problem of achieving the ideal level is the same for any of the virtues (Figure 2.5).

In addition, emphasis on virtues can change over time. In Aristotle's time, wisdom, justice, and courage were the most highly valued universal virtues. In today's diverse range of societies and cultures, many of which live in close proximity to one another, there is often little agreement about what virtues should be valued, let alone how

FIGURE 2.4

The four major ethical systems (virtue ethics, deontological ethics, teleological ethics, and ethical relativism), along with the various theories that are categorized under each of these major systems.

Virtue ethics
An ethical system that is based on the idea that a person's life should be committed to the achievement of an ideal or ideals.

FYI

Virtue ethics promotes adhering to a higher standard, but does not easily define when someone has reached the ideal level for that standard.

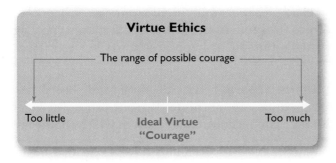

FIGURE 2.5

The challenge with virtue ethics: What is the ideal amount of a particular virtue (in this case, courage)?

FIGURE 2.6

Deontological ethics has three subcategories—rights theory, modern rights theory, and justice theory.

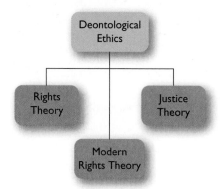

they are practically executed. If there is a conflict between an individual's most valued virtues and those of the common society, there is a significant risk of value conflict.

DEONTOLOGICAL ETHICS

Deontological ethics, which has its root in the Greek word *deon*, or "duty," is known as a nonconsequentialist ethical system (Figure 2.6). It focuses on the action itself, regardless of the result that it produces (Mallor, Barnes, Bowers, & Langvardt, 2010). Taken to the extreme, a person whose belief system is based in deontology would say, "I will/will not do X because doing otherwise would be wrong—I do not care what the consequences are to me or to anyone else." This area of ethics believes that certain universal principles apply to all ethical judgments, regardless of the specific details (Ghillyer, 2010). Actions are taken because of an obligation to a moral idea or principle, regardless of outcome. Deontological ethics differs from virtue ethics in that virtue ethics focuses on the specific virtues demonstrated by the *person*, while deontological ethics focuses on the *principle*.

Rights Theory. Although there are several forms of **"rights theory,"** they each share the belief that certain human *rights* are fundamental and should be respected by all other humans. For example, the Declaration of Independence declares that all people have the right to "life, liberty, and the pursuit of happiness." A key element of many of the laws in the United States is the presumption that the individual has not only rights but also the expectation that they will not be imposed on or restricted by other individuals, entities, or the government. On the other hand, rights theory also assumes that for people to live together peacefully, they must be willing to give up some rights to receive certain protections in return (Brown & Sukys, 2009). For example, if an individual's pursuit of happiness causes harm to others (freedom from harm is another presumed right), then the individual's pursuit of happiness must be restrained in some fashion.

Modern Rights Theory. Strict deontological theory has a problem in that its duties are **absolute**. Persons can never lie and never cheat—although circumstances may exist in which some see lying and

---

Deontological ethics
An ethical system that focuses on the action itself, regardless of the result that it produces.

FYI

Virtue ethics focuses on the *person,* whereas deontological ethics focuses on *principles.*

Rights theory
A theory that states the belief that certain human rights are fundamental and should be respected by all other humans.

Absolute
Nonnegotiable or unchangeable.

---

cheating as appropriate to saving their life or the lives of others. This has resulted in a mixed deontological theory, known as modern rights theory, that ranks moral rights and rules. Operating under this theory, a person should adhere to a moral rule unless a greater right takes priority over it (Mallor et al., 2010).

Strengths and Weaknesses of Rights Theory. Rights theory works well when a society agrees to the definition of the rights. The theory facilitates democratic societies because the definition of the rights can be integrated into the laws of the society and, thereby, become universally understood.

Rights theory has several weaknesses, however, including disagreement about the rights, their relative values, and the costs associated with allowing the exercise of rights. The right to free speech, regardless of how distasteful or repulsive we find the speech, is a fundamental right in our culture. However, exercising this right has caused damage to relationships between different groups within the society, and society has incurred immense expense associated with the court system in debating and litigating these rights.

Justice Theory.

While rights theory has a long history, spanning hundreds of years, **justice theory** is a relatively new entrant in the field of ethics. Justice theory's most articulate advocate is John Rawls, who wrote *A Theory of Justice* in 1971. Justice theory is very similar to rights theory in its first and most important principle—the Greatest Equal Liberty Principle. This principle states that each person has an equal right to basic rights and liberties (Mallor et al., 2010). According to Rawls, the ideal situation is created (and true rights and justice will occur) when people freely and impartially consider the situation under *the veil of ignorance.*[1]

> **Justice theory**
> An ethical theory that includes seeking justice by ensuring that the prospects of the least fortunate are as great as they can be.

To a large degree, this philosophy is a means by which Rawls expressed his political beliefs. His position was that the world is the most just when the prospects of the least fortunate are as great as they can be. It is strong in that its basic premise of protecting the least advantaged in society is agreeable to virtually everyone and it is consistent with the teachings of most religious philosophies that encourage the assistance of those in need (Mallor et al., 2010). Justice theory and rights theory are similar in that they both seek to promote the rights of others and to protect those rights.

However, justice theory varies from rights theory because justice theory usually attempts to define the outcome. Rawls sought equality of result, instead of equality of opportunity. As an example in the field of business, if a company was considering two sites for a new plant, the company would weigh the benefits and the costs associated with building the plant in each of the locations and then select the location most beneficial for the company. Under justice theory, the company would select the location that was most in need, with the purpose of raising the economic status of the people in the area.

> **FYI**
> The discussion about the right to health care in the United States is largely based on justice theory.

---

[1]The veil of ignorance means that the person puts aside everything that is specific to him or her (e.g., race, sex, intelligence, nationality, family background, and special talents). The theory is that if everyone did this, there would be unanimous agreement concerning rights and ethics (Hill & McShane, 2008).

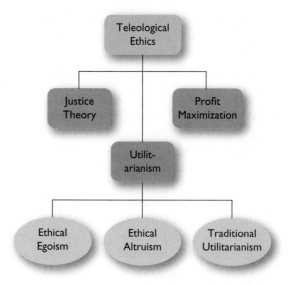

In the field of medicine, there is considerable discussion concerning the rights of Americans to receive access to health care. This would be a very important principle to those that espouse justice theory—all people, to the greatest degree possible, should have access to the same level and quality of care, regardless of their socioeconomic status or any other differentiating factor.

TELEOLOGICAL ETHICS

Teleological ethics

An ethical system that focuses on the results of an action, as opposed to underlying principles or rules.

FYI

Teleological ethics is concerned about *outcomes* or *consequences*. The objective is to arrive at the best possible outcome.

Teleological ethics is different from deontological ethics in its focus (Figure 2.7). Deontological ethics has as its primary focus the decision or the action, while teleological ethics focuses almost exclusively on the results or the outcome of a decision or action. Justice theory straddles the line between these two schools of thought, with a focus on both elements of a circumstance—the process *and* the outcome.

Another term for teleological ethics is "consequentialist" ethics. The most important consideration for this field of ethics is, "What is the outcome or consequence?" For a person who follows teleological/consequentialist ethics, an action is morally right (or ethical) if the consequences of the action are more favorable than unfavorable. This immediately brings a relevant question to the forefront—favorable or unfavorable to whom?

Utilitarianism. Utilitarianism is the most well-known and accepted teleological theory. There are three subdivisions of utilitarianism—each of which answers the identity of the recipient of the beneficial outcome.

>   *Ethical Egoism.* Ethical egoists are the ultimate in selfishness. They have no concern but achieving outcomes that benefit them. That which benefits them is what is "moral," although most observers would consider their behavior "immoral." Table 2.1 illustrates the differences between the beneficiaries in each type of utilitarianism.
>
>   *Ethical Altruism.* The difference between ethical egoism and ethical altruism is the recipient of the benefit. Altruism is the concern

Table 2.1 Beneficiaries in Types of Utilitarianism			
Ethical Theory	**Ethical egoism**	**Ethical altruism**	**Traditional utilitarianism**
Beneficiary	The individual	People other than the individual	Society as a whole

about the welfare of others. In this context, that which benefits others is the ultimate determination of "morality" for the ethical altruist. The most famous ethical altruist of all time would be Robin Hood. In his eyes, his actions were moral because they benefited the poor. Those from whom he stole would likely disagree with that assessment.

Traditional Utilitarianism. Persons who subscribe to traditional utilitarianism focus on the benefit to society, as a whole. This may cause them, on occasion, to take action that is not in their personal self-interest.

Utilitarianism is perhaps the clearest ethical theory to understand in principle. It is more challenging to put into practice because the member of a minority harmed because the "greater good" called for it would not likely be in favor of utilitarianism. In addition, sometimes it is difficult to identify what is "best" and it becomes extraordinarily difficult when attempting to do it for a group as large and diverse as an entire society.

Utilitarianism also has a weakness in that it does not consider either justice or law—only the greater good, as defined by the majority at that time. Deontological theories protect the rights of the individual, sometimes at the cost of the majority. Utilitarianism tends to favor the majority, sometimes at the cost of the individual or minority group. The fact that utilitarianism is not constrained by the law causes it to lose the benefits that the law offers. For example, the treatment of patients with HIV (or any other contagious disease) can be very expensive for society. Utilitarianism could theoretically state that it is in the interest of the greater good to quarantine everyone with the disease and withhold treatment. This would prevent the further spread of the disease and save massive amounts of money spent on treatment. This would achieve the goal of utilitarianism, but would be too unacceptable for most people to consider seriously as an alternative.

Profit Maximization. **Profit maximization** is another form of teleological ethics—the focus is on the results. However, the difference between profit maximization and traditional utilitarianism is the scope of the decision and the factors that are considered when making the decision. In utilitarianism, the goal of maximization relates to the satisfaction or dissatisfaction of the members of society. In the case of profit maximization, the goal must be obtained within the constraints of the law and the only concern is the individual company—not the entirety of society.

Profit maximization focuses on results, but given that it must work within the constraints of the law (based largely on rights and justice

Profit maximization
An ethical theory that focuses on results within the constraints of the law.

theory), it has significant features of both. In addition, the marketplace can control the behavior of some companies because they do not wish to experience a public relations disaster if unethical behavior is discovered and publicized. Companies have experienced boycotts, significant declines in sales, and increased costs associated with borrowing because of their behavior (Mallor et al., 2010).

Unfortunately, the singular focus on profits can cause individuals to forego their ethical standards to meet profit goals. Therefore, profit maximization is likely the traditional ethical framework that can most easily result in ethical failure.

ETHICAL RELATIVISM

Ethical relativism
An ethical theory in which the definition of "ethical" varies from circumstance to circumstance and person to person.

In recent years, a new ethical theory has gained momentum—**ethical relativism.** Under this theory, that which is "ethical" varies from circumstance to circumstance and person to person. It is commonly accepted in the United States because of the variety of cultures (and the associated ethical systems) introduced by immigrants coming to America (Brown & Sukys, 2009). When faced with widely differing cultures, values, and ethics, there is great hesitance to declare that one philosophy is superior to another, at the risk of offending members of a differing cultural community. Ethical relativism partially resolves that issue by stating that no one culture or ethical system is better than another—each person determines what is right and wrong for him or her, based on the person, his or her experiences, the circumstances, and any other factors relevant to the situation.

Situational ethics
A theory in which judgment can be rendered about a behavior only if the judge knows all of the relevant details associated with the situation.

Ethical relativism is completely incompatible with rights theory because there is no fixed standard of right and wrong. Taken to the extreme, no one can ever do, say, or think anything wrong because of the highly personal, individualized nature of the ethical process. Ethical relativism is commonly called **situational ethics.** In this theory, judgment can be rendered about a behavior only if the judge knows all of the relevant details associated with the situation. The most effective way to evaluate the behavior is to put oneself "in the shoes" of the other person and ask, "How would I behave if I were placed in that same circumstance?" This may help people view others with tolerance and patience, which is a desirable trait. However, the lack of a fixed standard, or even a definition of an acceptable outcome, makes ethical relativism a troubling concept in defining ethical behavior.

Thinking It Through 2.2

1. Is virtue ethics a viable ethical system for use by coders? Why or why not?

2. Is rights theory a valid tool for use in the practice of medical billing and coding? Why or why not?

3. Do all Americans have a right to health care? What does that mean? Who should decide?

4. How effective is the application of justice theory to the field of medical billing and coding?

5. In the task of medical billing and coding, is utilitarianism a practical ethical theory? Why or why not? If so, to what degree?

2.3 The Importance of Ethics for Individuals, Business, and Society

Ethics is a popular topic in American culture today, both in the general culture and, specifically, in the world of business. The primary reason for the intense focus on the topic of ethics is a remarkable series of major and public ethical failures documented in the media. Many of these companies and people (such as Enron, WorldCom, Nike, and Bernie Madoff) are household names—for all of the wrong reasons.

Unfortunately, the problem with unethical behavior exists not only in large and well-known corporations, but also has become a component of nearly every sector of society. Scandals involving politicians, pastors and priests, and illegal drug use in professional sports are in the newspapers nearly every day. This has created an enormous level of cynicism among the public. Pollster George Barna measured this doubt regarding human behavior when he asked the question, "Do you have 'complete confidence' that leaders from various professions would 'consistently make job-related decisions that are morally appropriate'?" The results are illustrated in Table 2.2.

Ethics is a serious issue when 86% of the American public is unwilling to place their complete trust in their most trusted leaders. Most other categories of leaders received significantly less support.

WHY ETHICS MATTER

Ethical standards are important for individuals and societies to function in a stable manner. Unless people have a set of ethical standards to which they adhere, their behavior and responses to others will be random and unpredictable. Some of the economic turmoil in recent years was the result of instability in the marketplace, driven by the fact that people did not trust major companies to do the right thing, did not trust government officials to do the right thing, and many did not trust their employer to do the right thing. Conducting oneself in an unethical manner damages the relationships between individuals and hampers the functioning of society as a whole.

> **FYI**
>
> Ethics matter because people need to rely on the consistent responses of others in dealing with difficult situations.

Table 2.2 Trust of the American Public in Leaders and Prominent Figures

	Complete	A Lot	Some	Not Much
Executives of large corporations	3%	9%	45%	38%
Owners of small businesses	8	33	41	13
Elected government officials	3	15	48	30
Ministers, priests, and other clergy	11	31	35	19
Teachers	14	39	34	10
News reporters and journalists	5	15	48	29
Producers, directors, and writers of TV and films	3	10	42	38

Source: Barna, 2002.

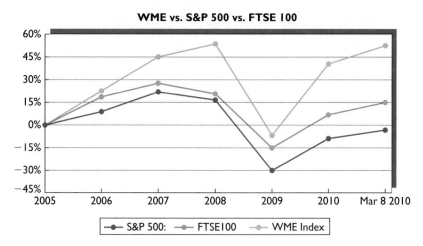

FIGURE 2.8

This chart compares the financial performance of the Standard and Poors 500, the FTSE 100 (an international index, based in the United Kingdom), and the World's Most Ethical (WME) companies, as determined by *Ethisphere* magazine.

WME vs. S&P 500 vs. FTSE 100

Source: Ethisphere magazine, 2010.

Ironically, research has shown that companies that behave in an ethical fashion on a consistent basis have better financial performance than companies that behave unethically (Figure 2.8).

Additional benefits to ethical behavior contribute to financial performance, but are not directly financial. According to Jim Blanchard, CEO of Synovus Financial Corporation, he created the company based on the same ethical principles that he held personally. To institutionalize the principles, he went so far as to create a People Development Component, a department specifically focused on appropriately treating the workforce. Blanchard stated that the measurable benefits include "lower turnover, fewer EEOC claims, and the disappearance of any kind of harassment issues. The benefits that can't be specifically measured are that you keep your best folks, your young emerging leaders want to stay, and people grow and flourish in an environment where they are not suppressed. So you're getting optimum and maximum growth at the highest level" (Maxwell, 2003).

It is unreasonable to expect that societal ethics will be any better than the ethics of the individuals who comprise that society. The ethics of the coding practices of a health system or provider office will be no better than the ethics of the providers and the individual employees at that facility. Therefore, it is vital to understand from a practical vantage point how ethics formation occurs.

HOW ETHICS ARE FORMED

Individuals do not develop personal ethical standards as they would develop knowledge of English, mathematics, science, or social studies. The study of metaethics and normative ethics are academic exercises, which can influence the development of personal ethics, but studying these disciplines will not make a person "ethical."

Development of Personal Ethical Standards. Personal ethical standards are developed, in part, by exposure to the environment and an individual's personal experiences. The path to the adoption of ethical standards is uniquely individual, although many will agree on the standards eventually adopted.

For most people, the leading factor in shaping personal ethical standards is the people who are in primary contact with the individual.

FYI

The ethics of a society can't be any better than the ethics of the individuals who make up that society.

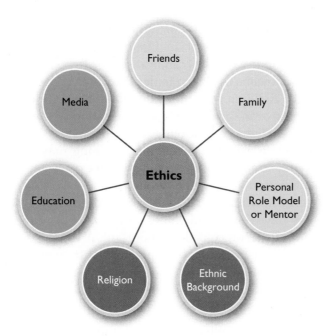

FIGURE 2.9
Many different factors influence a person's ethical development. Some, like friends, family, and role models/mentors, influence ethics through direct contact. Others are a function of traditions and beliefs to which they are exposed, such as ethnic background and religion. Elements in society, such as the media and educational philosophies, play a role as well.

This includes parent, siblings, and extended family. The reason for the significant influence of these people is the large quantity of time spent in the family context. Other people who influence ethical standards are friends, peers/classmates, and neighbors (Figure 2.9). Their influence increases significantly over time through the teenage years.

The influence of these people in shaping ethical standards can be either positive or negative. The standards of an individual will tend to moderate toward the general standards of the group. If a group of teenagers is involved in illicit drugs, alcohol, and other illegal activities, the dynamics of the group and peer pressure will likely influence the individuals within the group to adopt these activities as a legitimate pattern of behavior and their standards will change accordingly. The opposite can also occur—groups of students who are involved in community service, team sports, or other positive activities will likely adopt the ethics of that group.

Exposure to a suboptimal environment for ethical development in their family life does not mean individuals are destined to adopt those same standards. Many have taken this exposure to unethical behavior as a practical lesson in what *not* to do and have developed strong ethical standards in direct response to the negative behaviors they witnessed. Others who have experienced negative environments have had their ethical standards changed by the involvement of personal role models or mentors, who altered the course of the individual's life by allowing him or her to witness their ethical standards and the resulting behaviors.

Other factors that contribute to the development of ethical standards include the persons' cultural and ethnic background, their exposure to religious beliefs and systems, their educational experiences, and their exposure to various media outlets. Each of these can have a significant impact on how a person views the world and contributes toward the individual's determination of what is and is not acceptable behavior.

FYI

The fact that a person is exposed to a negative social environment does not condemn him or her to substandard ethics. In fact, some of the most ethical people have come from the most difficult environments.

The Roots of Personal Ethics. The exposure to all of these factors can produce different results in different individuals. For example, exposure to religious teachings can lead people to believe that behaving ethically is a means by which to demonstrate or live out their religious devotion. Religion may motivate others through fear of divine punishment now or in the afterlife, or anticipation of some present or future reward for living a virtuous life (Ghillyer, 2010). On the other hand, some people exposed to religious teaching may reject it altogether, basing their ethical behavior on human experience rather than a religion's definition of right and wrong.

Regardless of how individuals got to their destinations, when they get there, they have developed values and a value system. A **value** is a principle that a person considers important. A value system is a set of principles that the person has adopted as the framework for his or her behavior—the person's ethics. Not all values are equal. Sometimes there will be a conflict between two important values, but a choice must be made between the two. Examples include:

Value
A principle that someone considers important.

- Lying is wrong—but what if you were lying to protect the life of a loved one?
- Stealing is wrong—but what if you were stealing food to feed a starving child?
- Killing is wrong—but what if you had to kill someone in self-defense? (Ghillyer, 2010)

The value (worth) of a value is measured in two separate ways:

1. *Intrinsic value:* It is a good thing in itself and, whether or not it produces something good, it is pursued.
2. *Instrumental value:* It is something that is valuable because it can help reach another value. Money, in itself, is not valuable; however, money can be a tool to obtain something of value, such as financial security, shelter, food, and so forth.

Practical Personal Ethics. As indicated earlier, ethics is a challenging field of study because so many different definitions of *ethics* exist. To clarify the definition that we will use throughout the remainder of this book, the term *ethics* is categorized into one of the following four groups (Figure 2.10):

Simple Truth. This category includes those items that the majority of people would view as very straightforward in terms of right and wrong or good and bad. Many people would not consider this type of principle as an ethical issue until they see someone commit egregiously unethical behavior. In this case, "doing the right thing" seems clear. Placed in the form of a question, ethics asks, *What is the right thing to do?*

Individual Behavior. This category recognizes that a person's daily behavior is influenced by the values that he or she has developed over the years. This is a more personal form of ethics than simple truths, which are universally recognized. In this case, ethics asks, *How will I conduct myself in this specific situation?*

Personal Integrity. Personal integrity sees ethics and values from an external point of view, rather than an internal perspective. The

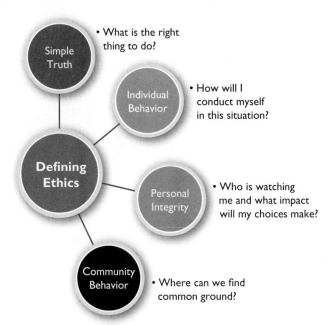

- Simple Truth
- What is the right thing to do?
- Individual Behavior
- How will I conduct myself in this situation?
- Defining Ethics
- Personal Integrity
- Who is watching me and what impact will my choices make?
- Community Behavior
- Where can we find common ground?

focus in this case is, What does my behavior say to other people? Someone is a person of integrity when he conducts himself in a manner consistent with his stated moral values and standards. Specifically, integrity is emphasized when the behavior matches the standards, even when there is significant financial or personal cost associated with maintaining that consistency. This form of ethics asks, *Who is watching me and what impact will my choices have on others?*

Community (or Societal) Behavior. Any collection of people in a given location will bring their set of values to the group. There is a tendency for people with common values to congregate together because of their shared values. However, as our communities and society become more diverse, it is increasingly likely that people with different values are going to be working together. In some fashion, agreement on basic ethical principles must be reached for the society to function effectively. In this case, ethics asks, *Where can we find common ground regarding our values and ethical principles?*

BUSINESS ETHICS

In his book *There's No Such Thing as Business Ethics,* author John Maxwell's thesis is that there should not be any distinction between the ethics that a person holds in his or her personal life and the ethics he or she displays in the conduct of business. However, the seeming frequency of ethical shortfalls in the business realm causes people to be skeptical concerning the general state of ethics in the business community. Although the failures of a few have tainted the reputation of the business community as a whole, the failures have not been without some benefit because they have brought the issue to light and reconfirmed the commitment of many to conduct their business in an ethical manner. Organizations that focus on ethics and compliance now commonly exist and one study showed that 68% of American companies have undertaken a formal ethics program (Ethics and Compliance Officer Association, 2006).

> **FYI**
>
> Business ethics involve all of the concerns associated with personal ethics, but also include additional issues because of the larger number of people (stakeholders) involved in the process.

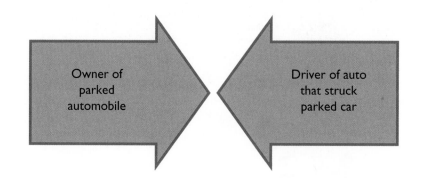

FIGURE 2.11
When a driver strikes an unattended parked car, the result is a conflict of interests. The interest of the owner of the parked car is to have his car remain in the same condition as it was when he left it. The interest of the driver who struck the car is ensuring that his insurance rates do not go up and that the police do not become aware of his multiple unpaid tickets. The driver feels that the damage to the car is minor and may not be noticed. However, he struggles with his conscience.

Stakeholder
A person with an interest in a company or organization.

The Difference Between Personal and Business Ethics.

When considering ethics in the business environment, we must account for all of the elements described concerning personal ethics to this point. However, there is a significant difference between personal and business ethics because there are usually multiple additional **stakeholders** in the process. Traditional personal ethics are generally limited to interactions between two parties or, in some cases, a relatively limited number of people (Figure 2.11). Even when personal ethical dilemmas occur within the context of larger groups, the number of different interests within the situation is usually limited. Business ethics involve a dramatically larger group of parties with widely different interests.

A stakeholder in the context of business is any individual, institution, or community that has a share or interest in a business operation. The stakeholders in any generic business can be identified as indicated in Figure 2.12.

When a business behaves in an unethical manner, it has the potential to affect negatively one or more of the other stakeholders. In extreme cases, it may affect all of them in different ways (Table 2.3).

FIGURE 2.12
The identity of the stakeholders that may exist in any type of business or medical practice.

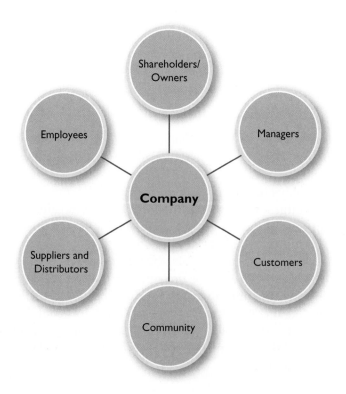

Table 2.3 Stakeholders and Their Potential Interest in the Organization

Stakeholders	Interest in the Organization
Shareholders or owners	• Investment decisions made on false or misleading information • Loss of value in the institution
Employees or managers	• Loss of employment • Insufficient funds to pay severance package or meet pension obligations
Customers	• Poor service quality
Suppliers or vendors	• Delayed payment for goods and services provided • Unpaid invoices if and when company goes bankrupt
Creditors	• Loss of principal and interest payments
Government	• Loss of tax revenue • Failure to comply with relevant legislation
Communities	• Unemployment of local residents • Economic decline

Source: Ghillyer, 2010.

In addition, not all stakeholders are equal. The interests of one stakeholder may not be comparable in importance or value to the stakeholder in question or the stakeholders as a group. Therefore, the concerns of all stakeholders may not receive equal consideration. This, by itself, could be an ethical concern (Figure 2.13).

The Conflict Between Personal and Business Ethics. Each business has a set of ethical principles by which it operates. In some cases these are formal and written, whereas in other cases they are informal and unwritten. The importance of ethics becomes very clear when an ethical conflict occurs between two stakeholders and one stakeholder has more power in the relationship, compared to the other stakeholder.

The power that is inherent on the part of the employer influences the nature and resolution of ethical issues. If the ethical standards of the employer are higher or more stringent than that of the employee, the employee who does not adhere to the employer's standards will be identified, disciplined, and possibly terminated. If the ethical standards of the employee are higher or more stringent than that of the employer, the employee has few options—most of which are not desirable in the eyes of the employee. This may tempt the employee to violate his or her ethical standards.

FIGURE 2.13
The process that must take place when competing, but incompatible, stakeholder objectives exist. The two steps denoted in orange are the areas where ethics play an extremely important role and ethical dilemmas have their most likely home.

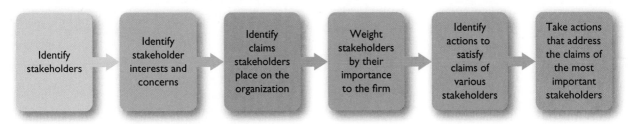

Source: Hill and McShane, 2008.

1. Do you agree that unethical behavior by an individual can have a significant detrimental effect on others or on society? If so, describe a personal experience or recent news story in which an individual's unethical behavior affected others. Summarize how that behavior came to negatively influence others.

2. Of the elements that influenced the development of your ethics, which had the most significant impact? Why was it the most significant?

3. Examine Figure 2.13, which addresses the situation when competing stakeholder interests are incompatible. Describe an example in which a stakeholder is more important than another stakeholder in a given situation. What makes that stakeholder's interest more important? Who determined whose interest had greater value?

2.4 Factors That Influence Business Ethics

In the context of business, including medical billing and coding, a number of factors influence business ethics (Figure 2.14). As described earlier, business ethics are more complicated than personal ethics because there are generally more stakeholders with varying interests involved in the process, and the actions of one stakeholder dramatically affect more people than a one-to-one personal interaction. Decisions in the business environment, by the nature of the transaction, influence a larger number of people. Consequently, it is necessary to understand the specific types of ethical factors that contribute to the ethical environment in which a person is functioning.

Occupational ethics
Standards that govern the manner in which members of a profession, trade, or craft conduct themselves while working within the context of their industry.

OCCUPATIONAL ETHICS

Occupational ethics are standards that govern how members of a profession, trade, or craft should conduct themselves when performing

FIGURE 2.14
Different types and sources of ethics all contribute to the formulation of the concept of "business ethics."

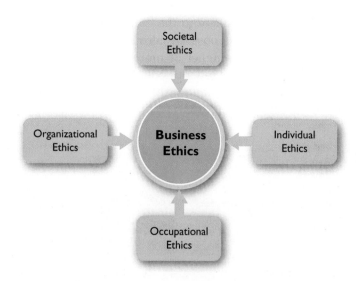

work-related activities (Frankel, 1989). These standards are unique to a particular industry and are not necessarily universally applicable in all circumstances. Some examples of industries with unique ethical standards include medicine, law, accounting, journalism, and direct marketing.

Within the coding industry, several organizations, including the American Academy of Professional Coders (AAPC) and the American Health Information Management Association (AHIMA) publish a code of ethics for members of their organization. (These are explored in detail in Chapter 10.) In general, the purpose of these codes of ethics is to encourage billing and coding professionals to engage in behavior that is of a higher standard than that which is required by the law.

ORGANIZATIONAL ETHICS

Whereas occupational ethics provides guidance for behavior among those within a given industry, **organizational ethics** provides ethical guidance for a company, its managers, and its employees. It provides instruction as to how company representatives should conduct themselves—it is more specific than occupational ethics. Either organizational ethics may establish a standard that is higher than traditional occupational ethics or it may provide more detailed instruction regarding appropriate behavior.

Ethics are important throughout an entire organization. However, the ethics of the top managers of an organization are crucial to the ethical direction of the corporation. If the ethics of the owners or top managers are questionable or inconsistent, it becomes difficult for the employees to whom they report to behave ethically. If employees fail to follow an instruction or refuse to engage in behaviors they personally find to be unethical, they may face the threat of discipline or termination. If unethical behavior is a hallmark of an organization, there is a substantial probability that the unethical behavior will spread to others who would have otherwise behaved in an ethical fashion.

Most ethical failures within organizations result when one of two things occur:

1. Individuals put their self-interest above that of the organization's published ethical guidelines.
2. The organization has created an environment in which ethical behavior is not highly valued and employees act accordingly.

Organizational ethics
Standards that govern the manner in which members of a particular company or organization conduct themselves in their role as an employee of the entity.

SOCIETAL ETHICS

Societal ethics are standards that govern how members of a society should deal with one another in matters such as fairness, justice, poverty, and the rights of the individual (Jones & George, 2009). Societal ethics come from the laws of a country, as well as customs, practices, and unwritten values and norms.

The ethics of a society can vary significantly among societies. Some societies believe very strongly in the importance of the welfare of each of their citizens. Therefore, they have relatively high tax rates that fund government programs to ensure that all citizens receive certain services, such as health care and significant retirement benefits. In other societies,

Societal ethics
Standards that govern how members of a society should deal with one another.

Ensuring Active, Engaged Compliance

A physician, whose coding practices were historically suspect, attended a presentation at a conference by a health care attorney. The attorney recommended that all attendees develop and implement a billing and coding compliance program to demonstrate the practice's good faith effort to Medicare, Medicaid, and other third-party payers to conduct themselves in compliance with all legal and ethical standards.

The physician told his office manager to write up a compliance plan, using some of the materials provided at the conference as a template. The physician asked the office manager to present a draft of the compliance program to him within a week. The physician looked at the draft, signed off as the compliance officer, and handed it back to the office manager.

1. Do you believe that this physician practice will engage in ethical behavior related to its coding? What is the basis for your belief?

2. What factors will influence this practice's (organization) success or failure in relationship to ethical behavior in coding?

Intractable
Unmanageable or impossible to resolve cooperatively.

FYI

The increased amount of interaction between different societies and cultures has emphasized the effect of differing societal ethics in creating conflict.

bribery is standard practice in "getting things done." This has created some problems for certain worldwide organizations that have to balance these competing societal ethical systems. How can a company work within a society where bribery is not seen as unethical when it is based in the United States, where bribery is not only unethical—it is illegal?

As the world becomes "smaller" and more integrated, certain societal differences become even more pronounced. In Western society, women's rights are very important and the ethical principle of treating all people fairly, both men and women, exists explicitly in many of our laws. However, in some other societies, women are viewed differently and there is no ethical motivation to ensure that they are treated in the same fashion as men. When people from different societies with widely varying ethical standards encounter one another, the opportunity exists for conflict and ethical dilemmas. Each society believes wholeheartedly that its approach is the "right" and "ethical" approach and, therefore, it has no obligation to change its position. Ultimately, the law of a given country has to establish the standard when the conflict is **intractable.** Yet, the law cannot necessarily change people's core ethical beliefs, which were formed, in part, by the culture in which they were raised.

Conflicting Cultures in the Billing Office

Stephanie went to work in the billing office of a physician who had emigrated from another country—one in which women's rights are not valued in the same way they are in the United States and where bribery is a common practice. The physician was very clear with Stephanie that it was her responsibility to obtain as much revenue as possible and that "playing with the rules" was not only acceptable, but also encouraged.

Stephanie was highly uncomfortable with this situation—it went so far that she became aware that the physician was submitting charges for services that he never provided. She attempted to speak to the physician about her concerns, but he exploded into a rage, stating, "How dare you question me! Don't ever talk to me about this again or you will be fired!"

1. How should Stephanie respond in this situation?

2. If the physician was asked about his behavior, he would indicate that he did absolutely nothing wrong—his behavior is consistent with his societal ethical norms. Explain how you would tell him that his standards are wrong.

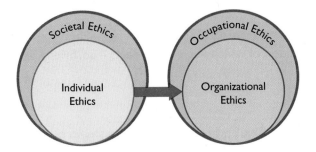

FIGURE 2.15
Individual ethics contribute to societal ethics, while organizational ethics contribute to occupational ethics.

Individual ethics are developed within the context of societal ethics. Each individual brings societal and individual ethics to the employer organization. As the employee becomes familiar with the organization and its ethical principles (and becomes familiar with occupational ethics if new to the industry; Figure 2.15), the individual will find either that his or her ethics are consistent with the employer and industry, or that his or her ethics are inconsistent with the work environment. The person will need to decide how to respond to the circumstance—leave the organization, modify his or her ethics, or seek to influence the ethics of the organization?

INDIVIDUAL ETHICS

Individual ethics are created within the context of the societal ethics in which the person was raised. That ethical framework is placed into the workplace world of occupational and organizational ethics.

Individual ethics are personal standards and values that determine how people view their responsibilities to other people and groups and how they should act when their own self-interests are at stake (Jones & George, 2009). The fact that a person is exposed to a particular society's standards does not mean that he or she automatically agrees with and/or conducts his or her life by those standards. In fact, some people completely reject the ethical standards to which they were exposed—they choose a different path. Either way, the standards to which they were exposed influenced how they arrived at the standards they ultimately follow.

The environment to which they were exposed, which includes family, peers, and those in the surrounding community, does not necessarily produce ethics that society, in general, would find acceptable. If a person were born into a family that was engaged in organized crime, the individual's concept of acceptable and ethical behavior could be substantially different from that of the average person. On the other hand, that person may find the behaviors to which he or she was exposed so unacceptable that the individual would reject the family's lifestyle and adhere to a different ethical standard.

Individual ethics
Personal standards and values that determine how people view their responsibilities to other people and groups and how they should act when their own self-interests are at stake.

Thinking It Through 2.4

1. Which of the ethical factors that contribute to the ethical environment in business is the most significant? On what basis do you form your opinion?

2. What is the primary issue currently affecting the health care industry that is influenced by societal ethics? On what do you base your opinion?

3. Have you ever had a circumstance in which your personal (individual) ethics conflicted with the ethics of your employer or other organization of which you were a part? If so, briefly describe the situation.

2.5 The Relationship Between Law and Ethics

A common misconception exists that the law and ethics are essentially the same. In a perfect world, ethics and law would always coincide. Unfortunately, we do not live in a perfect world. Law and ethics have a multilayered relationship and there are certain things that the law can do that ethics cannot do, and vice versa. The law, by definition, is the **codification** of rules of conduct, established by the government to maintain harmony, stability, and justice in the society (Brown & Sukys, 2009). It defines the legal rights and duties of the people under its governance and provides a way to enforce those rights through the courts and legislative system. In addition, the law provides a standard by which those in a society can agree to conduct themselves (see Table 2.4).

Codification
Formalized, written organization of rules or guidelines.

ETHICS AS A FOUNDATION FOR THE LEGAL SYSTEM

Laws not founded on a set of ethical principles will rarely succeed in reaching their objectives (Brown & Sukys, 2009). The reason why ethics is required as a foundation is that the law, in itself, is insufficient to cause people to do the "right" thing (Figure 2.16). The law does not provide an incentive for people to do the right thing—it simply provides a disincentive to *not* do the wrong thing. Unfortunately, for many people that disincentive is not sufficient to keep them from doing the wrong thing. In some cases, the risk of being caught doing the wrong thing is perceived as sufficiently low to justify the risk in engaging in the illegal activity. This is even more severe than the situation described

Table 2.4 Comparison of the Role of Ethics and the Role of Law

Ethics	Law
Develops and supplies standards for behavior, but can't enforce compliance.	Can enforce compliance with the standards.
Ethical standards change informally, generally over long periods of time.	Provides a means for laws to be formally modified.
Significant disagreements can exist regarding the source/type of ethical standards in use.	Universally recognized as a standard.
Facilitates the functioning of a society by serving as a framework for laws.	Facilitates the functioning of a society.
Indirectly promotes societal welfare by encouraging people to conduct themselves in certain ways.	Directly promotes societal welfare by rewarding/punishing behavior through tax laws.
Encourages individuals to resolve conflicts in a mutually satisfactory manner.	Protects rights of individuals and makes formal decisions in resolving conflicts.

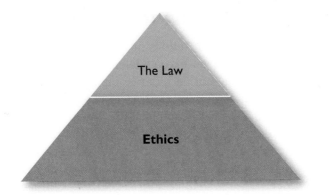

The Law

Ethics

FIGURE 2.16
Ethics must serve as the foundation for the law in order for there to be a true commitment to the following of the law. Without ethics, the law would collapse.

on page 34–35, where ethics are viewed only as a set of rules. In this situation, law without ethics is nothing more than potential punishment without a personal commitment to following any rules.

Ethics and law have a dependent relationship. The law requires ethics as a foundation to be effective. Ethics requires the law to serve as deterrent and enforcement tool. Neither is as effective independently as when they work together.

FYI

Law and ethics are often considered together, not because they are the same, but because they have an inseparable relationship.

Compliance Programs—Law and Ethics

Compliance programs are the American health care system's primary tool to strive toward compliance with the law. The challenge of compliance programs is that coding guidelines are not as firm as most laws. The law has the court system to settle different interpretations of the law; it is difficult to find an impartial avenue by which to resolve conflict in interpretation of coding guidelines. Therefore, health care providers are obligated to comply with ill-defined guidelines that have wide variations in interpretation, even among people who sincerely want to do the right thing. It is difficult to ensure that the practice adheres to the rules when the rules cannot be definitively identified.

In attempting to comply with guidelines that are not universally understood or applied, is there any hope for success for a compliance program when strong ethical principles do not preexist within the corporation? The answer to this question is, "Probably not." Just as the law is less effective when there are no underlying ethical principles, compliance programs are less effective when underlying ethical principles are absent.

Does that mean that compliance programs are not worthwhile? Absolutely not. They are valuable on three levels:

1. Compliance programs clearly communicate the expectations of the corporation to its employees. Employees who are committed to behaving ethically are supported in their efforts. Employees who are not committed to behaving ethically are not rewarded for their behavior. In fact, they may be disciplined or terminated. In summary, one purpose of a compliance program is to create an environment where behaving in compliance with the law is the expectation.

2. Compliance programs serve the same purpose as the law—they prescribe a method by which adherence to the program is monitored and measured. If there are variances from the standards of the program, there is a prescribed course of action to respond to that variance.

3. If there is determined to be a variance from legal standards by a government agency or other third-party payer, the existence of a compliance program may be helpful in mitigating potential liability. If there is an indication that the provider made a good faith effort to comply with the legal requirements associated with coding, but there was an inadvertent or unintentional violation of the law, the penalty imposed on the provider may be significantly reduced. If there was no effort to comply with the law or monitor the practice's compliance, the governing agency may impose more severe penalties because it is indicative of either a proactive intent to commit fraud or an indifference to doing the right thing.

ETHICS AS A CONTRIBUTOR TO THE LAW

Which is the higher standard—ethics or the law? Most generally recognize that ethical standards exceed legal standards. The fact that something is "legal" does not necessarily make it "ethical." On some occasions, the fact that something is ethical does not necessarily make it legal. However, the latter circumstance is far rarer than the former and is usually the result of a unique, complex situation.

Traditionally, laws are created as the result of an ethical breach identified by society. To formally indicate society's dissatisfaction with the unethical behavior, a law is created that specifically defines the behavior that is inappropriate and prescribes a penalty associated with the failure to comply with the law. In this way, ethics contributes to the formation of law.

Others disagree with this assessment, relying on the famous idiom, "Locks don't keep crooks honest; they just keep honest people honest." Another way to look at the relationship between law and ethics is that law is the boundary over which people should not cross; ethics is what encourages people to stay away from the boundary in the first place. People who ask only "Is it legal?" are really asking, "How close to the line can I get?" People who ask "Is it ethical" are really asking, "How can I get further away from the line?" (Figure 2.17).

In summary, ethical principles are superior to the law. The law tells people what they *cannot* do or what they *must* do. Ethics encourages people by informing them as to what they *should* do. Nonetheless, the law is necessary because not everyone adheres to strong ethical principles.

FIGURE 2.17

People's natural inclination is to see how close they can get to the law (as if it were a cliff) without going over the line (the red arrows). Strict adherence to ethical principles and standards serves as a magnet, pulling people away from the line toward a standard higher than the law (the yellow arrows).

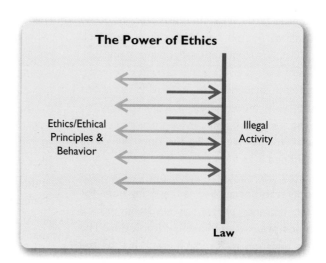

The Power of Ethics

Ethics/Ethical Principles & Behavior

Illegal Activity

Law

Thinking It Through 2.5

1. Examine Table 2.4. Where are ethics and the law most similar? Where are they most dissimilar?

2. Explain the statement "Ethics and law have a dependent relationship."

3. From a brief Internet search or review of recent news reports, identify a recently passed new law. What was the ethical issue that prompted the creation of that law?

2.6 The Range of Ethical Approaches to Individual and Corporate Behavior

Although many different sources for and theories about ethical behavior exist, individuals' and businesses' ethics are only as effective as the commitment they make to adhere to those ethics. The commitment to ethics can range from little to none, to a very intensive commitment to the highest ethical standard—with levels of ethical commitment existing between these two extremes (Figure 2.18).

OBSTRUCTIONIST APPROACH

The **obstructionist approach** to ethics describes the individuals or businesses that are aware of right and wrong and the basic principles of ethics, but choose not to follow them. They intentionally behave in a manner inconsistent with society's ethical standards and go so far as to intentionally commit illegal acts. The reason for adopting this approach is the belief that the individual or company will somehow benefit more by behaving unethically than ethically. On some occasions, a person does not intentionally start out with an obstructionist ethics framework in mind—a small infraction or a single poor choice that is in violation of his or her ethical standards is not addressed appropriately. The effort to hide the original small issue creates the need for further violation of ethical standards, which creates the need for further coverup, and so on. However, each additional choice to continue the coverup takes the person further from his or her ethical standards and the person in effect becomes obstructionist in behavior.

In the world of medical billing and coding, an extreme example of obstructionist ethics would be a person who establishes a durable medical equipment company, with the intent to defraud Medicare, Medicaid, and third-party payers by submitting claims for items and services never provided. Another example would involve a medical practice that discovers that one of its coders has been habitually overbilling the level of E/M services, resulting in tens of thousands of dollars of overpayments. While the practice did not initially intend to do this, it did not adequately monitor its employee. When it received notice of a routine chart audit, along with a list of charts to be reviewed, instead of admitting to the billing abuse it went into those charts and modified them to support the billing of the level of service that was

> **Obstructionist approach**
> An approach to ethics in which the individuals or businesses are aware of right and wrong and the basic principles of ethics, but choose not to follow them.

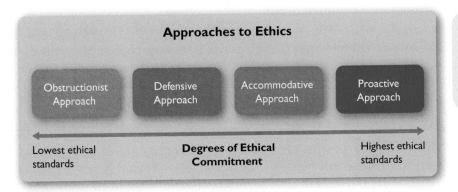

FIGURE 2.18
The range of methods in which individuals and businesses can approach ethics.

Source: Jones and George, 2009.

submitted. The decision to cover up the improper billing was obstructionist behavior on the part of the medical practice.

1. Identify three examples of obstructionist ethics in business in the last 20 years. Do you believe that they originally intended to conduct themselves in this fashion? Why or why not? If they did not, at what point did they become obstructionist in their behavior?

2. In the case of the medical practice in the previous example, what should it have done when it became aware of the improper billing?

3. Does your answer to question 2 change if the practice has virtually no money in the bank and it has maximized all possible sources of credit?

DEFENSIVE APPROACH

Individuals and businesses that conduct themselves using the **defensive approach** to ethics are ethical to the degree that they are required to do so by law, but they take no steps beyond the minimum standards of the law to be ethical. The defensive approach is more ethical than the obstructionist approach in that the ethics required by the law are considered.

Unfortunately, a large number of businesses in the United States operate in this fashion. They do what is legal—but no more than that. The operation that uses the defensive approach does things that many people would view as "not right," but they would not incur any legal penalty for behaving in this manner. A frequently cited example is the payment of very high salaries to CEOs, with large bonuses, at the same time that the company performance is declining and employees are laid off. High CEO salaries are not illegal, regardless of the company's performance, although in recent years lawmakers have made efforts to address this issue through revisions in the law and governmental regulations.

An example of defensive ethics in medical billing and coding would be a medical practice that implements a compliance program that defines the behavior that is and is not acceptable regarding the billing of services to patients and insurers. Although this practice has a compliance program, it does not engage in the activity required to monitor the quality of the billing and makes no specific effort to inform new employees of the compliance program. The program exists and it is available to any agency or insurer that wanted to see it. However, in reality, it does not affect the day-to-day billing and coding that occurs in this office.

1. It has been said that it is better not to have a compliance plan than to have a compliance plan and not follow it. What is your opinion of this sentiment? What are the risks and benefits of each option?

2. Would you reassign the categories if the compliance plan was established with no intent to ever follow it (as opposed to simply not following through on good intentions)? Why or why not?

ACCOMMODATIVE APPROACH

Individuals or businesses that use the **accommodative approach** to ethics are those that behave legally and ethically and do their best to balance the interests of different stakeholders, even in difficult situations (Jones & George, 2009). They want to do the "right" thing and, if faced with a choice that may harm the bottom line, they will act ethically—to the short-term financial harm of the company.

For both individuals and businesses, ethics can be categorized in one of five ways:

1. Always ethical
2. Mostly ethical
3. Somewhat ethical
4. Seldom ethical
5. Never ethical

Those that are accommodative in their approach to ethics would fit in category 1 or category 2, although they are always striving for category 1. In the case of business, a company that takes an accommodative approach is aggressive in dealing with employees who display ethical lapses, even if the action of the employee is not necessarily illegal. Although most people would claim to be in one of the first two categories, those in this category make a specific and concerted effort to be their best ethically.

In the world of medical billing and coding, an accommodative provider would be one that establishes a compliance program and follows through on all aspects of that plan. Regular monitoring, as prescribed by the plan, is carried out and adjustments and corrections are made as necessary.

1. Which is more likely to occur—a provider/employer with a higher ethical standard than the employee or an employee with a higher ethical standard than the employer? What is the basis for your answer?

PROACTIVE APPROACH

Individuals and businesses that engage in a **proactive approach** to their ethical behavior specifically go out of their way to conduct themselves in an ethical fashion. For companies, instead of being satisfied with conducting themselves ethically, they intentionally work to make doing the "right" thing part of the corporate culture. They become known throughout the marketplace as a company that is always ethical and treats all stakeholders fairly.

Proactive approach
An approach to ethics in which the individuals or businesses specifically go out of their way to conduct themselves in an ethical fashion.

An example of a proactive company in a billing and coding context would be one that routinely and regularly monitors its accounts receivable for credit balances. If a patient makes a prepayment for a given service and more is received from the insurance company than was originally expected (e.g., the patient met the deductible with expenses at another provider), this type of provider would send the refund check to the patient in a brief, defined period. It would not wait for the patient to request the refund—it would take the lead in the circumstance and issue the refund without prompting.

1. Why might a provider not be timely in issuing refund checks on overpaid accounts? Describe how the timing of refunds affects each of the stakeholders in the practice.

2. List the benefits and drawbacks of being proactive in issuing refunds quickly—in terms of economics and any other consideration that may come into play.

1. What is your opinion of the statement, "Individuals' and businesses' ethics are only as effective as the commitment they make to adhere to those ethics." Is it true? If so, why?

2. When examining the range of ethical behavior from "Always ethical" to "Never ethical," what do you believe is the most common response to this question? Why?

3. Is it reasonable to expect a medical practice to be proactive in its ethics? Why or why not? Is it sufficient to take an accommodative approach? Why or why not?

2.7 The Ethics System That Best Serves Billing and Coding

Throughout this chapter, we have discussed a number of belief systems and ethical theories. The broad array and widely differing scope of systems and theories appear to make defining an appropriate general ethical theory for life difficult, and defining one specific ethical theory for medical billing and coding nearly impossible. Although there are benefits to each of these systems/theories for the biller and coder, each also has drawbacks or elements that are troubling to one or more of the stakeholders in the process. So, what system is best for practical application for billers and coders within the medical industry?

THE GOLDEN RULE

FYI
The principle promoted by the Golden Rule is found in virtually every religion, culture, and philosophy in the world.

The best ethical system for application in the world of medical billing and coding is commonly known as the *Golden Rule.* This rule is by no means unique to Christianity. In fact, nearly every culture and religion around the world has a comparable principle within its teachings, as shown in Table 2.5.

THE VALUE OF THE GOLDEN RULE

The primary value of the Golden Rule is that any person can comprehend it, whether an elementary school child or the chief executive of the largest corporation. To determine whether an action is appropriate or to decide what course of action to take, all one must do is mentally place oneself in the other person's position—"If I were that person, how would I want me to behave in this case?" The answer to that question is likely the appropriate ethical response.

Another value of the Golden Rule is the fact that it is a principle accepted by most people. On what basis would a reasonable person indicate that he or she deserves to be treated better than someone else? If it is wealth or social status, a person could claim that he deserves to be treated better than someone in a lower social class who makes less money. However, that same person would also have to agree to be treated poorly by someone in a higher social class who makes more money. If the criterion for better treatment is talent, then the talented person could claim better treatment than less talented people—until someone else with more talent appears.

Table 2.5 Variations of the Golden Rule in World Cultures and Religions

Religion/Culture/Philosophy	Teaching
Buddhism	Hurt not others in ways that you would find hurtful.
Christianity	Therefore, whatever you want men (others) to do to you, do also to them.
Confucianism	Do not to others what you would not like yourself.
Grecian	Do not that to a neighbor which you shall take ill from him.
Hinduism	This is the sum of duty: do nothing to others which if done to you would cause you pain.
Humanism	Individual and social problems can only be resolved by means of human reason, intelligent effort, and critical thinking, joined with compassion and a spirit of empathy for all living beings.
Islam	No one of you is a believer until he desires for his brother that which he desires for himself.
Jainism	In happiness and suffering, in joy and grief, we should regard all creatures as we regard our own self.
Judaism	Whatever is hateful to you, do not to another.
Native American Spirituality	Respect for all life is the foundation.
Persian	Do as you would be done by.
Roman	Treat your inferiors as you would be treated by your superiors.
Shintoism	The heart of the person before you is a mirror. See there your own form.
Sikhism	As you deem yourself, so deem others.
Taoism	Regard your neighbor's gain as your own gain, and your neighbor's loss as your own loss.
Yoruban	One going to take a pointed stick to pinch a baby bird should first try it on himself to feel how it hurts.
Zoroastrianism	That nature alone is good which refrains from doing to another whatsoever is not good for itself.

Source: Mallor et al., 2010.

Those who are truly committed to the Golden Rule will always be able to find common ground with reasonable people (Maxwell, 2003). If an individual believes the Golden Rule, then he or she will take the time to learn more about the other person and understand the person's beliefs, particularly if there is a conflict that seems impossible to resolve. Resolution can generally occur when an individual truly understands the other person's position and is committed to responding, even if disagreement exists, in the same fashion in which he or she would like to be responded.

Finally, the Golden Rule is the ultimate win–win philosophy. Examine the position of two different people:

Person one: If I treat you as well as I desire to be treated, you win.
Person two: If you treat me as I desire to be treated, I win.

CHALLENGES TO THE GOLDEN RULE

There are two primary challenges to successfully living out the Golden Rule, particularly within the world of business.

Others Do Not Respond in Kind.   If a person is committed to treating others as they want to be treated, he or she is viewed as an ethical person. The challenge for this ethical person is dealing with people who do not respond in the same fashion. The other persons do

not consider the interests of others—they are interested in obtaining only what they want, regardless of the effect on others. The frustration for recipients of this type of behavior is that they cannot control the actions of others. If a person chooses to behave this way, there is no quick fix. An important concept to note is that the Golden Rule is not a conditional guideline—the instruction to treat others as you want to be treated is not waived if the other person fails to do the same.

It Is Easier to Ignore When a Corporation Is Involved. Corporations are often perceived as impersonal, faceless entities. As a result, an ethical individual many find it easier to conduct herself differently toward a corporation than toward a person with whom she has a personal relationship. Somehow, it is more acceptable to behave unethically toward a corporation than it is an individual. A key to successfully living the Golden Rule is to ensure consistency in application of the principle, regardless of the possible definitions of "them" in the phrase, "Do also to *them*."

APPLICATION TO THE WORLD OF MEDICAL BILLING AND CODING

The world of billing and coding presents challenges to individuals who wish to conduct themselves ethically. Keeping in mind the key principle of the Golden Rule, consider the following scenario: A patient asks a billing office representative to change the diagnosis on a claim because the insurance company denied the claim with the original (correct) diagnosis.

Consider the four points of view in this scenario, as depicted in Figure 2.19 and Table 2.6:

- The patient.
- The clinic employee.
- The clinic.
- The insurance company.

In billing and coding, occasionally parties to a transaction will ask another entity to act inconsistently with the Golden Rule. In these cases, the patient is asking the other parties to engage in behavior that they would not want to experience if the roles were reversed. When

FIGURE 2.19
There are six different ways in which the Golden Rule must be applied in a billing/coding scenario.

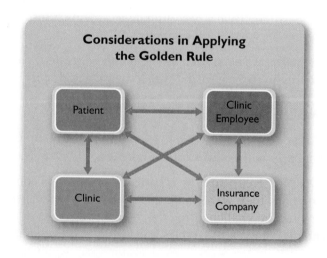

Considerations in Applying the Golden Rule

Patient

Clinic Employee

Clinic

Insurance Company

Table 2.6 Potential Interests of Parties in the Medical Coding Process

Entity	Desires of the Active Entity			
	Patient	Clinic Employee	Clinic	Insurance Company
Patient		Would like the patient to pay for the noncovered service	Would like to receive payment for services, while maintaining patient relationship	Desires that patients pay providers according to terms of insurance contract
Clinic employee	Wants employee to change diagnosis		Wants employee to obtain payment from patient	Wants clinic employee to be truthful in submitting claims
Clinic	Wants clinic to make employee change diagnosis	Wants to be supported in doing the "right" thing		Wants clinic to be truthful in submitting claims
Insurance company	Wants insurance company to pay for noncovered services	Has no specific request of insurer, given that payer has already made a determination	Has no specific request of insurer, given that payer has already made a determination	

Red—Requests that are not ethical/inconsistent with the Golden Rule.

this occurs, it is impossible for the Golden Rule to realize its full benefit and the win–win opportunity that is otherwise possible. Nevertheless, the other entities should not change their position because one of the entities did not follow the Golden Rule.

Thinking It Through 2.7

1. Would compliance programs be necessary if everyone followed the Golden Rule all the time? Why or why not?
2. List other entities that may be involved in the decision matrix in the health care arena.

CHAPTER REVIEW

Chapter Summary

Learning Outcomes	Key Concepts/Examples
2.1 Define the term *ethics* and differentiate between the various definitions assigned to the term. Pages 33–36	• *Ethics* and *ethical* have a broad range of possible definitions. The definition that a person chooses to use and the way in which he or she views ethics will shape how ethics affect his or her life. • There are three ways to see ethics: 　1. A field of study. 　2. A set of rules and guidelines. 　3. A set of personal beliefs and associated behavioral principles. • There are three categories of ethics: 　1. Metaethics 　2. Normative ethics 　3. Applied ethics

(continued)

Learning Outcomes	Key Concepts/Examples

2.2 Identify and discuss the various methods available to establish ethical norms. Pages 36–42	• Ethical standards are established in one of four ways:
	  1. Virtue ethics
	  2. Deontological ethics
	    • Rights theory
	    • Justice theory
	  3. Teleological ethics
	    • Justice theory
	    • Utilitarianism
	    • Maximizing profit
	  4. Ethical relativism has become more accepted in recent times.

2.3 Elaborate on the importance of ethics on personal, business, and societal levels. Pages 43–50	• The issue of ethics has become quite prominent in recent years, primarily because of the widespread awareness of massive ethical failures, both personal and in the business world.
	• Ethics are important because:
	  1. Ethical behavior allows society to function predictably and effectively.
	  2. There are financial and nonfinancial benefits to behaving ethically.
	• Ethics are formed in individuals through their exposure to the behavior of those around them.
	• The root of personal ethics is values. There are two types of values:
	  1. Intrinsic value—The value is good in itself, whether or not it produces a particular result.
	  2. Instrumental value—The value is good because it helps reach another value.
	• Ethics are categorized into one of four groups:
	  1. Simple truth—Uniformly accepted standards of right and wrong.
	  2. Individual behavior—An individual's interpretation and application of simple truth.
	  3. Personal integrity—The effect of a person's behavior choices on others.
	  4. Community or societal behavior—Identifying common ground regarding appropriate behavior.
	• The primary difference between personal ethics and business ethics is that there is a significantly larger group of stakeholders affected by ethical decisions in business.
	• A complicating factor in business decisions is that not all stakeholder interests are equal. A challenge is measuring that inequality and handling it appropriately.
	• There can often be conflict between personal and business ethics. Because of the variance in relative power in the business environment, this can create its own set of ethical dilemmas.

2.4 Distinguish between the factors that influence personal ethics and the factors that influence business ethics. Pages 50–54	• Four factors can influence business ethics:
	  1. Occupational ethics
	  2. Organizational ethics
	  3. Societal ethics
	  4. Individual ethics

2.5 Explain the relationship between law and ethics. Pages 54–56	• Law is the codification of rules of conduct, established by the government to maintain order in society. • Ethics is the foundation of the law. • Ethics and law are similar in many ways, but there are some things that ethics can do that the law cannot and vice versa. • Ethics is a higher standard than the law and, in most cases, is the first step in the creation of laws and rules.

2.6 Evaluate the range of ethical approaches in which individuals and companies can conduct themselves. Pages 57–60	• There are four ethical approaches that individuals and companies can use to conduct themselves:
	  1. Obstructionist approach
	  2. Defensive approach
	  3. Accommodative approach
	  4. Proactive approach

Learning Outcomes	Key Concepts/Examples

2.7 Describe the system of ethics that best serves the practice of medical billing and coding. Pages 60–63	• The Golden Rule is the best ethical system for application to the field of medical billing and coding. The principle appears in some form in nearly every society, cultural, and religious system.
	• The Golden Rule is valuable because:
	  1. Anyone can comprehend it.
	  2. It is a principle accepted by most people.
	  3. It is possible to find common ground with reasonable people.
	• There are challenges to applying the Golden Rule:
	  1. Others may not respond in kind.
	  2. Some have difficulty applying it to entities within the corporate world.

End-of-Chapter Questions

Multiple Choice

Circle the letter that best completes the statement or answers the question.

1. **LO 2.1** All of the following can affect a person's definition of ethics *except*

   a. Personal experience

   b. Family and peer influence

   c. Formal or informal training in ethics

   d. The scope of a person's vocabulary

2. **LO 2.1** Which of the following is the correct ordering of types of ethics, from most theoretical to most practical?

   a. Metaethics, normative ethics, applied ethics

   b. Normative ethics, metaethics, applied ethics

   c. Applied ethics, metaethics, normative ethics

   d. Normative ethics, applied ethics, metaethics

3. **LO 2.1** Which of the following is most important regarding a person's ethics?

   a. Beliefs

   b. Words

   c. Actions

   d. Relationships

4. **LO 2.2** Virtue ethics focuses on _____, while deontological ethics focuses on _____.

   a. The person, principles

   b. The person, outcomes

   c. Principles, outcomes

   d. Outcomes, the person

5. **LO 2.2** Each of the following are forms of utilitarianism *except*

   a. Traditional utilitarianism

   b. Ethical altruism

   c. Ethical achievement

   d. Ethical egoism

6. **LO 2.2** Another term for ethical relativism is

   a. Situational ethics

   b. Relative utilitarianism

c. Ethical altruism

d. Judgmental ethics

7. **LO 2.3** Why has ethics been brought to the forefront of discussion in the world of business?

a. The universal belief that ethical behavior is more profitable

b. Massive ethical failures on the part of major corporations

c. Encouragement by prominent authors to be more ethical

d. Fear that ethical failures will result in the destruction of corporations

8. **LO 2.3** Personal ethical standards are developed by

a. Academic study

b. Exposure to the surrounding environment

c. Corporate training

d. Working with others to arrive at consensus

9. **LO 2.3** Which of the following factors is *not* a contributing factor to the development of ethics?

a. Cultural and ethnic background

b. Religious beliefs and systems

c. Exposure to various forms of media

d. Attendance at a private school

10. **LO 2.3** What is the biggest difference between personal and business ethics?

a. Business ethics standards are lower.

b. There is no difference.

c. Business ethics generally have more stakeholders.

d. Personal ethics generally have more emotional issues attached.

11. **LO 2.4** Which of the following is *not* specifically a factor that contributes to business ethics?

a. Organizational ethics

b. Occupational ethics

c. Individual ethics

d. Situational ethics

12. **LO 2.4** Societal ethics originate in all of the following, *except*

a. The laws of the country in which the society exists

b. Personal/individual standards

c. Practices within a society

d. Unwritten rules and traditions

13. **LO 2.5** Which of the following is *not* a characteristic of ethics?

a. Significant disagreement can exist regarding its source and use.

b. It has an enforcement component.

c. It develops and supplies standards for behavior.

d. It serves as a framework for laws.

14. **LO 2.6** The minimum acceptable approach to ethics is

a. Obstructionist

b. Defensive

c. Accommodative

d. Proactive

15. **LO 2.7** The best ethical system for use in the billing and coding world is

a. Rights theory

b. The Golden Rule

    c. Justice theory

    d. Consequentialist ethics

Short Answer

Use your critical thinking skills to answer the following questions.

1. **LO 2.1** Summarize the relationship between metaethics, normative ethics, and applied ethics.

2. **LO 2.1** Look at the definitions of *ethics* on page 33. Which definition do you more closely identify with? Why?

3. **LO 2.2** Compare and contrast virtue ethics, deontological ethics, and teleological ethics.

4. **LO 2.2** Discuss the primary weakness of virtue ethics.

5. **LO 2.2** What is the most significant weakness of strict rights theory? How has this been overcome in modern rights theory?

6. **LO 2.2** Discuss the primary weakness of utilitarianism.

7. **LO 2.2** Why is ethical relativism an appealing concept in the United States?

8. **LO 2.3** Discuss why there is so much distrust within American society today.

9. **LO 2.3** The research shows that companies that are ethical are more profitable than the average company. Why do you believe so many businesses are willing to behave unethically?

10. **LO 2.3** Discuss why all values are not equal.

11. **LO 2.3** Describe the conflict that exists when the ethical standards of an employee are different than those of the employer.

12. **LO 2.4** Do an Internet search and locate the ethical guidelines for a specific professional group not mentioned in the chapter. Provide an example of a behavior that the group discourages that is not illegal.

13. **LO 2.4** Discuss why the ethics of the top managers of an organization have such a significant impact.

14. **LO 2.4** Explain the relationships between individual–societal ethics and organizational–occupational ethics.

15. **LO 2.5** Discuss the ability of the law to serve as an incentive for ethical behavior.

16. **LO 2.5** Which has the higher standard—ethics or law? Explain your position.

17. **LO 2.6** Is a defensive approach to ethics adequate? Why or why not?

18. **LO 2.7** Discuss the key features of the Golden Rule that make it an attractive ethical system.

19. **LO 2.7** Discuss the two primary challenges in applying the Golden Rule.

Applying Your Knowledge

Case Study 1

At the beginning of this chapter, the story of Sandra Hobson was presented. Sandra was faced with an extremely difficult set of choices, each with different ethical implications.

To complete your analysis of this case, answer the following questions:

1. Apply each of the ethical theories presented in the chapter to this situation. What would Sandra do if she followed a strict interpretation of each theory? What would be the possible outcome for her professionally and what would be the outcome of the employees in her department?

2. Describe how the Golden Rule could be applied to this case. What are the challenges with applying it and how could they be overcome?

3. Put yourself in Sandra's shoes. What would you do in this case? Why? What is the most difficult element of the decision for you?

Case Study 2

Two years ago Kathy, a 57-year-old female, was laid off from the employer for whom she had worked since graduating from high school. She was disappointed because she believed that, in exchange for her many years of loyal service, her employer would be loyal toward her, even when the company experienced economic problems. She was especially troubled when she heard that the CEO of the corporation had received a sizable bonus from the company board because of the cost savings he had achieved through the company-wide layoffs.

Kathy was despondent because she didn't know how she could find another job that would have the same salary and benefits that she had previously—especially given her age. Although age discrimination is not legal, she knew that finding a new job wasn't going to be easy. She decided that she had to obtain a new skill set to start a new career. Her family physician, who she respected greatly, recommended that she become a medical biller and coder. After investigating her options, Kathy enrolled and graduated from an accredited medical office program at the local community college.

After graduation, Kathy quickly obtained a position in the office of a reconstructive surgeon, working in the billing office. She was responsible for coding for services, entering the charges, submitting them to third-party payers, and following up with the payers on denied claims.

Early in her tenure, Kathy discovered that there was often confusion among the payers concerning what should and should not be paid. Some services, which were required to restore a patient's physical functioning, were denied as "cosmetic" procedures. Other services, which were purely cosmetic procedures, were reimbursed by the payer, even though the practice had made special effort to ensure that the payer understood it was an elective procedure.

Kathy brought this matter to the attention of the office manager. She was told that she was obligated to fight the incorrect denials for the noncosmetic procedures, as the patients were entitled to benefits for those services. In the cases in which cosmetic procedures were improperly paid, Kathy was told to "just accept the payments," because it was the payer's fault if they couldn't figure out how to process claims and it helped offset the hassle associated with the improperly denied claims. In fact, Kathy had a conversation with a representative of one of the payers, who said, "If the claim was paid based on the information submitted, then you can assume the payment was correct."

Kathy did not feel right about the situation. However, she had mixed feelings because she needed this job and did not know how she would find another one if she "made too many waves" about this issue.

1. Several times in this scenario, law and ethics intersect. List those circumstances and provide a brief description of the issues.

2. How might Kathy's personal history have an effect on her opinions and possible actions?

3. Assess the circumstances in the reconstructive surgeon's office. Are illegal activities occurring? Are unethical activities occurring? If so, what are they?

4. If you were Kathy, what would you do in this situation?

Many businesses reflect their ethical standards in their mission and/or vision statement. Most companies, including hospitals and health care systems, publish these statements on their websites for the benefit of their employees and their patients.

Identify a health care organization in your geographic area, with which you are familiar, that has its mission and/or vision statement on its website. Examine this statement and answer the following questions:

1. Is there anything in the statement that makes reference to ethics or ethical standards? If so, summarize the elements that refer to ethics.

2. Review the information provided in this chapter and compare it to the selected statement. Based on the information provided in this chapter, what normative ethical standards are most significant to this organization? What elements in the statement cause you to believe this?

3. Based on your personal experience or through reputation, is the ethical component of the mission statement consistent with reality? Explain why or why not.

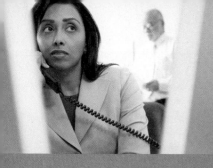

3

Why Ethical Dilemmas Occur

LEARNING OUTCOMES

After completing this chapter, you will be able to:

3.1   Develop a working personal definition of *ethical dilemma.*

3.2   Define the reasons why people do not always behave
       ethically.

3.3   Describe the roots of unethical behavior in the business
       setting.

3.4   Explain the reasons why unethical behavior can continue
       even when the behavior is potentially damaging to the
       individual or company.

3.5   Identify concrete personal tools to help in the problem-
       solving process when facing an ethical dilemma.

3.6   Apply ethical decision-making principles to case studies in
       billing and coding.

CASE STUDY

Enrique was a new coder at Overlook Family Practice, a small practice with three physicians—one owner and two employed physicians. He had just completed a coding program at the local college and passed his certification examination on the first try. He was very excited about the new job as he and his wife were expecting a baby in about three weeks.

Enrique was one of four people in the office who were assigned to administrative tasks—the receptionist, the office manager (who also performed medical records and receptionist duties), and his coworker in the billing office. Enrique worked closely with the other employee in the billing department, learning the particulars of how things were done in this practice. For the first two weeks, it appeared that this was the job of his dreams—everything that he imagined working in the health care industry would be.

One of Enrique's responsibilities was to cover his coworker's responsibilities in her absence. The coworker was going on vacation in a few weeks and he needed to be prepared to handle her duties. One of her duties was to post payments from the insurers and to refile claims as necessary to obtain payment on denied claims. Because of the demographics of the area, a significant portion of their patient base was covered by Medicare and this was the first payer for which Enrique was trained in posting. He was surprised when he was told by his coworker that when patients had Medicare coverage, but did not have a secondary insurer, that he was just to write off the balances as the Medicare patients were not supposed to receive statements. He asked his coworker why Medicare patients were not billed. She simply replied, "I don't know—that's just the way that I was told to do it."

As the day continued, they encountered some Medicare denials because the diagnosis code did not support the procedure that was performed. For these claims, the coworker pulled out a three-ring binder, which had selected pages from the Medicare coverage manual. When she found the guidelines that showed which diagnosis codes supported the medical necessity of the CPT code in question, Enrique saw that there were red X marks next to one or two of the diagnosis codes. His coworker went into the billing system and replaced the diagnosis code with one of the marked codes from the binder. She then prepared the claim for resubmission. Enrique asked her about what was going on. The coworker replied that she was told to "do whatever it takes to get paid for Medicare claims." Enrique indicated that he wasn't sure this was right—did the patient really have the condition that was assigned? His coworker did not know; this was just what the person before her did.

Enrique went home that night deeply troubled. He had become aware of two serious violations that day—an across-the-board policy of waiving Medicare copayments and submission of false diagnosis codes to Medicare. He talked to his wife and decided that he could not tolerate the situation. He was going to speak to the office manager the next day.

Early the next morning, before the clinic opened for the day, Enrique went into the manager's office. He asked to speak with her and she agreed. He started by saying, "I was learning about Medicare payment posting and claim refiling yesterday and . . ." She cut him off and shouted, "What is it with you people? Just do your job as you're told! The person who was here before you just wouldn't follow instructions! A word to the wise—just do your job as you are told and let me worry about everything else!" With that, she got up and left and the meeting was over.

Enrique went back to his desk, more troubled than before. He thought about what he knew concerning Medicare rules and regulations, and he remembered his class in ethics. It did not feel right—nothing about the situation felt right.

Enrique did not feel like eating at lunch—he took a walk instead to think more about the situation. He had always felt that doing the right thing was important, but he had never been in a position where he had so much responsibility. He could not afford to lose this job, and he certainly could not afford to lose his health insurance.

Enrique never imagined that he would encounter an ethical dilemma so early in his career. He decided that he would think about the situation over the weekend. On Monday, he would make a decision about what to do next.

1. What are the factors contributing to Enrique's dilemma?
2. Who created the dilemma?
3. What are the possible solutions to this dilemma?

Introduction

Ethical behavior can be defined as having two components or parts:

1. A *fundamental belief* in certain values, principles, or guidelines that are intended to govern choices, actions, and behavior.
2. A *commitment to conduct* oneself in a manner that is consistent with the beliefs, values, principles, or guidelines identified in component 1.

The second part of the ethical behavior definition—acting on your values and beliefs—is essential to behaving ethically. Have you ever known persons who swore they were honest or had certain values, but then acted in the opposite way? When there is a difference between a person's stated values and their behavior, an *ethics gap* exists (Figure 3.1).

FIGURE 3.1

An ethics gap occurs when there is an inconsistency between a person's beliefs and values and his or her conduct. When a person behaves ethically, there is a connection between his or her beliefs and values and conduct.

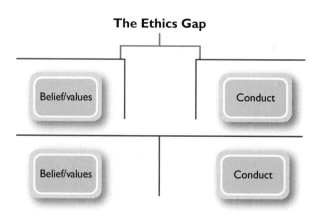

The Ethics Gap

Belief/values — Conduct

Belief/values — Conduct

Holding values but acting contrary to them can be worse than not professing your values at all. It is important, therefore, to keep both of these elements in mind.

3.1 Defining *Ethical Dilemma*

Many different possible definitions of *ethical dilemma* exist. Some examples, each with a different focus or emphasis, are listed in Table 3.1.

None of the definitions in Table 3.1 are satisfactory in defining an ethical dilemma in every possible circumstance. In some cases, although there is no lack of agreement on the principles, it is a simple matter of struggling with doing what the person knows to be "right" according to his or her beliefs and values. In other cases, the options are clear—it is an issue of choosing to do right. Finally, there is not always a third party involved in the ethical dilemma—it is sometimes an individual issue. For our discussion, we will define **ethical dilemma** as an occasion when a person is at a point of decision concerning a conflict between his or her *values* and the *action* he or she will ultimately take.

John Maxwell (2003) presented a comparable definition of *ethical dilemma* in his book *There's No Such Thing as 'Business' Ethics*. Maxwell wrote, "An ethical dilemma can be defined as an undesirable or unpleasant choice relating to a moral principle or practice" (p. 5). Another related method of defining *ethical dilemma* is to place the focus on the decision-making process, as illustrated in Figure 3.2.

Because being in an ethical dilemma can feel unpleasant (such as being caught between two tough choices), sometimes people make a quick decision without considering the future effects. The guilt from making a decision that does not feel right can seem like a better outcome than the anxiety of having to make that decision.

The reason that the decision-making process is the defining element for an ethical dilemma is that choice is the foundation of the second element of ethics—the will to do that which is consistent with ethical belief. In other words, are my ethical beliefs and values more important than whatever circumstance is challenging them at this time? If the answer is yes, the person agrees to encounter whatever possible

> **FYI**
>
> There are two parts to behaving ethically: (1) having values and beliefs that are important to you, and (2) behaving consistently with those beliefs.

> **FYI**
>
> Ethical dilemmas occur when behaving consistently with your beliefs and values is challenging or uncomfortable.

Ethical dilemma
An occasion when a person is at a point of decision concerning a conflict between his or her values and the action he or she will ultimately take.

Table 3.1 Definitions of *Ethical Dilemma*

Definition	Focus/Emphasis
A situation in which there is no agreement over exact accepted principles of right or wrong	Lack of agreement on principles
A situation in which there is no obvious right or wrong decision, but rather a right or wrong answer	Lack of agreement on options
A quandary people find themselves in when they have to decide if they should act in a way that might help another person or group, even though doing so might go against their own self-interest	Acting against self-interest Acting in the interest of others

Ethical Decision Points

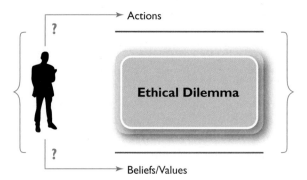

FIGURE 3.2

When individuals are at a point of decision concerning a conflict between their values and beliefs and the actions they will ultimately take, they have an ethical dilemma. Once they choose a specific behavior, the dilemma is resolved. If they act inconsistently with their values and beliefs, they may face the same circumstance again since no resolution occurred in their previous decision.

FYI

Ethical dilemmas are not unique to individuals. They exist within businesses of any size and are usually more complex than the ethical dilemmas of individuals because of the larger number of stakeholders involved.

adverse outcomes result from that choice. If the answer is no, then the person indicates that he or she does not have the will to do something that is consistent with his or her ethical beliefs and values.

Ethical dilemmas are not exclusive to individuals—companies and organizations of any size can also encounter dilemmas. The decision-making process can appear more complex than for that of the individual, but the essential elements remain the same: Does the company have principles and values to which it adheres? Does it have the will to conduct itself in accordance with those values (Figure 3.3)?

The presence of ethical values, conflict, and difficult choices are all requirements for ethical dilemmas. If a decision or choice is easy or straightforward, then no dilemma exists. Similarly, if a person or organization has no core values or beliefs, then no dilemma exists. Dilemmas may exist for those that encounter the person or entity with no core values or beliefs, but that occurs only because the behavior of the unethical person/entity conflicts with their own values and beliefs.

FIGURE 3.3

Multiple components contribute to the creation of an ethical dilemma. These factors include the presence of various values and beliefs, the desire to live according to those values and beliefs, and some sort of conflict.

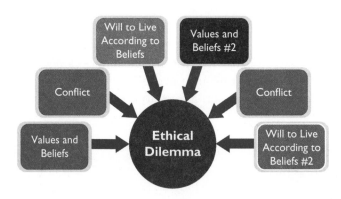

Thinking It Through 3.1

1. Do you agree with this textbook's definition of *ethical dilemma?* Why or why not? If you disagree, how would you change it?

2. Which is more difficult—defining values and beliefs or behaving consistently with them? Why?

3. Why is the presence of difficulty necessary for a dilemma to exist?

3.2 The Reasons Why People Behave Unethically

There has to be some reason why people behave unethically. It is unreasonable to believe that people would engage in a behavior unless there was a benefit, either real or perceived, in doing so. The question then becomes, What are the factors that cause people to choose unethical behavior when faced with an ethical dilemma?

A number of elements in business (and coding in particular) contribute to the development of dilemmas that result in unethical behavior. However, before we address them it is necessary to understand the factors that can influence every individual, regardless of role or place in life, to engage in unethical behavior.

THE ROOT AND INFLUENCES OF PERSONAL UNETHICAL BEHAVIOR

Several circumstances can create the temptation to engage in unethical behavior. However, the bottom line is usually the same—responsibilities, needs, and desires are viewed as more important than ethical standards and values. When it is difficult or impossible to fulfill responsibilities or meet specific needs *and* behave consistently with ethical standards and values, unethical behavior results when the responsibility or need takes priority.

In a hypothetical case in which a billing professional is asked by her manager to violate her moral principles by reporting procedures that weren't provided or by falsifying diagnoses, there is a combination of two decisions and four possible outcomes (Figure 3.4):

- *Ethical behavior—good outcome.* In this circumstance, the billing professional tells the manager that she is unwilling to engage in the behavior. The manager recognizes the fact that the action for which he is calling is wrong and commends the employee for her stand. An alternative, but similarly desirable, outcome could be that the billing professional is fired for failing to follow instructions and is hired the next day by a competing practice at a substantial salary increase.
  - Underlying thoughts/beliefs—Values are so important that the risk of ethical behavior outweighs the potential bad outcome that may occur. Fortunately, the bad outcome does not occur.

- *Unethical behavior—good outcome.* In this case, the billing professional tells the manager that she is unwilling to engage in the

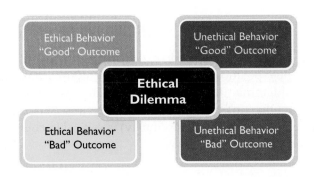

FIGURE 3.4

The matrix illustrates the possible scenarios that can occur when faced with an ethical dilemma.

requested behavior. The manager threatens the employee with termination. After evaluating the circumstances, the billing professional determines that she cannot afford to be without the job and agrees to engage in behavior that is not acceptable to her moral values. The outcome is good only in the sense that the employee retains her position, benefits, and security. Generally, these types of good outcomes supply short-term solutions and will likely have negative ramifications in the future.

- Underlying thoughts/beliefs—Responsibilities and needs are of greater importance than the values. The short-term benefits are positive, although there may be ongoing psychological struggles regarding the decision that was made. There is also a belief that the unethical behavior will never be discovered, although it often becomes public.

- *Ethical behavior—bad outcome.* The billing professional tells the manager that she is unwilling to engage in the requested behavior. The manager threatens the employee with termination. The billing professional refuses and is fired. She is unable to find another job and is at risk for losing her home.

  - Underlying thoughts/beliefs—The values are so important that even though a bad outcome is a likely or certain result, the person agrees to endure whatever hardship results from the choice not to engage in unethical behavior.

- *Unethical behavior—bad outcome.* The billing professional agrees to engage in the behavior requested by the manager, either willingly or unwillingly. The behavior of the company becomes known and the company is destroyed. The employee is out of a job and is in possible personal legal jeopardy.

  - Underlying thoughts/beliefs—Responsibilities and needs are of greater importance than the values. There is a false belief that there will be benefits, but the behavior is discovered so quickly that no benefits are actually realized.

Ideally, whenever there is a conflict between values and beliefs and the resulting behavior, people would always choose to be consistent with their values *and* there would be a positive short-term outcome. If this were the case, everyone would choose to behave properly, there would be no bad outcomes, and there would be no more ethical dilemmas. Unfortunately, arriving at a desirable outcome for all parties can be quite difficult—three out of the four possible behavior–outcome pairs are undesirable. This dynamic creates the abundance of ethical dilemmas that individuals face.

INFLUENCES THAT AFFECT ETHICAL DECISION MAKING

Mitigate
To make less severe or to minimize damage.

Since ethical dilemmas continue to exist, people are always attempting to improve their position and/or **mitigate** potential damages when faced with a dilemma. Resolving ethical dilemmas is never easy, but understanding the underlying goals and desires that inform these decisions (consciously or subconsciously) is critical in comprehending the foundation for these decisions.

The factors that influence ethical decision making are (Figure 3.6):

- Pressure
- Pleasure
- Power
- Pride
- Priorities

Pressure.   Most people like to be liked and there is usually underlying pressure (direct or indirect) to behave in such a way to facilitate "being liked." If a person makes choices that will cause people to be displeased or angry with him or her, the objective of being liked is not being fulfilled. A goal similar to "being liked" is "fulfilling expectations." If a person is successful in the endeavor in which he or she is engaged, expectations are set at a baseline level. Each time success is achieved, the baseline keeps increasing. At some point, it seemingly becomes impossible to continue improving and there has to be some way to alleviate the pressure. One way to resolve the pressure is to take ethical shortcuts.

For example, if an employee who is responsible for managing accounts receivable receives an "Employee of the Month" award due to his performance, he will be proud of his accomplishment. He will not want to have that award be tarnished by having others see or think that his performance has declined. Three months later, the accounts receivable for which the employee is responsible increased dramatically. This is unacceptable to the employee, so to "resolve" this problem he simply writes off some of the balances, instead of attempting to refile the claims or otherwise attempt to collect the charges. This shortcut allows the employee to maintain the appearance of his excellent performance level without actually doing the work necessary to maintain that level (Figure 3.5).

Ethical shortcuts allow the person to keep the perception of continuously improving performance without actually experiencing the pain of doing so. It allows people to appear to keep their commitments,

> **WARNING**
>
> Companies often create ethical dilemmas for employees (and themselves) by establishing improper "reward" systems. Great care must be taken when developing bonus systems that do not put too much pressure on the employees, while protecting the long-term interests of the company.

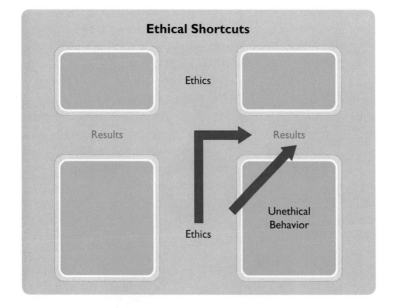

FIGURE 3.5

Often the pressure to perform causes people to take ethical shortcuts. Shortcuts are easier, and they suggest ongoing performance improvement that would not be possible if ethical standards were being followed.

satisfy others' opinions, and seem to keep promises when, in fact, they are not.

Pleasure.   People sometimes engage in unethical behavior because of the pleasure that it can produce. People cheat on their spouses because of the excitement and pleasure associated with being found attractive and desirable by another person, regardless of the wreckage that is created within their family and with their children. Others mischaracterize the nature of their deductions on their income tax forms so they can retain greater sums of money than they are entitled to. This allows them to buy some luxury item that they otherwise could not afford.

The decision to forego pleasure is a matter of discipline. Does the person have the discipline necessary to say no to temporary pleasure, in exchange for the long-term benefits of adherence to ethical guidelines and the integrity that accompanies it? In today's world, the issue of discipline and pleasure deferment is a greater challenge than it has been in the past. Significant research has shown that generations in which the majority participated in enforced, nonvoluntary discipline such as military service demonstrate more discipline in their business dealings (M. Lewis, 2002).

Power.   People seek power for a variety of reasons. Some seek it for the altruistic features—it enables them to do good for others. Some seek it for personal gain and the benefits that power can bring to them. However, power can be a corrupting force, regardless of the original intentions of the person. John Maxwell (2003) wrote, "For many people, having power is like drinking salt water. The more you drink, the thirstier you get" (p. 80).

Unethical actions can be driven by the desire to obtain or retain power. One means by which to obtain or retain power is to create a distorted image that may not necessarily be based in reality. A person may attempt to control his or her **subordinates** through fear of retaliation when the person does not really have the authority to take the threatened actions. Another method of creating a distorted image to maintain power is for a manager to impress his or her supervisor

Subordinate
An employee who reports to a particular individual.

FIGURE 3.6
Several elements of a person's life, by virtue of having inappropriate influence, can produce unethical behavior when ethical dilemmas arise.

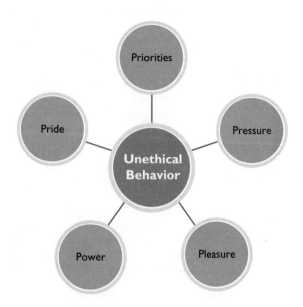

by providing incomplete or misleading information about the department's performance.

The attempt to manage an image to maintain or achieve power is a highly risky decision, compared to simply managing one's character, which is the fundamental root of an individual. If image management is the objective, the person is always concerned that someday, somehow other people will "see behind the curtain." The temptations associated with power will not be so great if the individual's character and commitment to values is so firm that it does not waiver. A coder who seeks to achieve a higher position in management may be tempted to deflect blame for a problem on an innocent coworker to protect his or her own image and not harm the coder's opportunity for a promotion, as opposed to admitting errors and accepting responsibility.

Pride. Nineteenth-century writer John Ruskin said, "Pride is at the bottom of all great mistakes" (quoted in Maxwell, 2003, p. 83). If Ruskin is correct, then it is not surprising that pride could be an issue in relationship to unethical conduct and behavior. Pride is either the personal belief that you are better than others or the desire that the opinion of other people toward you not be negatively reduced below a certain level.

If the Golden Rule is a desirable and viable model for ethical behavior, then pride is not compatible with that model. How can you treat others in the fashion they wish to be treated if you are primarily concerned with either defeating or impressing them? Pride, by its definition, focuses on the individual, which makes consideration of others a secondary concern. If the focus is on the individual, then time and energy will be spent maintaining his or her image, which may require behavior that is inconsistent with a person's ethical beliefs and values. Pride can also blind a person to his or her own weaknesses, the needs of others, and the potential ethical pitfalls that may exist.

Priorities. According to the research of management expert Jim Collins, the most successful companies are those that "have built a set of core values and lived by them" (quoted in Maxwell, 2003, p. 86). This is also the case for the individual. An individual will be most successful when she actively prioritizes her life according to her core values. When she simply reacts to the circumstances that surround her—most of which cannot be controlled—then it is difficult for her to navigate the challenges that life often presents.

Without defined value priorities there is no sense of control, which can lead to unethical behavior. Behaving unethically can restore a sense of control, regardless of how tentative or unstable that control may be.

WARNING

Pride is often confused with confidence or self-assurance. Make sure that the line between the desirable characteristic of confidence does not become blurred with the undesirable and, potentially harmful, characteristic of pride.

Thinking It Through 3.2

1. Describe how a person might come to believe that behaving unethically can be the best option.
2. Which influence listed in this section do you believe is the most powerful? Why?
3. Discuss the role of discipline in ethical behavior.

3.3 The Roots of Unethical Behavior in Business

The struggles that individuals face in ethics and ethical behavior are the very foundation of the struggles faced by businesses. This is true because businesses and organizations of any size are made up of people, and it is impossible for those people to check their personal ethical issues at the door when they arrive at work each day. Five additional elements contribute to ethical dilemmas for organizations and businesses (Figure 3.7). They exist both because of the interactions of humans within the organization or business as well as the outside pressures that exist within the marketplace. These elements are:

- Immoral leadership.
- Employees with poor personal ethics.
- Unethical organizational culture.
- Unrealistic performance goals.
- Failure to consider ethical issues.

IMMORAL LEADERSHIP

The quality of leadership is a serious issue related to ethical dilemmas within the workplace. When the people highest in an organization, such as doctors, administrators, managers, or supervisors, either do not have a strong ethical foundation or are willing to abandon what they do have without much consideration, it creates ethical dilemmas for those who report to them within the organization, such as clinical staff, front office staff, and billing personnel. Because of the unequal

FYI

You cannot separate the ethics in your personal life from those in your professional life. Many have tried to do so, and find it to be a very unpleasant and uncomfortable experience.

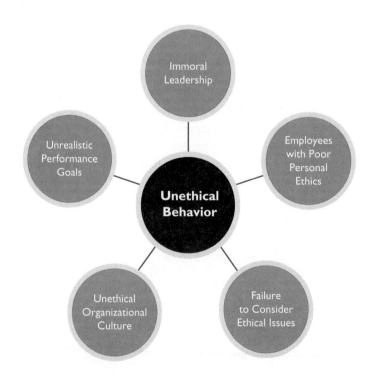

FIGURE 3.7
Additional elements can contribute to unethical behavior in the workplace because of the complexity of employer organizations and the influence of the marketplace on the organization's behavior.

power that exists between leader and employee, having a meaningful conversation regarding the employee's concerns can be extremely difficult. Frequently, there is little opportunity for the employee to participate in a give-and-take that weighs the pros and cons of engaging in a particular course of behavior. Instead, there is significant "top-down" pressure to do whatever the "boss" wants.

Additionally, it seems that the risk of unethical behavior is higher within organizations because if the boss is promoting/requesting the unethical behavior, the odds increase that it will come about. A leader committed to ethical behavior that matches his or her ethical values will not put the employees in the position of violating their own ethical principles—at least not without the opportunity to discuss their concerns.

Another difficulty with immoral leadership is that, at a minimum, it provides a poor example for the employees. It suggests to the employees that unethical behavior is acceptable. This can lead to unethical behavior from employees who were not previously inclined to engage in unethical behavior.

EMPLOYEES WITH POOR PERSONAL ETHICS

This is the opposite end of the spectrum from immoral leadership, but it can have a negative result on the conduct of an organization. The leadership may be committed to appropriate ethical behavior, but if care is not exercised in the selection and monitoring of employees, the ethical values (or lack thereof) brought to the organization by the employees can infect it so that the employer can appear to have poor ethical standards. Either way, the result is undesirable.

UNETHICAL ORGANIZATIONAL CULTURE

Individual leadership can have a significant impact on organizational culture, but institutions—particularly larger institutions—can develop a culture of their own that is independent of the individual manager, either positive or negative. In addition, if the organizational culture is tolerant of unethical behavior by the individual, it develops a self-perpetuating environment that will continually spiral into more and more unethical behavior, unless some factor stops the spiral.

UNREALISTIC PERFORMANCE GOALS

This can be directly related to the unethical organizational culture. If employees are asked to perform tasks that are impossible in the ordinary course of events, they may feel that they have no option but to take ethical shortcuts. Unfortunately, the organization may also encounter the "law of unintended consequences" by focusing too much on short-term performance goals. When employees receive bonuses or other recognition or compensation based on short-term performance, acts are encouraged that may not be in the long-term interest of the company. In addition to promoting unethical behavior, they are harming the long-term health of the organization.

STOP WARNING

Even though you are likely not in a leadership position now, at some point you may be and you need to be prepared.

STOP WARNING

It is important to make your employer aware of the unethical behavior of your coworkers. Your coworkers can create a negative impression of your company, which can harm you and your employer.

FAILURE TO CONSIDER ETHICAL ISSUES

Sometimes, when issues are complex or pressure is high, leaders of an organization may not realize the dilemma in which they are placing their employees, nor do they fully comprehend the effect of their requests. The fault occurs when a complicated ethical dilemma is solely viewed as a straightforward business issue (Hill, 2008). A decision based strictly on economic logic may result in an unethical outcome unless the ethics of the action are intentionally considered.

Thinking It Through 3.3

1. Which of the five contributors to ethical dilemmas that are unique to business do you think occurs most frequently? Why?

2. What possible steps can businesses take to avoid focusing so narrowly on short-term outcomes? How can this affect the occurrence of ethical dilemmas?

3. Describe how an organization can develop a culture of its own.

3.4 Why Unethical Behavior Continues to Occur

Given that there is significant evidence that engaging in unethical behavior does not produce the desired results in the long term, why do people continue to violate their ethical standards? Psychologist and management consultant Saul Gellerman (1989) identified four commonly held rationalizations that can lead to misconduct. These rationalizations are the beliefs that individuals tell themselves to make deviating from their ethical standards psychologically acceptable.

- If an activity is within reasonable ethical and legal limits, then it is not *really* illegal or immoral.
- If an activity is in the individual's or corporation's best interest, the individual is expected to undertake the activity.
- If an activity is safe, it will never be found out or publicized.
- If an activity helps the company, the company will condone it and even protect the person who engages in it.

THE ACTIVITY IS WITHIN REASONABLE ETHICAL AND LEGAL LIMITS

If an activity is within reasonable ethical and legal limits, then it is not really illegal or immoral. A simplified statement of this belief is that if everyone else is doing it, then it must okay. This reverse form of peer pressure is very powerful in that it provides an otherwise ethical person the permission to do something that is incompatible with his or her values.

STOP

WARNING

If we tell ourselves the same information enough times, we begin to believe it.

This false belief illustrates the importance of understanding and committing to ethical principles and the weakness of the law and the legal system in promoting ethical behavior. Those who adhere to this belief claim that if a given activity is not specifically prohibited by the law, then it is legal and thereby acceptable. Throughout this book, ethics is promoted as a "higher" standard than the law.

The weak ethics associated with this belief easily expands the scope of "acceptable" behavior because an individual can always find new ways to act without breaking the "letter of the law." As indicated, the law is always catching up with people's behavior, so there is always sufficient room for questionable behavior.

Adhering to this philosophy in essence drives the behavior of the marketplace to the **lowest common denominator.** If a behavior is acceptable because "everyone" is doing it, then as long as *someone* is doing it the behavior becomes acceptable. Unfortunately, because of human nature it is more common for behavior standards to be lowered by the community than to be raised by the community.

Lowest common denominator
The lowest common standard within a group.

Unethical behavior can spread like a virus throughout the medical community because medical practices often hire employees from other medical practices. Therefore, the unethical conduct at one practice can become unethical conduct at another practice.

It is not difficult to see how this philosophy can spread through different medical organizations. Because of the specialized nature of billing and coding, new employees for a specific practice are often recruited or hired from a pool of applicants that have previous experience in billing and coding. For example, consider an employee who joins a practice that has high ethical standards. The employee states, "We did X successfully at my previous practice—why don't we do it here?" Unless the person comes from a practice that adheres to strong ethical guidelines, the lower standard of the previous practice could negatively affect the new practice.

THE ACTIVITY IS IN THE INDIVIDUAL'S OR CORPORATION'S BEST INTEREST

If an activity is in the individual's or corporation's best interest, the individual is expected to undertake the activity. Leaders within organizations are charged with the responsibility of serving the best interest of the organization *and* all of its stakeholders. If a behavior that is unethical, but not illegal, is available that will result in huge profits to the shareholders, most of the shareholders (of whom there are usually many) will expect the leader to protect their financial interests.

For instance, in a hospital billing office one of the insurance payment posters discovers that the largest payer is overpaying the most frequently billed service by 70% above the rate called for by the contract. She brings this information to her peers who say, "What, are you crazy? Why would you even bring this up? Just post it and be quiet." She decides to take it to her supervisor, who says the same thing only in terms that make it seem more legitimate. At the end of the quarter, the hospital administration announces that billing office employees will receive bonuses based on their collection percentage, compared to the previous year. The extra payments dramatically increased the collection percentage and all of the employees in the billing office received bonuses.

The extra payments continue and, as time goes on, it becomes more difficult for the employee to think about informing the insurer because it would result in reduction in the hospital's bottom line and would reduce the bonuses for the people in her department. In addition, it might result in the need to issue a sizable refund to the insurer, which would further hurt the hospital's financial status.

THE ACTIVITY IS SAFE

The activity is safe because it will never be found out or publicized. Every time an organization or individual engages in unethical behavior that is not discovered or punished, it implies that the behavior is acceptable and is a risk worth taking. This emboldens the unethical entity or person to continue the behavior and, perhaps, move into more unethical behavior.

Compliance program
An organization's written plan for ensuring compliance with ethical rules and legal regulations.

Some companies try to address this issue by doing internal audits or random checks, in accordance with their **compliance program.** These are effective to some degree in that they can discourage unethical behavior, or at least make the person or persons doing the behavior think twice before continuing it. However, the reality of today's human resources climate makes it difficult to discuss the ethical failures of people within the organization. The organization may have legitimate concerns about possible lawsuits if an employee's wrongdoing is made known—so it addresses the problem with the person but does not make the corrective actions public. However, this can be counterproductive. Part of correcting unethical behavior is taking steps to prevent it from happening again. One way to do this is to address the behavior publicly.

When faced with the prospect of being caught doing something wrong, often we attempt to blame someone else or at least distract attention away from ourselves.

THE ACTIVITY HELPS THE COMPANY

If an activity helps the company, the company will condone it and even protect the person who engages in it. This belief is enmeshed with a conflict over the issue of loyalty. If the employee is faced with the decision about acting unethically, her sense of loyalty to the company may encourage her to take the action because it benefits the company. However, repeated historical examples illustrate that the loyalty often does not extend the other direction. Whenever unethical or illegal action takes place within the corporation, it is common for the company to claim that the employee was acting on her own and it was not authorized by the company.

In medical billing and coding, the physician/provider whose name is on the claim form is ultimately responsible, both legally and ethically, for the information on the claim. Therefore, unethical behavior on the part of a biller or coder is the responsibility of the provider because he or she either knew or *should have known* that the billing was improper. Ironically, it is often the provider who encourages the biller/coder to submit claims unethically or illegally. In most cases this occurs either because the provider believes that he or she will not be found out or does not understand the risks associated with engaging in this behavior.

WARNING

If an activity helps the company, the company will condone it and even protect the person who engages in it.

Thinking It Through 3.4

1. Which of the four rationalizations do you believe occurs most commonly? Which have you personally experienced the most often?

2. Do you believe that there is risk associated with discussing an employee's ethical failings with other people within the organization (e.g., the person's peers)? What are the risks?

3. If ethical failings are discussed throughout the organization, what are the potential benefits in doing so?

4. How should the risks versus benefits be evaluated?

5. In your opinion, do compliance programs achieve their desired goals? Why or why not?

3.5 Practical Tools for Analyzing and Resolving Ethical Dilemmas

To analyze and solve ethical problems as they arise and to successfully negotiate problems in the future, it is a good idea to develop a concrete decision-making process to apply when you face an ethical dilemma. The steps in developing this process follow.

GENERAL GUIDELINES FOR MAKING ETHICAL DECISIONS

When solving ethical problems, it is necessary to analyze all possible solutions from every possible angle—even those which are clearly unethical. This is necessary because unethical actions are often taken without fully considering the ramifications of those actions. It is much better to consider unethical behavior as a hypothetical exercise, rather than finding it necessary to remove oneself from a situation in which a bad choice was made and adverse results followed.

To evaluate a situation and determine the ethical course of action, individuals must take the following action steps:

1. What are the facts?
2. Who are the stakeholders?
3. What are the alternatives?
4. How do the possible choices affect me? My employer? Society as a whole?

Step 1: What Are the Facts?   This question is so obvious that many people overlook it. Decisions are made without gathering *all* the facts, which then eliminates important considerations or possible alternative solutions. Fact-gathering can go undone because of a perceived familiarity with the situation or industry, busyness, laziness, or a desire to avoid facts that are not consistent with the desired outcome.

Step 2: Who Are the Stakeholders?   When analyzing situations, the temptation is to look at the situation through the lens of "How does it affect me?" and "How does it affect those people who have the power to affect me?" While that is a valid consideration—one with which we have the most interest—a sole focus on that consideration will ignore the interests of other people, the company, other firms, and society as a whole. This can lead to unethical actions because the fallout of decisions can expand beyond the obvious scope to affect individuals far beyond the immediate players. Your choices can affect, sometimes negatively, other people who may never have been considered as part of your decision-making process (Figure 3.8).

FYI

It is a good idea to consider unethical options when trying to solve an ethical dilemma. By thinking through the unethical alternative, you might be discouraged from choosing that option.

FIGURE 3.8
A comprehensive decision-making process can help individuals analyze a situation to determine the appropriate ethical action.

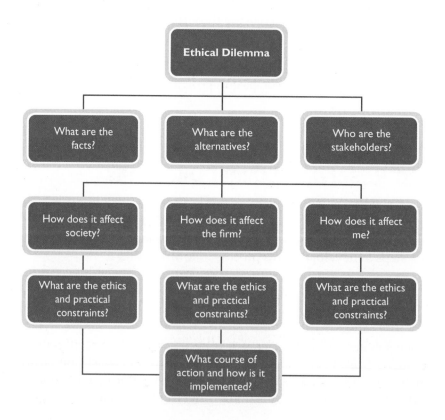

Step 3: What Are the Alternatives? Often, difficult circumstances are presented as either/or choices. Particularly in the case of ethical dilemmas, it seems that there are only two options—both of them undesirable. By failing to examine all alternatives, less undesirable options are not considered. There may be an option that is ethical, achieves the objectives of the parties involved, and does not have negative ramifications for other people.

Step 4: How Do the Possible Choices Affect Me? My Employer? Society as a Whole? There are mixed elements in considering how a decision affects one personally. The two extremes are:

1. A fear of appearing selfish—can a decision that benefits me personally be ethical?
2. An unlimited opportunity—I will take advantage of this situation to achieve maximum benefit for myself.

Between those two ends of the spectrum, there are many other points in between. In fact, there is no specific "rule" that indicates if an individual benefits from a situation that it is automatically unethical. Each case must be examined individually and decisions made based on the merits of the situation.

If all alternatives are examined, including their ethics and the practical constraints of carrying out the alternatives, then the odds of arriving at an ethical, yet acceptable solution are greatly increased.

PERSONAL CONSIDERATIONS IN RESOLVING ETHICAL DILEMMAS

Given that billing and coding usually occurs within a professional or corporate environment, much of the discussion concerning ethics has focused on that setting. Yet, the individuals who work within the environment bring their own personal issues with them to the process. Therefore, consideration must be given to personal characteristics that influence personal ethics when reviewing larger ethical dilemmas. How does the individual prepare himself or herself to be ready for a difficult ethical dilemma?

Take Responsibility for Actions. Those who claim that they do not have any power to change a situation ensure the correctness of their faulty belief. Ethical dilemmas occur, and will continue to occur, as long as people accept a philosophy of "victimhood." Each person has the ability to behave ethically on a consistent basis—no one can force him or her to be unethical.

In some cases, unethical behavior occurs because of the tendency to point fingers and shift blame. Leaders of all types can take responsibility for their actions and can guide organizations positively toward ethical conduct, raising the ethical "tide" of all "ships" in the organization and industry. Those who not only accept responsibility but also embrace it put themselves in a position to grow in leadership and responsibility. Winston Churchill stated that responsibility is "the price of greatness" (quoted in Maxwell, 2003).

Develop Personal Discipline. When individuals fail to be disciplined through the entire course of their lives, it is completely unreasonable to expect that they will be disciplined in the middle of a particularly difficult circumstance. The undisciplined person will often find himself or herself in difficult situations for which a shortcut seems to be the only viable solution. The shortcut invariably takes the person through unethical territory.

Know Weaknesses. A person will never overcome his weaknesses unless he has identified them, analyzed them, and taken specific steps to address them. A person who is not detailed-oriented may have difficulty if she is responsible for following up on unpaid insurance claims. She may be tempted to cover her shortcomings or the errors that result from her shortcomings. Instead of expending energy trying to hide negative outcomes because of the presence of weakness, energy is better spent establishing tools to help accommodate and account for the weakness before the weakness creates an issue.

Align Priorities with Values. Integrity is described as making your beliefs and your actions line up (Maxwell, 2003). When someone intentionally does something that is inconsistent with what he or she states, there is an absence of integrity. Yet, when someone does not consider his or her behavior and unintentionally is inconsistent with his or her belief system, there is still an adverse effect on the person's integrity (Figure 3.9).

Admit Wrongdoing Quickly and Ask Forgiveness. All people make mistakes and sometimes choose unethical behavior. It becomes a more serious problem when additional unethical behavior is used to cover the initial infraction. Integrity is strengthened and enhanced when people of character admit their wrong quickly. The comment is often made that "it is easier to ask for forgiveness than permission." However, this philosophy is not particularly ethical.

Take Extra Care with Financial Issues. Henry Ford stated, "Money doesn't change men, it merely unmasks them. If a man is naturally selfish or arrogant or greedy, the money brings that out—that is all" (quoted in Maxwell, 2003, p. 100). In the world of medical billing, the opportunity for inappropriate diversion of funds is very great. Although it is not discussed often, because practices are embarrassed

FIGURE 3.9
When beliefs and actions are not aligned, it is difficult, if not impossible, to have integrity.

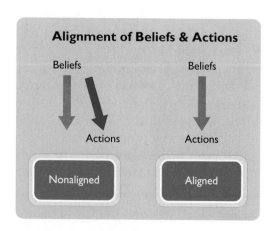

Alignment of Beliefs & Actions

Beliefs → Actions — Nonaligned

Beliefs → Actions — Aligned

to admit that they were swindled, many practices experience embezzlement by employees—from administrators to file clerks. Usually, the embezzlement occurs because appropriate safeguards are not put in place to ensure proper accounting. Ethical employees will not only respect safeguards, they will insist on them to guard their own integrity. Even if they are not tempted to take money that does not belong to them, the presence of safeguards removes any possibility of false allegations against them.

Thinking It Through 3.5

1. Have you previously considered your decision-making process when in the middle of an ethical dilemma? If so, how does it compare to the model provided?

2. Of the recommended action steps to maintaining strong ethical behavior, which do you believe is the most important? Why? Which do you believe is the most difficult to sustain consistently? Why?

3. What do you think of the recommendation to actively consider unethical alternatives? Why might this be helpful? Why might this be harmful?

3.6 Case Studies of Ethical Dilemmas in Billing and Coding

The best method of grasping the concepts regarding ethical dilemmas is to look at specific case studies. The principles discussed to this point can be viewed in light of real-world circumstances. The scenarios can also demonstrate circumstances that seem to be an ethical problem that, in fact, may not be a problem.

CASE 1: IT'S JUST A LITTLE BIT MORE

An obstetrics/gynecology (OB/GYN) practice performs a significant number of folliculograms (CPT code 76857) as part of its infertility practice. However, it learned that by doing a few more measurements during the course of the ultrasound exam, it could bill for a complete pelvic ultrasound exam (CPT code 76856). The reimbursement for 76856 is, on average, 21.6% higher than the reimbursement for 76857.

A routine medical record audit by the insurance company brought this practice to light. The insurer requested a refund for the difference between 76857 and 76856 for all 76856 codes billed in the past 18 months. The practice defended its actions, indicating that the medical record detailed all of the information needed to bill 76856. The insurer stated that, while the medical records documented a 76856 procedure, the extra measurements were not medically necessary to accomplish the intended purpose of the ultrasound exam. The insurer notified the clinic that if payment was not received by a particular date, it would begin withholding payments on future claims to offset the overpayments from the past. The clinic notified the insurer that

CODING TIP

Providing extra, but unnecessary, care simply for the purpose of billing a higher level of service is unethical if the care provided is not medically necessary.

it was considering a report to the state's department of insurance or other legal action.

1. Is there any unethical behavior taking place in this scenario? By whom?
2. What is your opinion of the proposed resolution of this case? Is it appropriate?

CASE 2: PAYABLE DIAGNOSIS, PLEASE

A patient who had a previous tubal ligation would like it to be reversed. If the doctor uses the appropriate diagnosis (ICD-9 code V26.51—Tubal ligation status), the claim will be denied because of a specific contractual exclusion. The doctor likes this couple and tells the billing personnel to find a "payable" diagnosis, like ICD-9 code 628.2—Infertility, due to tubal factors.

The billing personnel tell the physician that they find this an inappropriate coding approach. The physician replies by reporting that when the patient had the tubal ligation, she was in an abusive relationship. She had no way of knowing that she would remarry into a stable relationship. The patient cannot afford the procedure or any infertility treatment if she has to pay out-of-pocket.

1. If the billing personnel follow the physician's request, is this an ethical problem? Why or why not?
2. Does the mitigating information about the patient change the scenario in any way?
3. What might be some possible ways to address the concerns and issues of all parties involved?

CASE 3: IT'S ABOUT THE SAME—ISN'T IT?

A surgeon removed a large abdominal (12-cm) cystic teratoma through a laparoscopic approach. The coder used CPT code 49329—Unlisted laparoscopy procedure, abdomen . . . because there is no code to precisely describe the procedure. The insurance company denied the claim, desiring more information, even though medical records were sent with the original claim. The surgeon, who is highly involved in his accounts receivable management and is somewhat knowledgeable in coding, says, "Just bill 49205—that will get paid." Unfortunately, this code is for an "open" procedure. However, it is the correct code for the procedure if it had been done through an open incision.

The surgeon's billing staff is opposed to the coding change because the American Medical Association's *CPT Assistant* specifically indicates that this is not appropriate (American Medical Association, 1999). The physician responds that this is a covered benefit for the patient under the insurance plan and this payer has historically been difficult to work with in resolving outlier cases.

1. What elements of this case may have features of an ethical dilemma?
2. What is your opinion of the physician's justification of his "solution"?
3. What is the most ethical way to resolve this situation, or is the proposal recommended satisfactory?

CASE 4: WE TRIED TO AVOID THE ETHICAL DILEMMA

The patient seeks a high-dollar medical service that is often not covered by his insurer. According to practice guidelines, the provider's representative calls the insurer to confirm benefits and is told that diagnosis of the patient's condition is covered but treatment is not.

As a result, the provider's representative asks the patient to pay the balance for treatment before service begins. The patient asks the provider to code the treatment services as diagnostic services (using symptoms diagnosis). The provider, who has gone through this scenario before, absolutely refuses to mischaracterize the diagnosis codes.

The patient has a **flexible spending account (FSA)** that will reimburse him for services not covered by insurance. However, to obtain that FSA payment a denial must be received from the insurer. The physician's office submits the claims to get the denial for the patient, but the insurer unexpectedly pays for the services. Two days before the provider actually receives the funds, it receives a phone call from the patient, who received an **explanation of benefits (EOB)** from the insurer. The patient wants to receive a refund of the money that he paid since the insurer "covered" this service. The patient insists that if he does not receive the refund immediately, he is going to call his attorney.

1. At this point, have any ethical dilemmas occurred?
2. Is it an ethical problem for the provider's office to comply with the patient's request? Why or why not?
3. Do the circumstances change if the provider calls the insurer and the insurer's representative insists that the claim payment is correct? Does this solve the problem? Are more ethical problems created? Explain.

CASE 5: PICK A DIAGNOSIS—ANY DIAGNOSIS

The patient comes in for a routine gynecological exam. A claim is filed to the insurer as CPT code 99395 with a diagnosis of V72.31. The claim is denied because routine services are not covered under the policy. The patient calls and states that she came in for **dysmenorrhea** (625.3). She wants it to be refiled as CPT code 99213 with a diagnosis of 625.3.

The patient tells the provider that the insurance company told her that if the office had "coded it right," the claim would be paid. The coder checks the patient's chart and sees that the "annual exam" note form was used. In the "complaints" section, dysmenorrhea was noted as "2" on a 10-point scale. There was no indication of any treatment or significant counseling related to the dysmenorrhea.

The patient is a long-time, loyal patient whose insurance had paid for annual exams in the past. She loudly tells the billing representative, "I am not going to pay the bill. I am going to speak to the doctor and 'have you fired,'" adding, "you are incompetent!"

1. What are the ethical issues in this situation?
2. Does the situation change if the physician has just discussed his dissatisfaction with the billing representative about complaints he received from patients regarding her "refusal" to help them? Why or why not?
3. What are some possible solutions to this problem? Do any of them not violate ethical principles?

Flexible spending account (FSA)
A benefit program that allows employees to put money away on a pretax basis to cover out-of-pocket health care expenses, such as copayments, deductibles, and other noncovered medical services.

Explanation of benefits (EOB)
The form provided by a third-party payer to both providers and patients, informing them of the way in which a particular claim was processed. The formal name for the version supplied to providers by insurers is Remittance Advice (RA).

Dysmenorrhea
Painful menstrual periods.

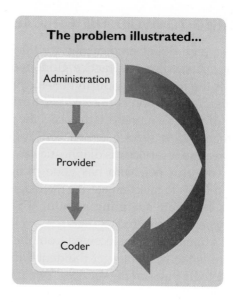

The problem illustrated...

Administration

Provider

Coder

CASE 6: WE NEED TO SOLVE A PROBLEM

Capitated
A third-party reimbursement program that compensates providers on a per-patient basis, not on a production basis.

Carved out
Designated as separately payable and therefore not covered by an agreement.

A new HMO comes to town. It agrees to assign patients to your practice and pay you a **capitated** rate for "routine" services. Non-routine services are **carved out** and are payable on a fee-for-service basis. Six months later, your practice's finance committee decides that they committed to a terrible deal, stating "We've got to increase revenue" (Figure 3.10).

Meanwhile, the practice's coder sees a dramatic drop in the number of routine services being billed—every person who comes in seems to have a problem. Some research by the coder reveals that the charts really do not support the "problem-based" services.

1. What are the possible ethical dilemmas in this scenario?
2. Is it okay for reimbursement matters to affect the way a service is coded? The patients do describe these complaints—what is wrong with coding them?
3. Is this situation changed if the provider's financial stability (and ongoing existence) is in question?

CASE 7: TO BILL OR NOT TO BILL?

A patient undergoes a hysteroscopy with polyp removal (58558). This particular service has a 0 day global period, according to the Medicare fee schedule. It is the physician's standard practice to see the patient back in one week for follow-up. The physician submits an E/M charge for that service (9921x).

The physician's coder is not comfortable with this practice because the CPT code book indicates that surgical codes (including this one) include "typical postoperative follow-up care" (American Medical Association, 2010). She feels that since every patient has this service, it is not appropriate to bill for the separate E/M code.

1. Is this an ethical dilemma? On what basis do the parties involved in this situation make their case?
2. What factors could affect your decision in this case?

1. What elements do all of these cases have in common?

2. Pick one of the cases and analyze it in detail, using the tools provided in Learning Outcome 3.5. Following your analysis, what would you do to resolve that situation?

3. Select one of the cases and identify the fundamental philosophical flaw that created the ethical dilemma.

CHAPTER REVIEW

Chapter Summary

Learning Outcomes	Key Concepts/Examples
3.1 Develop a working personal definition of *ethical dilemma*. Pages 73–74	• There are two component parts to ethical behavior: 1. Fundamental beliefs or values, which are of great importance to an individual. 2. A commitment to conduct oneself in a manner consistent with those beliefs and values. • Although a significant number of different ways in which to define *ethical dilemma* exist, this textbook focuses on the decisions that must occur when there is a conflict between the values and the commitment. • Ethical dilemmas are not exclusive to individuals, but can exist within companies, organizations, and society as a whole.
3.2 Define the reasons why people do not always behave ethically. Pages 75–79	• On a personal level, anytime a person faces an ethical decision, he or she must select one of at least two options, which can result as in as many as four different scenarios. 1. Ethical behavior—good outcome: The person does what is consistent with his or her values and likes the outcome. 2. Unethical behavior—good outcome: The person acts inconsistently with his or her values and, at least in the short-term, avoids the negative consequences that acting consistently with values might have produced. 3. Ethical behavior—bad outcome: The person acts consistently with his or her values and experiences negative consequences as a result. 4. Unethical behavior—bad outcome: The person acts inconsistently with his or her values and does not avoid the bad consequences. • The temptation to select unethical behavior occurs because individuals must deal with: 1. Pressure 2. Pleasure 3. Power 4. Pride 5. Priorities

Learning Outcomes	Key Concepts/Examples
3.3 Describe the roots of unethical behavior in the business setting. Pages 80–82	• All of the ethical dilemmas faced by individuals also occur in business. Businesses face five other elements in the ethical decision-making process: 1. Immoral leadership. 2. Employees with poor personal morals. 3. Unethical organizational cultures. 4. Unrealistic professional goals. 5. Failure to consider ethical issues before making decisions.
3.4 Explain the reasons why unethical behavior can continue even when the behavior is potentially damaging to the individual or company. Pages 82–85	• Even in the light of the pitfalls of unethical behavior, it continues to occur because unethical decisions are rationalized in one of four ways: 1. Everyone is doing it. 2. The employee must act unethically if it is good for the stakeholders or the corporation. 3. Nobody will notice. 4. The company will protect the employee who behaves unethically.
3.5 Identify concrete personal tools to help in the problem-solving process when facing an ethical dilemma. Pages 85–89	• To successfully recognize and resolve an ethical dilemma, four action steps must be taken that ask: 1. What are the facts of the situation? 2. Who are the stakeholders (or potential stakeholders)? 3. What are the alternative solutions? 4. How does my decision affect me? My employer? Society at large? • To behave ethically on a consistent basis, a person must be able and willing to: 1. Take responsibility for actions. 2. Develop personal discipline. 3. Know weaknesses. 4. Align priorities and values. 5. Admit wrongdoing and seek forgiveness. 6. Take extra care when working with financial issues.
3.6 Apply ethical decision-making principles to case studies in billing and coding. Pages 89–93	• The case studies include scenarios involving: 1. Providing more service than is medically necessary. 2. Providing misleading diagnoses in an attempt to receive payment for noncovered services. 3. Approximating CPT code selection. 4. Resolving conflict between the payer and the patient. 5. Identifying "payable" diagnoses. 6. Using coding to "solve" poor contracting decisions with coding. 7. Inappropriately billing for postoperative services.

End-of-Chapter Questions

Multiple Choice

Circle the letter that best completes the statement or answers the question.

1. **LO 3.1** What are the two key components of ethical behavior?

   a. Beliefs and conduct

   b. Values and ethics

   c. Circumstances and conduct

   d. Beliefs and values

2. **LO 3.1** The focus of the definition of *ethical dilemma* is on

   a. The decision-making process
   b. The choice selected from the dictionary
   c. The behavior of the individual
   d. The behavior of the organization

3. **LO 3.1** Ethical dilemmas are exclusive to

   a. Individuals
   b. Organizations
   c. Corporations
   d. They are not exclusive

4. **LO 3.1** When people face an ethical dilemma, they may do one or more of the following *except*

   a. Make a choice to match their actions to their beliefs
   b. Choose an action inconsistent with their beliefs
   c. Experience psychological stress until the dilemma is resolved
   d. Take an action that provides permanent relief from further ethical dilemmas

5. **LO 3.1** What is the foundation of the second element of ethics?

   a. Values
   b. Choice
   c. Behavior
   d. Circumstances

6. **LO 3.2** Most people engage in unethical behavior because

   a. They are inherently unethical
   b. It always produces a good result
   c. They believe there is some benefit in doing so
   d. They have not been taught proper morals

7. **LO 3.2** When considering the ethical matrix of possible decisions and outcomes, how many possible decisions and possible outcomes exist?

   a. Two possible decisions, three possible outcomes
   b. Two possible decisions, four possible outcomes
   c. Three possible decisions, four possible outcomes
   d. Three possible decisions, three possible outcomes

8. **LO 3.2** Which decision–outcome combination has this underlying thought/belief: "The values are so important that even though a bad outcome is a likely or certain result, the person agrees to endure whatever hardship results from the choice not to engage in 'unethical behavior'"?

   a. Ethical behavior—good outcome
   b. Ethical behavior—bad outcome
   c. Unethical behavior—good outcome
   d. Unethical behavior—bad outcome

9. **LO 3.2** The decision to forego pleasure is primarily a matter of

   a. Leadership
   b. Determination
   c. Choice
   d. Discipline

10. **LO 3.2** Which of the following is *not* compatible with the Golden Rule?

    a. Pride
    b. Power

    c. Priorities

    d. Pressure

11. **LO 3.3** The "law of unintended consequences" occurs when there is (are)

    a. An unethical organizational culture

    b. Unrealistic performance goals

    c. Employees with poor personal ethics

    d. Immoral leadership

12. **LO 3.4** If individual behavior occurs because "everyone is doing it," the behavior of the marketplace will

    a. Go to the lowest common denominator

    b. Rise to a higher level

    c. Not be affected

    d. Go to the highest common multiple

13. **LO 3.5** Which of the following is *not* one of the four initial steps or considerations in the ethical decision-making process?

    a. What are the facts?

    b. Who are the stakeholders?

    c. What are the possible outcomes?

    d. What are the alternatives?

Short Answer

Use your critical thinking skills to answer the following questions.

1. **LO 3.1** What is the purpose of core values, principles, and guidelines?

2. **LO 3.1** Discuss the element that is the foundation of the second element or component of ethics. Do you agree or disagree?

3. **LO 3.2** Analyze the statement, "Dilemmas would not exist if the potential for 'bad' outcomes were not real." Do you agree or disagree? Why?

4. **LO 3.2** What would it take for ethical dilemmas to disappear? Why?

5. **LO 3.2** Discuss the reasons why people seek power and how this could influence the medical biller/coder.

6. **LO 3.3** Discuss the reasons why there are elements associated with ethics in business, in addition to those faced by individuals.

7. **LO 3.3** In your opinion, which of the five elements associated with ethics in business is the most serious? Why?

8. **LO 3.3** Ethical dilemmas are created for employees when the leadership of an organization is immoral. Discuss what role disparate power plays in creating these dilemmas.

9. **LO 3.4** Evaluate the statement, "If everybody does it, it is not immoral." Do you agree? Why or why not?

10. **LO 3.4** How does the "everyone does it" philosophy spread quickly through the medical community?

11. **LO 3.4** Discuss why today's human resources climate makes it difficult to discourage unethical behavior.

12. **LO 3.5** Is an individual's ethical decision important, regardless of his or her place in a corporation? Explain your answer.

13. **LO 3.5** Is it possible for a decision to be ethical if the person making the decision is in the middle of an ethical dilemma and receives personal benefit because of the decision? Why or why not?

14. **LO 3.5** What do you believe is the most significant personal consideration in resolving ethical dilemmas? Why?

Applying Your Knowledge

Reexamine the case of Enrique at the beginning of this chapter, reading it in light of the information that you have learned in the chapter. Pay particular attention to the following questions in the scenario:

1. Who are the parties involved in this ethical dilemma?

2. What factors may be contributing to this dilemma?

3. What do you think is the most desirable possible outcome in this case?

Continue your analysis of the case in the following exercises:

1. Create a table with the parties involved listed in the left-hand column and the different factors that could be influencing each of them listed across the top of each column. Identify the influences affecting each individual by marking the corresponding boxes. Does this change the way that you view this case?

2. What ethical issues that are unique to business seem to be at work at Overlook Family Practice?

3. Using the chart on page 86, analyze this case by identifying the causes, stakeholders, alternatives, and effect on society.

4. Based on the information you have in the case study, which personal factors seem to be influencing Enrique in his consideration of the situation?

Internet Research

The Internet provides a wealth of sample ethical dilemmas for consideration. Some sites simply provide a scenario, but do not provide any insight as to the actual outcome of the situation. Other sites provide input as to the decisions that were made.

The best way to identify these sites is to use a search engine to look up the terms "ethical dilemma samples" or "ethical dilemma case studies." Some recommended sites include:

- University of Southern California—Levan Institute Ethics Resource Center
  http://college.usc.edu/dilemmas-and-case-studies/

- Institute for Global Ethics
  www.globalethics.org/dilemmas.php

- The Friesian School
  www.friesian.com/valley/dilemmas.htm

Although these cases may not necessarily involve medical coding, select one that is of interest to you. Summarize the details of the case and then outline the key factors as follows:

1. Who are the parties involved? What factors are influencing them?

2. If it is a case involving a business context, what unique business factors come into play?

3. Using the chart on page 86, analyze the case.

4. Which personal considerations may come into play?

5. If you were in the place of the primary character in the case, what would you do? On what factors would you base your decision?

PART TWO

Ethics in Coding

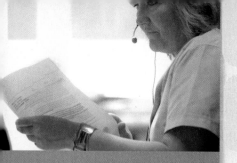

4

Coding, Ethics, and Third-Party Financing

LEARNING OUTCOMES

After completing this chapter, you will be able to:

4.1   Describe the unique elements of the U.S. health care payment system that produce and promote the opportunity for ethical dilemmas.

4.2   Identify the stakeholders in business transactions and the medical coding process.

4.3   Evaluate the role played by each stakeholder in the medical coding process.

4.4   Analyze the position of stakeholders who face specific ethical dilemmas related to third-party reimbursement.

CASE STUDY—PART 1

D r. Niels Lauersen, a well-known obstetrician/gynecologist who provided care to numerous celebrities at his Park Avenue office in New York City, faced one of the most severe penalties ever levied against an individual doctor because of his billing practices. The authorities accused Dr. Lauersen of insurance fraud and related charges and he faced a sentence of more than 25 years if he received the maximum sentence for the charges (Steinhauer, 2001).

The government alleged that Dr. Lauersen defrauded insurance companies by submitting claims for expensive fertility treatments not covered under the patient's insurance contract. According to the suit, filed in federal district court in Manhattan, Dr. Lauersen billed insurance companies for covered gynecological procedures to mask fertility procedures that were not covered. For example, the insurer would be billed for an ovarian cyst removal (CPT code 58925) when the procedure actually performed was an oocyte (egg) retrieval (CPT code 58970) (Steinhauer, 2000b). The government's case stated that Dr. Lauersen received approximately $4 million in fraudulent payments over a 10-year period.

1. What factors might have caused prosecutors to pursue charges against Dr. Lauersen, as opposed to other physicians or providers?
2. What mitigating factors might legitimately explain Dr. Lauersen's billing patterns?
3. What do you think was the outcome of this case?

Introduction

All people face ethical dilemmas in a variety of settings, whether those settings are academic, occupational, or personal. Individuals in the field of medicine, and specifically medical coding and billing, face all of those same challenges, *plus* some unique issues that are directly attributable to the structure of the U.S. third-party payer system.

4.1 The Unique Elements of the U.S. Health Care Payment System

A BRIEF HISTORY OF U.S. HEALTH CARE ECONOMICS

Fully understanding the basics of health care economics is critical in understanding both how and why ethical dilemmas exist in relationship to coding. Coding is an activity that both facilitates collection of data for public health reporting and, more importantly, facilitates reimbursement. Therefore, coding has a direct relationship with reimbursement and is a fundamental part of U.S. health care economics.

Which came first—reimbursement or coding? History shows that the answer is reimbursement. In fact, before the middle of the twentieth century there were no codes at all to report the delivery of medical

---

FYI

Medical coding did not exist until much later in the development of the U.S. health care system. There were no health insurance companies until the 1930s.

Commodities
Articles of trade or commerce; something useful that can be turned to commercial or other advantage.

services. This is true because, prior to 1930, there were no insurance companies and no one to whom services were reported. Coding was unnecessary.

Before insurance companies existed, reimbursement for health care was very different. Medical services were **commodities**—viewed no differently than food, clothing, farming supplies, or any other purchased good. Patients paid the doctor or the hospital directly for the services they received and payment took various forms—cash, trading of goods, or provision of services. Most physicians, particularly in the 1800s, were not wealthy and usually had second jobs to supplement their income.

The Early Twentieth Century. The situation changed in the early 1900s. In 1910, the American Medical Association (AMA) supported the publication of an exposé that revealed that the majority of medical care in the United States was shoddy and substandard. As a result, 45% of the existing medical schools closed while the number of new medical school graduates dropped by 35%. Soon, prices for medical services began to rise because of a shortage of physicians, as illustrated in Figure 4.1. According to traditional economic theory, when demand increases at the same time that supply decreases, prices will go up.

To complicate the situation, improvements in public health, such as water purification, better waste management, development of pharmaceuticals, and improvements in medical treatment, further drove up demand. People were living longer, which caused them to require and consume more medical care (Figure 4.2).

As expected in standard economic theory, the increase in price and income for physicians solved the problem of physician supply. The

FIGURE 4.1

As the supply of doctors decreased (blue line) in the early twentieth century, demand increased significantly (left to right) which increased the cost of medical services (green line).

Supply and demand in the early twentieth century

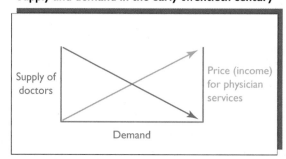

FIGURE 4.2

Life expectancy increased significantly in the twentieth century, with the fastest increase occurring in the first half of the century.

Life Expectancy

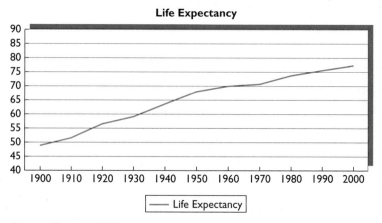

Source: Shrestha, 2006.

increased opportunity for income and the rise in prestige for medical professionals led many to become doctors. Unfortunately, the economics of the country began to change, as the United States descended into the Great Depression. There were plenty of doctors and hospitals with better and more effective treatments available, but few could pay for their services (Achenbaum, 1988).

As medical providers began to struggle economically, the concept of **prepaid** health plans was born. Hospitals began to offer programs to patients where, for a fixed fee (premium), they would supply all of the patient's medical needs. This served a twofold economic benefit—hospitals and physicians could expect a steady stream of income through the premium, while patients could define and control the costs associated with their health care. All parties viewed **risk pooling** as a win–win situation. All members of the group pay a relatively small amount in exchange for coverage of the potential undesirable event.

At the same time that hospitals developed prepaid health plans, commercial companies also began to market insurance products using the same principle. For a fixed monthly fee, the insurer would cover the health care expenses of the patient. Since the insurer did not have the resources of a hospital and medical personnel, the insurer contracted directly with providers to deliver services on its behalf. In exchange, insurers would pay the providers directly.

Wage controls and **price controls** associated with World War II limited the ability of employers to attract and retain employees. Employers began to offer health care benefits, because these benefits were exempt from wage and price limitations. In 1941, Chrysler offered 100% coverage for hospitalization services. In other companies, employees made relatively small premium contributions through payroll deduction. As time went on, other automakers increased their benefits to compete for employees, resulting in higher levels of coverage at lower cost to the employee. As this practice spread into other marketplace sectors, a significant pattern of health care inflation emerged.

The 1950s, 1960s, and 1970s. By the 1950s, health insurance benefits were a routine part of labor–management negotiations as more and more Americans were covered through employer-based plans. To control the increasing costs in the 1960s and 1970s, insurers began to negotiate their reimbursement to providers, offering to pay **usual, customary, and reasonable (UCR) rates.** In paying according to this UCR fee schedule, insurers agreed to pay providers the lesser of the provider's billed charge or the UCR rate. The UCR rate was usually established by ranking the charges of all providers (usually by specialty) from highest to lowest and selecting a percentile rank (e.g., 60th percentile). If a provider's charge was below the 60th percentile, it received payment for the billed charge. If its charge was higher than the 60th percentile, it agreed to accept the 60th percentile level as the payment (Figure 4.3).

This system was logical for insurers in that it guaranteed that they would pay no more than a certain amount for each procedure. The problem was that providers soon realized two things (Figure 4.4):

1. If prices go up, reimbursement goes up, regardless of the actual cost of delivering the care.
2. Every provider should ensure that its prices are above the UCR rate allowed by the insurer, or else it is "leaving money on the table."

Prepaid
Paid for prior to requiring the service.

Risk pooling
The joining together of a group of people in anticipation of a possible undesirable event, such as injury, illness, property damage, or death. All members of the group pay a relatively small amount in exchange for coverage of the potential undesirable event.

COMPLIANCE TIP

Concerns about compliance became an issue when additional parties were introduced to the health care system. When medical services were originally a direct transaction between patient and provider, reporting was not necessary. The primary purpose of compliance programs is to ensure that reporting is consistent with the services actually delivered.

Wage control
A limit on rising wages.

Price control
A limit on rising prices.

FYI

A number of efforts were made to control health care costs in the last half of the twentieth century. None were particularly successful, and many resulted in outcomes that were completely unforeseen.

Usual, customary, and reasonable (UCR) rate
Amount determined to be paid for a service by third-party payers.

FIGURE 4.3

In this example, a provider that billed $25 for an office visit received payment of $25 from the insurer. A provider that billed $75 for the same service received $55, the amount identified as the UCR rate.

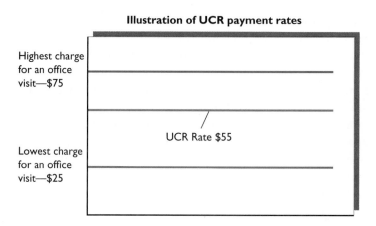

Illustration of UCR payment rates

Highest charge for an office visit—$75

UCR Rate $55

Lowest charge for an office visit—$25

FIGURE 4.4

An example of the medical hyperinflation that occurred when a provider increases its prices and the UCR rate is adjusted higher. Even though the payers tried to combat the increase by establishing a lower percentile for the UCR, the total health care cost for this service increased dramatically.

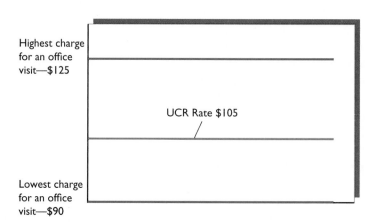

Highest charge for an office visit—$125

UCR Rate $105

Lowest charge for an office visit—$90

Medicare
A government-funded insurance program for persons who are elderly or disabled and those with certain severe diseases.

Medicaid
A government-funded insurance program for low-income children, their caretaker relatives, pregnant women, infants, and other individuals below certain income levels.

Health maintenance organization (HMO)
A health care system in which patients receive health care through a formal management process—often coordinated by a primary care physician.

This medical inflation trend continued into the 1960s, at which time the Medicare and Medicaid programs were established. Legislators recognized that millions of seniors did not have the financial means to pay for their medical services, the price of which was increasing significantly. The **Medicare** program was established by the federal government to provide coverage to persons who are retired or disabled, allowing access to the health care services that they needed. The federal government also facilitated funding of state-operated **Medicaid** programs for those near or below the poverty line so that they could access needed medical care. Because of these programs, demand for health care services increased substantially since people who previously could not afford the services now had access to them.

In the 1970s, the government encouraged growth in the health care industry by providing grants and loans to students studying medicine. The process succeeded, and many more doctors graduated from medical school. Unfortunately, at this time, there was a trend toward specialization, so the ranks of primary care physicians did not increase at the same rate that the number of specialists increased.

HMOs in the 1970s. During the following 20 years, various actions attempted to control the rising costs of health care. One major effort to control costs was the introduction of **health maintenance organizations (HMOs)**. HMOs were intended to control costs in several different ways. First, HMOs attempted to control cost by emphasizing, encouraging, and covering preventive care. The theory was that if patients received less expensive preventive care, serious illness could be identified and treated before it was necessary to engage in expensive and invasive treatments.

Second, many early HMOs were designed with a "gatekeeper" model. Patients chose or were assigned a primary care physician (PCP) who was the gatekeeper for their specialty medical care. The theory was that unnecessary care would be reduced because a medical professional would be making the decisions about which treatments were necessary, rather than the patient.

Third, HMOs controlled costs by limiting their provider panels. By delivering care through a relatively small group of providers, the HMO negotiated a lower reimbursement rate with the provider, in exchange for increased patient volume from patients directed to the provider by the HMO.

Although there was an element of success in cost control through HMOs, a number of unintended consequences resulted from their use. First, patients became insulated from the real cost of their care. To attract patients to the HMO model (which placed limitations on the patient's freedom), HMOs introduced the **copayment** concept. For example, a patient might pay $10 for an office visit, $5 for a prescription, $50 for a visit to an emergency room or, in some cases, $10 for global obstetrical care. This highly affordable care (from the patient's perspective) masked the real cost of the service and patients took advantage of the fact that they could receive substantial amounts of medical care for relatively little personal cost.

Copayment
A fixed amount that must be paid as part of the patient's insurance agreement each time a patient visits a provider.

The second unintended consequence was that administrative tasks in the provider office increased dramatically. Primary care physicians had to review and approve specialty care for their patients—usually with no additional reimbursement for their time and effort. Specialists had to ensure that **referrals** or **preauthorizations** were in place before they delivered treatment or they risked losing reimbursement for the services they delivered. Administrative staff size in physician offices increased while reimbursement for services decreased, shrinking the profit margins of many physician practices. Physicians complained that more money was being spent "pushing paper," which had no positive impact on the health of their patients.

Referral
Preapproval of a service by a patient's primary care physician, intended to ensure that no unnecessary services are approved.

Preauthorization
Referral provided directly by the insurance company to the physician who desires to provide a service, usually an expensive diagnostic test or surgery.

The third unintended consequence is that HMOs were largely unsuccessful at controlling patient behavior and the related expense. Many patients resented not being able to see "their" doctor and resented the requirement to see a physician on the HMO panel. As patients began to move away from the HMOs because of the lack of choice, HMOs loosened their rules to make their product more palatable to patients. Open-access HMOs and preferred provider organizations (PPOs) allowed patients to see any provider on their panel without a referral. Out-of-network benefits allowed patients to have more choice by letting them see any provider, although they had more out-of-pocket cost if they saw a nonnetwork provider. However, insurers lost a major tool in their effort to control cost, because HMOs and PPOs insulated patients from the cost of health care while weakening the insurer's best weapons in controlling costs (Figure 4.5).

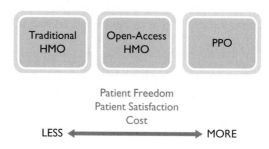

FIGURE 4.5

The relative strengths and weaknesses of traditional HMOs and PPOs in terms of satisfying patients and controlling costs.

During this period, the power in health care economics shifted away from providers and toward insurers. Insurers became more aggressive in limiting reimbursement and fixing payment rates at lower levels. Providers, many of whom previously enjoyed a comfortable lifestyle and significant salaries, faced increased costs and decreased take-home pay. Many had a difficult decision—retire or join a larger group?

Supply and demand curve
A curve reflecting that as demand increases, supply decreases, resulting in higher prices. Conversely, if supply exceeds demand, then prices will fall.

Revenue cycle
The period between when a product or service is delivered until the time that payment for that product is received.

TODAY'S HEALTH CARE ECONOMICS

Health care economics in the early twenty-first century do not follow the pattern of traditional economic theory. Traditional **supply and demand curves** do not apply to health care. **Revenue cycles** are much longer in health care than in traditional business and, to a large degree, are out of the control of the provider. Due to the events that transpired during the history of the U.S. health care system, insurers generally

Case Study—Part 2

Dr. Lauersen's first trial ended in 2000 with a mistrial because jurors, after deliberating for more than six days, could not reach a verdict. One juror stated that she "simply did not believe insurance companies" (Steinhauer, 2001). Newspaper accounts reported a "circus-like" atmosphere due to the presence of numerous former patients of Lauersen, along with their children, who turned the courthouse hallways into a "day care center" (Steinhauer, 2000a). The fiercely loyal patients turned out to support the doctor in appreciation for the care he had delivered to them in the past.

Before his second trial, Dr. Lauersen lost his New York medical license due to allegations of "imminent danger to public health" (Steinhauer, 2000a). In addition to the insurance fraud accusations, the medical board accused him of negligence and incompetence related to the care of his patients, including improperly performed surgeries and several deliveries in which the babies either died

or suffered permanent injury. Lauersen and his attorneys vehemently denied that he did not meet the standard of care for his patients. They responded to the charges by alleging that the medical board had a long-term vendetta against Dr. Lauersen and this was simply another attack. The board also accused him of witness tampering related to the fraud charges because he encouraged patients to lie regarding their understanding of the billing arrangements, resulting in charges by the medical board of fraudulent practices and moral unfitness.

1. What is your opinion of the juror's statement that she "simply did not believe insurance companies"? What might be the reasons for her position?

2. Dr. Lauersen's patients were very loyal to him. How do you think this affected the judicial process?

3. Do the charges of negligence and incompetence affect your opinion of this case at this point?

have substantially more power than providers in determining reimbursement levels and, ultimately, provider profitability.

A fundamental principle of business is that, to be successful the business must be profitable. To be profitable, a business must have adequate **cash flow** and **revenue.** In normal business circumstances, an entity has the ability to manage and improve its revenue stream by:

1. Selling more products (provided an adequate profit margin exists on each unit).
2. Increasing its profit margin on each unit by reducing costs.
3. Differentiating its product from others in the marketplace to convince consumers that its product supplies enough value to justify the consumer paying a higher price for the product.

Unfortunately for providers, none of these methods are particularly effective in increasing revenue in the U.S. health care system.

Because health care is not a commodity, unlike shoes or fast food, it generally cannot be marketed and sold as a commodity. For example, the orthopedic surgeon cannot do more hip replacements (which usually have a good profit margin) by suggesting that every person who walks in the door with the slightest hip problem have a hip replacement. In fact, significant controversy erupted in political circles in 2009, when President Barack Obama suggested that physicians performed certain surgeries to make additional income, even though they were not medically necessary (Klukowski, 2009).

Increasing the **profit margin** on services is also difficult to do in the health care industry. The most significant area of cost in the vast majority of medical practices is staff salaries. While providers can capture some savings through skillful vendor negotiations, nothing can begin to compare with the costs associated with staffing the clinic. Some clinics have attempted to work with fewer staff members, or with lesser-qualified or credentialed staff, in an effort to save money. Most regret the decision because the adverse impact on patient care is substantially greater than the short-term savings realized in staff salaries. In fact, in a counterintuitive finding, the Medical Group Management Association (MGMA) annual cost survey consistently reports that the most successful medical practices (in terms of profitability) are those that spend more on staff salaries than the less successful practices.[1]

Differentiating one practice from another is, in theory, not very difficult. The first practice may advertise that its physicians trained at the top medical schools or are experts in a particular new procedure. However, practices that attempt this often find that patients do not share their same values. In fact, many practices are frustrated to find that patients select providers not based on the providers' qualities but rather on their willingness to accept payment from their insurer.

In the auto business, this would be considered absurd. The price of a premium performance sports car is dramatically higher than that of

Cash flow
A balance calculated by subtracting cash payments (expenses) for a specific period from cash receipts over that same period.

Revenue
The total amount of money received by a company before any deductions, such as expenses, are made.

Profit margin
Total revenue minus the total expenses in producing that revenue.

---

[1]The hypothesis behind this consistent finding is that better-performing groups have the ideal number of staff members, which promotes the highest levels of patient satisfaction (increasing patient volume), the highest levels of employee satisfaction (increasing productivity), and the highest levels of throughput (increasing work volume). Practices that attempt to take shortcuts in terms of staffing or staff salaries often save in the short term but lose in the long term because key performance measures are adversely affected.

a 15-year-old minivan, and most purchasers would expect to pay that premium price. However, what if the purchaser did not care about the driving experience and was simply interested in getting from point A to point B? Even though driving the expensive sports car is far more pleasurable than driving the old minivan, the cost of driving the minivan is significantly less and that is the controlling factor in the purchaser's decision-making process.

Top-level physicians experience this same frustration. Historically, because of the third-party payer system in the United States, every doctor providing the same service—regardless of skill level, experience quality provided, or consistency of outcome—receives the same payment as the marginal physician who provides poor service and has poor outcomes. This makes reinvestment in capital equipment and other items difficult, which then tends to diminish improvements in patient experience and outcomes in the future.

Similarly, even if a dramatic increase in demand occurred in a given geographic region, payment levels would not rise because supply and demand curves do not apply—the payer controls the reimbursement. Many rural areas, which have large Medicare populations, have experienced a substantial shortage of providers because even though there is great demand and little supply, the provider receives only as much as Medicare will allow. In fact, even physicians who choose not to participate in the Medicare program cannot charge patients more than 115% of the Medicare-allowed amount for that geographic region ("Medicare Glossary," 2008). Therefore, providers that have no control over their profit margin elect to move to some other location, with more favorable economic circumstances (Figure 4.6).

What is the provider to do? All of the traditional options of generating revenue seem to be unavailable or impractical. It is this environment that has created the circumstances in which coding can be used as a tool to increase revenue and profitability. However, the provider that does not adhere to firm ethical principles is easily tempted to cross the boundary into unethical behaviors related to coding.

FIGURE 4.6

In traditional economic theory, when demand goes up, price (reimbursement) goes up. However, when insurers define the reimbursement rates, reimbursement stays the same, regardless of demand.

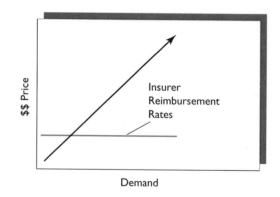

$$ Price

Insurer Reimbursement Rates

Demand

Thinking It Through 4.1

1. What part of the history of health care in the United States do you think contributes most to ethical problems in the coding and reimbursement process?

2. To what degree does the structure of health care economics create potential ethical problems? Explain your answer.

3. If the health care system had developed differently, do you believe that prices for health care would be higher or lower than they are currently? Would access to care be greater or less than it is now? What are the ethical considerations associated with health care cost and access?

4.2 The Stakeholders in Business Transactions and the Medical Coding Process

To understand the environment and some of the dynamics that create potential ethical problems in health care and coding specifically, consider another commonly provided service: auto repair. This case illustrates that even very simple transactions can be more complicated than they seem.

STAKEHOLDERS IN BASIC BUSINESS TRANSACTIONS

A man noticed that the yellow check engine light was illuminated on his car dashboard. As he was new in town and he did not know anyone who could provide a personal recommendation, he located the nearest auto repair shop that appeared capable of performing the required service. After examining the car, the repair shop representative told the man that his car required a lengthy list of repairs totaling $1,823.43. The man, shocked at the total given that his car did not seem to have any major problems, agreed to the repairs because he did not feel that he had any better alternative at the time. After paying the bill and receiving the car, it operated as it did before the repairs, except the yellow light was no longer on.

This example illustrates what appears to be a straightforward transaction between two parties: one person who has a need and the other person who has the ability to meet that need. Table 4.1 demonstrates the possible objectives of the two parties in this simple transaction.

Unfortunately, not all simple transactions of this type have positive outcomes because the parties could have different objectives, as illustrated in Table 4.2.

Table 4.1 Complementary Objectives of Parties in Car Repair Transaction	
Car Owner's Objectives	**Garage Representative's Objectives**
Obtain repairs in an inexpensive manner	Satisfy the customer's needs in a cost-effective manner, while making a satisfactory profit in the process
Obtain repairs within a reasonable period with minimal inconvenience	Deliver the service in an efficient manner
	Satisfy the customer to the extent that the customer will return for future service needs

Table 4.2 Conflicting Objectives of Parties in Car Repair Transaction

Car Owner's Objectives	Repair Shop Representative's Objectives
Obtain repairs in an inexpensive manner	Generate as much profit as possible by recommending unnecessary repairs and using substandard parts while charging for premium parts
Obtain repairs within a reasonable period with minimal inconvenience	Overestimating the amount of time needed to perform a task to maximize the "labor" component of the billing; work slowly to "fill" the amount of time
	Facilitate future service by providing "kickbacks" to tow truck drivers who divert cars requiring repair to the shop

Business model
The plan of how a business creates and delivers value.

WARNING

Many times, when a transaction seems very direct and straightforward, there are factors that can significantly complicate it. Consider the position of the other persons or entity. What objectives might they have that do not seem obvious?

Publicly traded
Shares sold on a public stock exchange.

FYI

The health care industry has changed dramatically in the last part of the twentieth century, with several health insurers becoming publicly traded in the 1980s. More recently, pharmaceutical companies began advertising in major media outlets, a practice that was not practical until the FDA revised its rules in 1997.

In this case, it seems that the objectives of the two parties are in opposition to each other. The car owner is unhappy, but the repair shop representative does not particularly care because his **business model** has no regard for ethical concerns. The customer will not go back to this repair shop, but again, the repair shop representative does not care because his business model does not require repeat customers.

Usually, the situation is not this obvious to customers. The customers may suspect that they were cheated, but they do not know for sure. Distrust can exist even when the immediate personal experience seems positive. The reasons that there may be distrust include:

1. Bad personal experiences by the customer in the past.
2. Knowledge of bad experiences in the past by other friends, relatives, and neighbors.
3. A lack of knowledge of how an automobile works, making the customer unable to personally evaluate the quality or fairness of the service.
4. A presupposition by the customer that many business people are unethical.

In addition, the situation can be more complex than it appears on the surface. Instead of a business transaction conducted between only two parties, Figure 4.7 illustrates how other, unseen parties may influence this same transaction. If this repair shop is part of a **publicly traded** national chain, several other interested parties want to see increased profitability. Often, the pressure brought to bear from above can be so great that it tempts an ordinarily ethical person to "cut corners" to increase the revenue. Pressure to increase revenue and/or sacrifice ethics can be created unintentionally. In this case, suppose that the mechanics received incentives to increase productivity by receiving commissions on the work they do. However, if a specific mechanic increases productivity by performing unneeded repairs or receives a disproportionate share of the work because he is a friend of the person charged with distributing the work, the best interest of the customer and coworkers is adversely affected.

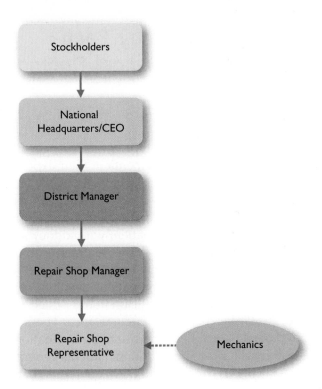

FIGURE 4.7

In a basic transaction between a repair shop representative and a customer, several other parties who are unseen to the customer can influence the nature of the transaction.

THE PARTIES INVOLVED
IN HEALTH CARE TRANSACTIONS

As illustrated, although the transaction between a customer and an auto repair shop seems simple on the surface, it can be more complicated than it appears. On the other hand, in the U.S. health care system, the transaction between provider (business) and patient (customer) appears substantially more complicated and, when fully analyzed, has elements and nuances that almost invite fraud, abuse, and ethical violations. To comprehend this complex environment you must understand the parties involved and their individual positions in the process.

Health care has more stakeholders than the average business transaction. Virtually every health care transaction has at least the following parties involved:

1. The patient (customer).
2. The employer (a customer, but also with business concerns).
3. The provider (business).
4. The third-party payer (business).

Thinking It Through 4.2

1. Do you believe that health care transactions are more or less complex than the example cited in the car repair case study? Why?

2. Have you personally had an unsatisfactory experience in a business transaction? If so, has it affected the way that you view other business transactions? How?

3. Of the four parties in the average health care transaction, who do you think has the most difficult position in the process? Why?

4.3 The Role Played by Each Stakeholder in the Medical Coding Process

THE PATIENT

Patients who arrive at a provider's office to receive medical care have a universal desire for at least two elements in their experience. First, patients desire a high quality of care. They want to have their medical needs addressed by a skilled professional who delivers the most appropriate treatment that will have the greatest benefit, once a risk versus benefit analysis is considered. A patient with kidney stones could receive treatment involving surgery or the treatment could consist of nothing more than waiting to see what happens. Both are appropriate treatments for this condition, but the patient usually does not have sufficient knowledge to make the decision about which treatment is appropriate for his or her particular circumstance. The patient relies on the provider to lend his or her expertise to the evaluation and treatment process and make a recommendation. Patients generally assume that the provider will recommend and deliver the care that is least invasive to achieve a positive outcome.

Second, patients also expect to receive treatment in a convenient and timely manner. Studies have shown that patients are generally willing to sacrifice convenience and endure long waits to see who they believe is the provider best able to serve them. However, there is a limit to this patience and, eventually, patients will change providers if the experience associated with their care does not meet a minimum standard. In fact, more recently, providers have taken a proactive approach to incorporate better customer service in their health care delivery processes. Some have gone as far as to incorporate customer service principles from the retail industry into their employee training and operational protocols, as well as adopting a retail-branding philosophy (Hinson Neely, 2006). The service quality expectations of patients are increasing simultaneously with these changes.

Increasing Expectations.   A more recent trend in patient expectations is the desire to pay as little as possible for the service, with the least possible amount of work on their part. The expansion of insurance coverage in the United States produced this trend. Through their insurance coverage, many patients are often personally responsible only for copayments and small **deductibles.** They see the cost of health care as equal to the amount they must personally pay—not the total cost of the service they desire to receive. The primary reason that this occurs is that patients frequently do not understand the fundamentals of health care finance and are insulated from the actual cost of the service. Therefore, a patient presented with a choice between a generic antibiotic (generic copay $10; total cost $15) and a new antibiotic that he or she saw on a television commercial (brand name copay $25; total cost $300) will often choose the new, brand name drug. The reason is simple—the price difference is only $15 and the perceived value of the new drug is worth the $15 difference.

Deductible
The financial responsibility of the patient that must be met prior to the patient's insurer making any payments for the patient's medical services.

WARNING

Providers can engage in unethical actions because many patients do not understand coding and the billing process. Patients who understand when they are being cheated in other business transactions may not have the same level of understanding in a health care transaction.

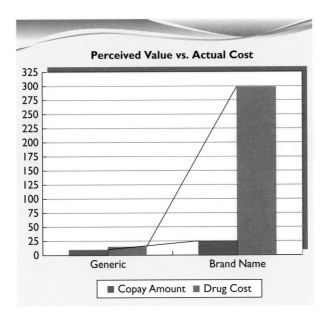

Perceived Value vs. Actual Cost

Legend: ■ Copay Amount ■ Drug Cost

However, the fact that the new drug costs 20 times more than the proven generic drug is either unknown to the patient or is not a concern to the patient because it does not affect his or her personal finances (Figure 4.8).

Decreasing Responsibility.   Moreover, because patients either have little understanding about insurance products or have developed an **entitlement mentality** about insurance, they frequently resist attempts to make them take responsibility for understanding their insurance coverage. Often, providers are expected to know exactly what is and is not covered by the patient's insurance policy, what laboratory obtains the maximum benefit for the patient, and which specialists the patient can see that will minimize his or her personal financial liability. Efforts by providers to explain the seemingly infinite variety of coverage that is available and the futility of attempting to understand every patient's insurance coverage are often rebuffed with a response of "It's your job to know about my coverage." Patients generally take this position because of their own lack of understanding (Figure 4.9).

Entitlement mentality
The belief that a person deserves or has a right to a benefit.

THE EMPLOYER

One often-overlooked party in the U.S. health care system is the employer of the patient. The employer is frequently, the party that purchases the coverage that provides insurance to the patient. The employer defines the benefits that it wants to provide and negotiates with the insurers to determine the coverage level and cost of the insurance that employees receive.

Employers originally became involved in the health care system due to wage and price controls in the 1940s (see page 103). Their purpose in doing so was to attract and retain high-quality employees. Therefore, employers do want to provide the best possible health insurance coverage to satisfy employees adequately (Figure 4.10).

FYI

Employers buy most of the commercial insurance in the United States. The patient frequently has no choice about the type of coverage he or she receives and often has little understanding about that coverage.

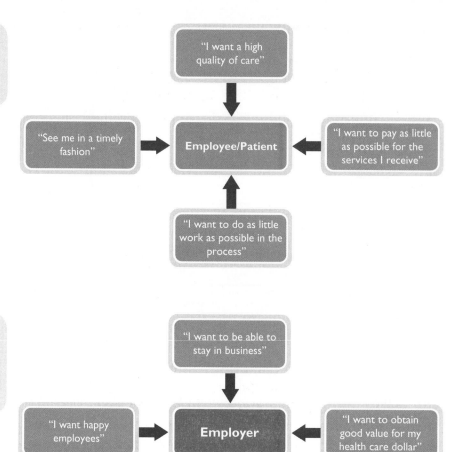

FIGURE 4.9

In the health care process, a patient often has multiple interests.

"I want a high quality of care"

"See me in a timely fashion"

Employee/Patient

"I want to pay as little as possible for the services I receive"

"I want to do as little work as possible in the process"

FIGURE 4.10

Health care employers have their own set of interests related to the health care system.

"I want to be able to stay in business"

"I want happy employees"

Employer

"I want to obtain good value for my health care dollar"

At the same time, they face the struggle of the skyrocketing costs of health insurance. Over the decade from 1999 to 2009, insurance premiums for employer-sponsored plans increased 131%, or four times more than the inflation rate for the rest of the economy (National Coalition on Health Care, 2009). This has placed many businesses, particularly small businesses, in economic jeopardy because they cannot afford the increased overhead costs. Employers have the unenviable task of balancing economic realities with employee satisfaction. Many employers have reduced benefits while others have completely dropped employee coverage.

One tool that employers have used in the past to control their cost is to increase the employees' share of the health care premium expense. As a result, the amount paid by employees for their health insurance premium is projected to increase substantially over the next few years (National Coalition on Health Care, 2009). Many employees respond to this prospect with complaints and protests, claiming that their wages have not increased sufficiently to allow them to afford additional premium expense.

THE PROVIDER

Defining *provider* in terms of this discussion is very important. The term is not limited to the physician—it involves the physician and several other key parties employed by or affiliated with the physician. The situation is complicated by the fact that not every party affiliated with the provider has the same interests or objectives, which can create conflict and pose potential **ethical challenges.**

It is reasonable to presume that the overwhelming majority of providers of medical care in the United States desire to provide the highest possible quality of care to their patients. Sensational stories of exceptions notwithstanding, medical professionals care about their patients and, in many instances, have long-standing relationships that extend over many years. This is true of all medical providers and is not limited to physicians. When describing providers, we must also incorporate nurse practitioners, physician assistants, certified nurse midwives, genetic counselors, chiropractors, podiatrists, and dozens of other health care professionals not listed here. Unfortunately, many of these providers often do not have the same level of commitment to accurate coding that they have for ensuring high-quality care to their patients.

The fact that health care professionals spend many years in training to perfect their diagnostic and treatment skills but have little or no education related to coding seems counterintuitive, because coding drives the business of medicine. A physician, no matter how technically proficient, cannot successfully stay in business if his or her coding is not performed correctly and optimally.

In the U.S. health care system, physicians and other health care professionals are not able to practice successfully unless they have appropriately trained and functioning support staff. The support staff can have many titles and have a broad range of training and technical expertise. Clinically, the staff could range from medical assistants, to nursing assistants, to registered nurses (RNs), to radiology and/or ultrasound technicians. Administratively, this could include front desk personnel, medical records personnel, surgery schedulers, billing clerks, medical coders, collection personnel, and so on. Although changes in many of the formal training programs are expanding the range of coding education provided, many of these people do not have adequate (or any) training in medical coding. This is problematic because they are often the parties physically delivering the services to the patients. It is difficult to envision how they can select the correct codes if they do not have at least a basic understanding of procedure and diagnosis codes.

Compounding the issues related to proper administrative function—specifically, correct coding—is the fact that the delivery of appropriate medical care can seem to conflict with ensuring that patients are satisfied customers. For example, a physician may feel that a particular treatment is the best alternative to address the patient's medical needs. However, the patient's health insurance plan does not cover the particular treatment and the patient cannot otherwise afford the treatment. The physician, wanting the patient to receive the appropriate treatment (and in today's highly competitive environment, also wanting to retain a customer), tells the coder to find a code that would make the service payable. This can easily create conflict within the office between the physician and the coder, if the coder believes that the code selected does not accurately describe the service provided.

During the past century, medicine has become more of a business, with larger practices requiring additional layers of administration

Ethical challenge
A situation in which the right or consistent action may produce an uncomfortable or undesirable result.

CODING TIP

Most U.S. medical schools provide little or no training in coding or reimbursement. All newly graduated physicians who go into practice should seek or receive coding training as soon as possible. This can dramatically improve the practice of ethical coding.

COMPLIANCE TIP

Any compliance program (see Chapter 11) must include the opportunity for employees to express their concerns about ethical practices within a health care organization. The varying degrees of power that exist in a health care organization can create intense pressure to take action that violates the employee's ethical beliefs.

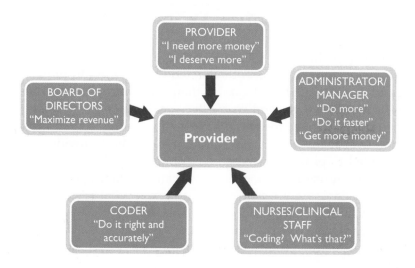

FIGURE 4.11
Within the provider's practice, the interests of various parties must compete.

and professional management, such as medical directors, chief financial officers, marketing directors, and so forth. These additional professionals may also have an adverse effect on the coding process because the physician may feel an additional pressure to perform and to have constant increases in productivity. The managers, board of directors, and others may push the provider organization to cut corners in coding to ensure that maximum possible level of revenue (Figure 4.11).

Providers that are not part of large practices and are, in effect, owners or operators may more directly feel the pressures imposed by the economy at large or by specific issues related to third-party reimbursement. They may not need a board of directors or administrators to place pressure on other employees to maximize all possible revenue sources. Physicians will hear complaints from patients to the effect, "The billing office is billing incorrectly. If they had used diagnosis xxx.xx, my insurer says the claim would have been paid!" Because they want to ensure patient satisfaction, the billing office staff often receive the directive to change the diagnosis.

Finally, provider income has been steadily dropping over the past 20 years because of increases in Medicare and Medicaid populations and minimal increases in Medicare, Medicaid, and other third-party payer reimbursement. Providers must work harder to achieve the same income levels that they previously experienced, with nearly 73% of primary care physicians reporting that their practices are not growing and their profit margins are shrinking (Merritt Hawkins & Associates, 2008). This is naturally frustrating for providers, and there may be a temptation to identify any way possible to keep reimbursement at previous levels. This can include unethical decisions related to coding.

THE CODER

The coder, although an integral part of the provider organization, is considered separately here because of the perspective the position requires. The primary objective of the diligent coder (and certainly a certified coder—see Chapter 10 for more information) is the selection and assignment of the procedure codes that most accurately describe the

COMPLIANCE TIP

The purpose of compliance programs is to ensure that billing and coding is done appropriately. Sometimes the program accomplishes this by discouraging intentional incorrect coding. On other occasions, the compliance program makes people aware of policies to prevent unintentional incorrect coding.

services provided. Similarly, coders have an equal stake in selecting and assigning the diagnosis codes that most accurately describe the reasons for the services provided. This skill requires careful study and thoughtful analysis and is honed through years of experience. Coding is a unique position in the administrative arm of provider organizations in the U.S. health care system because it carries with it an opportunity for professional designation and recognition that most other administrative roles do not provide. Coders unquestionably play a vital role in the revenue cycle of any provider organization (see Chapter 9). However, they are different from physicians or administrators in that the financial ramifications of their coding decisions are not or should not be their *first* consideration. Their primary objective is coding accuracy.

However, coders do not work in a vacuum. There is a direct and inextricable connection between coding and reimbursement. Coders must perform their task in an accurate *and* timely fashion. For example, a coder who selects and assigns codes with 100% proficiency will not be employed very long if he or she processes only 10 claims per day. Coding must be done accurately *while* meeting defined productivity guidelines. On the other hand, unreasonable productivity requirements can easily result in inaccurate coding. Some may allege that grossly unreasonable production requirements are almost a tacit endorsement of improper coding methodologies, which drive inappropriate provider reimbursement.

Coders also face the challenge of understanding third-party payer rules and guidelines. While the **Health Insurance Portability and Accountability Act (HIPAA)** of 1996 requires third-party payers to use selected code sets (CPT and HCPCS for procedures; ICD-9-CM for diagnoses), HIPAA does not require payers to adhere to the rules and guidelines of the organizations that publish these code sets. Therefore, payers have the option of establishing certain coding requirements that providers must follow for a claim to be considered "payable" by the insurer. Coders find themselves in the position of determining whether they should follow the standardized coding rules and guidelines issued by the code set publisher or follow the rules and guidelines issued by the payer that is responsible for payment for a given patient.

Finally, coders are in the difficult position of trying to satisfy conflicting demands of physicians, administrators, third-party payers, and patients. Often, coders are seen as the solution to a reimbursement problem because they have the ability to change a code to make a service payable. Theoretically, the patient is happy because the insurer paid for the service. The physician is happy because (1) he or she received payment, (2) the patient is happy, and (3) the payer is often unaware of the "creative" coding that took place. The coder often is not happy with the outcome of this situation because decisions and behavior took place that are inconsistent with the ethical duty associated with his or her position.

THE THIRD-PARTY PAYER

In the U.S. health care system third-party payers are often maligned, a view recognized by the industry as early as 2004, when one industry

Health Insurance Portability and Accountability Act (HIPAA)
A law allowing patients to obtain health coverage without underwriting or pre-existing condition limitations when a person changed jobs. Other elements of the law include security regulations, code set definitions, and the requirement of filing claims to insurance electronically.

BILLING TIP

Although HIPAA requires all payers to use the specified code sets, it does not require consistent interpretation of those code sets. Health care organizations must be aware of the varying payer billing rules and guidelines to receive appropriate payment.

The Effect of ICD-10 on Ethics and Coding

Two primary elements determine whether a service is covered by a third-party payer—the procedure codes and the diagnosis codes. In the case study at the beginning of the chapter, the government alleged that Dr. Lauersen misled the third-party payers in his choice of procedure and diagnosis codes, resulting in payment for noncovered services. One element that contributes to the ability of providers to mislead payers is the fact that ICD-9 is not adequately detailed. On many occasions, providers have no choice but to use codes that describe conditions as "other specified," meaning that the provider knows the condition, but there is no corresponding ICD-9 code to report that condition. In other cases, providers must use "unspecified" codes, meaning that either the physician does not know the exact nature of the condition or no code accurately describes the condition. Sometimes,

providers take advantage of this lack of clarity to either commit fraud or mask the true nature of the condition or treatment.

If providers intend to commit fraud, they will continue to do so. However, ICD-10 makes that a little more difficult because of the dramatically larger number of codes and the specificity required by the code set. Providers will not be able to hide as easily in the "unspecified" or "other specified" diagnosis codes in ICD-9. Payers will likely require providers to use the specific codes that are available and, as a result, dishonest providers must actively commit fraud, as opposed to "bending the rules." ICD-10 will be an important component in addressing ethical challenges related to diagnosis coding because its very detailed nature makes those dilemmas less easy to ignore or accept.

De facto arbiter
A decision maker that was not specifically assigned a task, but became the decision maker through a chain of events or by default.

FYI

Payers determine what is covered or not covered, as well as what services can and cannot be billed together. Payers do not have to follow CPT billing guidelines, which has led to provider accusations of unethical practices on the part of payers.

Administrative costs
The costs of real estate, employee salaries and benefits, advertising, and other costs separate from the production of salable items.

publication reported that a Harris poll found that 36% of those surveyed thought insurers did a good job for their consumers and only 30% thought that managed care companies did a good job. This was down 19 and 21%, respectively, over the preceding seven years ("Pharmaceutical and Health Insurance Companies Seen in Negative Light by Public," 2004). Regardless of how they are perceived or labeled, third-party payers are the **de facto arbiters** of correct coding in the health care system because they control the payment for services. They define what is covered or not covered and determine what procedure and diagnosis codes providers must use to designate a covered service.

The ability of payers to define covered services is very important because it is a key function in their business model. Third-party payers establish premiums based on statistical analysis of the anticipated cost of paying for the services the people they cover will ultimately receive. That cost includes the actual claim expenses, the **administrative costs** of operating the company, and sufficient additional income to either return a dividend to investors or have enough funds to ensure continued operations. A critical component of that analysis is accurately defining the services that they will be providing. If they establish a premium at a certain level based on the assumption that a particular type of treatment is excluded from coverage and, subsequently, they pay $100 million in claims for that treatment, their profit will be, at best, reduced and possibly they will experience a financial loss. Therefore, it is in the payer's interest to process and pay claims/benefits according to the contractual terms between the patient and the payer on which the premium determination was based (Figure 4.12).

To be successful, a payer must also provide satisfactory service to its insured and the employer groups to which it markets its policies. A payer that does not deliver a minimum level of customer service will have extreme difficulty retaining market share and attracting the new business required to keep it a viable entity. Many claim that insurers do not care about their policyholders, seek to deny claims whenever possible, and are focused solely on profits. While there certainly are demonstrated cases of unethical conduct by payers, the vast majority of payers are simply paying claims according to the terms of the insurance contract. The lack of understanding on the part of the patient/ employee is often the driving force in the conflict between payers and patients.

A controversial recent development in the area of health insurance in the United States is that many insurance companies/payers are now publicly traded companies. These corporations generate massive quantities of cash in selling stock in their company. In exchange, shareholders expect to receive a return on their investment in the

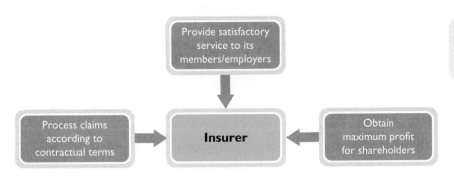

FIGURE 4.12
An illustration of the third-party payer's interests.

Case Study—Part 3

In Dr. Lauersen's second trial, the prosecution based its case on reams of documents that showed that Lauersen billed the insurers of patients who had insurance coverage for fertility treatments differently than the insurers of patients who did not have the coverage. Dr. Lauersen's defense to this evidence was that the insurance companies were immoral and greedy in denying needed medical treatment to patients to facilitate their dream of having a family. He also claimed that many times he performed "dual procedures" in which he would perform a covered procedure to correct a congenital or structural abnormality at the same time that he would perform a fertility-related procedure. This blurred the line between the covered and noncovered procedures. Lauersen claimed that he simply was seeking to obtain the insurance benefits to which the patient was entitled (Steinhauer, 2001).

Ultimately, the jury found Dr. Lauersen guilty of insurance fraud, sentencing him to 7 years, 3 months of incarceration, a $17,500 fine, and ordering restitution of approximately $3.2 million. After serving 4 years, the court reduced his sentence to 5 years, 10 months, primarily due to his age (68 years old). The judge observed that Dr. Lauersen had served the public good by bringing many babies into the world and that New York law had been subsequently revised to require insurers to cover some of the fertility treatments for which Dr. Lauersen submitted claims and received payment (Preston, 2005). However, the judge also noted that the doctor had never taken responsibility for his crime.

1. In considering the prosecution's evidence and Dr. Lauersen's defense, which do you believe has the stronger argument?

2. Are you surprised by the jury's verdict in the second trial? Was the penalty too much, too little, or about right?

3. Does the fact that this case, in part, effected change in the New York laws regarding fertility coverage change your opinion about the case?

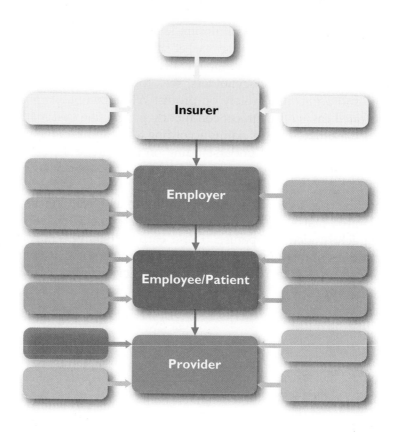

FIGURE 4.13
There are many different voices, with many different objectives and opinions, in health care transactions.

Insurer

Employer

Employee/Patient

Provider

Stock option
A contract giving an individual the right to purchase stock in a given company at a given price.

Deferred compensation
A form of compensation in which payment is delayed until a later date.

company. CEOs and other insurance executives receive **stock options** and **deferred compensation** based on stock prices and meeting target goals. Many have questioned whether the objectives of the shareholders and the objectives of the policyholders are mutually compatible. Regardless of one's position on this issue, shareholder satisfaction is an important concern for payers that are publicly traded companies.

In summary, four different parties are involved in the health care financing process: the patient (the customer), the employer (also a customer), the provider (a business), and the third-party payer (a business). Moreover, employers, payers, and providers often have complex organizations with many competing internal demands and issues that exist without regard to the relationship with the other parties (Figure 4.13). Many of the issues and conflicts that exist, both internally and externally, have been solved incorrectly and unethically by modifying the codes reported in the billing process.

Thinking It Through 4.3

1. Do you agree with the assertion that the health care industry is significantly more complex than the average business environment? Why or why not? If so, which factor do you believe contributes the most to its complexity?

2. What recommendations do you have to increase the level of understanding between the various parties involved in the health care financing process?

3. Of the four parties in the health care financing process, which do you believe has the greatest propensity for unethical behavior? On what do you base your opinion?

4.4 Thoughts and Behaviors of Stakeholders in Health Care

The number of parties involved in health care transactions and the nature of the relationships between the parties dramatically increase the complexity of the transactions. Although a seemingly simple transaction between a customer and an auto repair shop can be surprisingly complex, the issues increase exponentially in a health care transaction. One reason is the widely varying objectives of all the parties involved. Each party desires certain actions from other parties and all of them desire certain outcomes. It is impossible for all of these objectives to be coordinated, aligned, and absent of conflict.

Part of the reason for conflict in the process is the separation that exists between the various parties (Figure 4.14). In the physician–patient relationship, for example, the process is straightforward until it comes time to submit a claim for the service to a third-party payer. At that point, the payer becomes intimately involved in the previously private relationship between physician and patient. The payer often has the right to impose requirements on the provider, on behalf of the patient, to obtain maximum benefits for the patient. The provider may have to contact the insurer to have a service preauthorized or "preapproved." The provider may have its choices limited when referring the patient to another provider for a consultation or diagnostic test—the patient may not have benefits if an "out-of-network" provider sees him or her. When it comes time to submit a claim, the provider has to consider carefully the payer's reimbursement rules to ensure that the patient obtains the benefits to which he or she is entitled.

Interestingly, many of the parties in this process did not voluntarily choose to be in a relationship with the other parties. For example, the patient often has no choice regarding the insurer that provides the

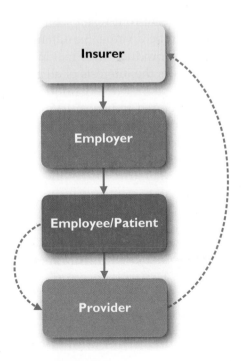

FIGURE 4.14
Relationships between parties in health care transactions are often not direct and are complicated by other entities that have an interest in the process and its outcome.

Market share
The percentage of the total number of possible enrollees insured by a given company in a given marketplace.

coverage. That is a decision made by the patient's employer. Similarly, patients often do not choose providers because they are the "best" or the most convenient. They sometimes select a provider that has a contract with the insurer (whom they did not choose) and is willing to accept a reduced rate of reimbursement. Likewise, providers often do not contract with certain insurers by choice. They sometimes must make the decision based on the insurer's **market share.** Not having a contract with the payer would result in an insufficient number of patients to keep the practice operational.

CAUSES OF ETHICAL DILEMMAS IN HEALTH CARE AND CODING

Ethical dilemmas in business are not uncommon, as indicated by the number of books published on the topic and recent high-profile examples of ethical lapses. The U.S. health care system has all of these traditional ethical dilemmas, and more. The primary reason for these additional ethical dilemmas is because health care is complex, as illustrated in the preceding sections. That complexity creates conflict and provides additional opportunities for ethical dilemmas to occur in an effort to avoid or, in some fashion, resolve the conflict.

Beyond the common causes of ethical dilemmas, which are discussed in detail in Part 1 of this book, four separate, identifiable causes increase the probability of an ethical dilemma arising from the medical coding process.

1. Conflicting interests.
2. Name-calling.
3. Lack of understanding or education.
4. Lack of relationship or alignment of objectives.

Conflicting Interests.   The ideal business transaction is one in which the interests of all the parties are aligned. In common language, this transaction is known as a win–win deal. For example, consider the retailer who is able to make a profit when selling a product at a price that the consumer finds to be a value. Simultaneously, the manufacturer is able to produce the product while making a satisfactory profit for the business. In this case, the interests of all parties are aligned, as illustrated in Figure 4.15.

However, the model pictured in Figure 4.15 is not always possible and, in the case of health care economics, it can sometimes be literally impossible. Consider the following scenarios in which interests are not aligned.

> **FYI**
>
> Sometimes ethical dilemmas result because not everyone can achieve their goals simultaneously. A patient wants to receive maximum benefits, while the payer wants to achieve maximum profitability, while the provider wants to receive maximum payment.

Third-Party Payer	Employer
Desires adequate profit because expenses are increasing. Chooses to raise premium rates by 30%.	Does not want (and cannot afford) a 30% premium increase due to increasing overhead costs and declining revenues.

Third-Party Payer	Patient
Desires adequate profit as expenses are increasing. Chooses to raise premium rates by 30%. Reduces or eliminates certain benefits.	Desires to have insurer pay for now noncovered benefits. Angry that additional premium costs have been deducted from paycheck.

Third-Party Payer		Provider	
Increases utilization review and preauthorization procedures to help control cost increases.		Angry that additional staff is required to fulfill payer documentation and claim filing requirements.	
Freezes or reduces reimbursement to providers to help control cost increases.		Angry that payer does not seem to recognize that overhead cost increases can't be absorbed while reimbursement declines.	
Third-Party Payer		**Payer Shareholders**	
Takes actions necessary to ensure adequate shareholder return.		Dissatisfied with payer performance. Places pressure on company executives to perform better.	
Patient		**Provider**	
Desires third-party payer to cover costs for services. Believes provider can address this problem by changing codes.		Desires to code correctly *and* satisfy patient (internal conflict).	
Employer		**Patient/Employee**	
To control cost increases, changes benefit plan and increases employee share of premiums.		Angry that previous benefits no longer exist. Feels as though he or she is paying more for less.	

Many other possible permutations of competing and conflicting interests exist in the health care marketplace, when the only parties considered are the patient, the provider, the employer, and the payer. However, on a larger **macroeconomic** scale, when other parties are considered the situation is even more complex.

Macroeconomic
Pertaining to an economy at the highest level, such as that of an entire nation or a particular sector of the economy.

Name-Calling. In the health care financing debate, there are cases where the argument devolves into name-calling, when one party in the process maligns the other party. When this occurs, the parties either ignore or devalue the validity of the other's position to the point that there is no constructive communication. Examples of name-calling in the health care arena include:

- "Greedy insurance companies."
- "Dishonest and greedy doctors."
- "Lazy and dishonest patients."
- "Employers take profits on the backs of employees."

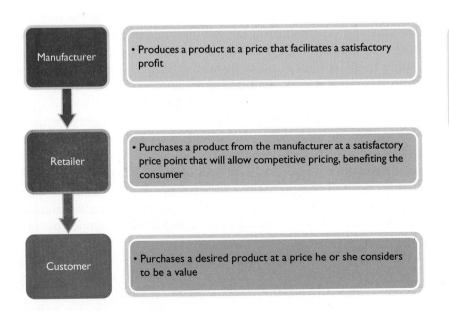

FIGURE 4.15
In this business transaction model, the interests of all parties are aligned, allowing everyone to achieve their objective.

Manufacturer
- Produces a product at a price that facilitates a satisfactory profit

Retailer
- Purchases a product from the manufacturer at a satisfactory price point that will allow competitive pricing, benefiting the consumer

Customer
- Purchases a desired product at a price he or she considers to be a value

The problem is that there are instances in which these characterizations are proven true. However, it is not appropriate or accurate to assign automatically this characterization to anyone with whom there is disagreement.

Specifically in the area of coding, increasing numbers of insurers and even the federal government are asking patients to identify potential cases of fraud and/or billing abuse on each explanation of benefits (EOB) that they send to patients. While in theory this is a practical way to identify the inappropriate coding of unethical providers, it may actually cause more problems than it solves.

For example, Dr. Horowitz is a cardiologist with University Cardiology Associates. An ambulance took Mr. Franklin to the Emergency Department of University Hospital because of chest pains. In evaluating Mr. Franklin's chest pain, the emergency room physician ordered a 12-lead electrocardiogram (EKG) to help evaluate his chest pain. Although the EKG appeared normal, hospital policy required it to be read by a cardiologist. The next day, Dr. Horowitz reviewed Mr. Franklin's EKG readout and provided an interpretation. Dr. Horowitz billed 93010-26—EKG interpretation only.

The provider submitted a claim to Mr. Franklin's insurer, Medicare, which paid the claim and sent an EOB to Mr. Franklin. Mr. Franklin did not recognize Dr. Horowitz's name, since he had never met him. Mr. Franklin assumed that this must be a fraudulent claim of some sort and called the number on his Medicare EOB. Medicare sent an inquiry letter to University Cardiology Associates to begin an investigation of the allegation of billing fraud.

Dr. Horowitz's **billing protocol** was totally appropriate and ethical. However, he and/or his practice will have to spend time defending their correct billing practices because the patient believes his insurer (in this case, Medicare) told him to report suspected fraud. These calls are getting more common because politicians and other public figures are depending on savings from identifying billing fraud and abuse to fund many other activities in the health care arena (Moore, 2009).

Lack of Understanding or Education.

Closely linked with the issue of fraud accusations provoked by political battles is the fact that many allegations of inappropriate billing are driven by the fact that coding is not simple. Things that appear to be inappropriate or unethical are actually correct in many instances. Simply stated, accusations are made because coding rules and guidelines are not understood by patients and, sometimes, even government agencies.

The federal False Claims Act (FCA) is the government's primary tool in identifying inappropriate coding and combating the associated fraud. The penalties associated with "knowingly submitting false or fraudulent claims" are severe, with fines of between $5,500 and $11,000 per violation and the possibility of also repaying an amount three times greater than what was improperly received. Since 1986, the Department of Justice has collected more than $15 billion under the law (Senterfitt, 2007).

Dr. R. D. Prabhu was audited because he submitted claims at a level higher than that of his peers. The government did not provide any evidence of misconduct, but demanded the refund of a substantial

<hr />

BILLING TIP

Patients may not understand the difference between "professional" and "technical" services. A physician may bill for professional services (e.g., interpretation of tests, etc.) without ever physically seeing the patient. The patient may not be aware of the nature of the services.

Billing protocol
The specific pattern and guidelines for billing medical services to insurance companies.

amount of payment. When Dr. Prabhu questioned the audit, charges were filed against him under the FCA.

The basis of the government allegation was that the physician and his practice knowingly submitted claims for simple pulmonary stress tests performed as part of a pulmonary rehabilitation program. Pulmonary stress tests were covered under the Medicare program; pulmonary rehabilitation programs were not covered. The government claimed that Dr. Prabhu was attempting to hide the noncovered services by using a covered CPT code. In addition, the government allegations also included a claim that Dr. Prabhu's documentation was inadequate and that he did not provide all of the services necessary to bill for the CPT code. He faced a possible financial penalty of $22 million if the government prevailed.

During the trial, Dr. Prabhu demonstrated that the Medicare guidelines regarding coverage of pulmonary rehabilitation programs were unclear and that the government had misinterpreted the rules published by the American Medical Association for the CPT code. He also presented the testimony of a number of coders whose interpretation of the rules and opinion of the documentation quality seriously conflicted with the government's interpretation. In fact, testimony was given that even government auditors disagreed on the interpretation of the rules.

The judge in the case ruled in Dr. Prabhu's favor, indicating that there was no evidence of his intent to knowingly submit a false claim. Unfortunately, the physician expended great amounts of time, energy, and money in defending himself against these charges (Akin, Gump, Strauss, Hauer & Feld, LLC, 2006).

In this particular case, the federal government—an institution that arguably has a broad knowledge base about coding and coding issues—brought charges of ethical failure and fraudulent claims against a physician that eventually were proven inaccurate. If the government is unable to clarify adequately what is and is not ethical coding behavior, we must ask the question: How can any layperson who is not familiar with coding understand and identify an unethical or illegal action related to coding?

Unfortunately, if individuals are inclined to be unethical they will take advantage of the complex rules and general lack of knowledge, hoping that their unethical behavior will be difficult if not impossible to detect. In many instances only the most extreme cases of fraud are identified and prosecuted; but sometimes parties who do not have unethical intentions are caught in the middle of ethics allegations.

Lack of Relationship or Alignment of Objectives. The most significant factor that influences ethical dilemmas is a lack of relationship between the parties involved (Figure 4.16). This was demonstrated on two levels by Stanley Milgram, the social psychologist who conducted experiments in the 1960s to determine how far subjects would go in inflicting pain on other people. The subjects of his research were led to believe that there were people connected to a device on the other side of a wall. The subjects were told to turn a dial—the further they turned the dial, the more they heard screams of pain from the other side of the wall. (In reality, there were actors on the other side of the wall and no actual pain was inflicted.)

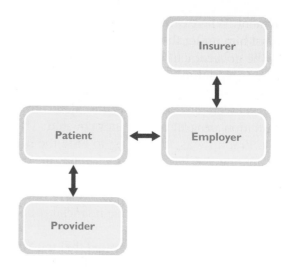

Milgram's research was shocking in that a remarkable number of test subjects were repeatedly willing to turn the dials all the way, eliciting screams of pain. When faced with the dilemma of following instructions from the researcher or refusing to inflict pain on someone else, many chose to follow the instructions (Card, 2005).

Two key elements of Milgram's research apply to our discussion of ethics. First, it is unlikely that the subjects would have followed the instructions and inflicted the pain if they personally knew the person on the other side of the wall. Similarly, if the subjects had been able to see the pain they were inflicting, they likely would have been less willing to participate in the process. Therefore, a lack of connection to the other party seems to be a contributing factor to an individual's willingness to violate his or her personal code of conduct.

Second, Milgram learned that there is a distinct difference between individual responsibility and organizational responsibility. People seem more willing to put aside their personal ethics and standard decision-making frameworks if there is an organizational objective to be met. Milgram called it the **"erosion of agency"** within organizations (Card, 2005). He postulated that although these people, as individuals, would never willingly inflict pain on others, in an organizational context, they were "doing their job," which, in some fashion, psychologically justified their actions.

When focusing this discussion on coding ethics, several parties are affected by the lack of a relationship that exists in the process. First, patients generally do not know individuals at the insurance company. When acquiring benefits to which they are not contractually entitled, they do not see it as stealing, but rather they justify it by saying that "the insurer won't miss it" or "it's a big company and they make too much profit."

The provider's attitude can be similar to that of the patient in that there is often not a personal relationship: The insurer is a depersonalized entity. However, added to that can be a general, underlying sense of anger regarding decreasing reimbursements and increased administrative paperwork. By violating the principles of coding ethics to obtain additional reimbursement, the provider's attitude can be, "I'm just getting paid what I deserve—I was underpaid to start!"

Erosion of agency
The theory that people are more likely to allow their moral position or beliefs to slip when they are acting on behalf of another party (agency), such as an employer.

Case Study—Part 4

After Dr. Lauersen's release from a federal detention center in Pennsylvania in 2006, he continued to fight to regain his medical license. One of his attorneys said that he did not understand why the jury sympathized with the insurance companies instead of his client. According to the attorney, Lauersen treated rich and poor patients alike, not turning away anyone because of their inability to pay (Hartocollis, 2006).

Lauersen continues to seek support in his appeal to the medical board on his website (**www.nielslauersenmd .org**), where he asks patients to e-mail stories of how he helped them. Numerous patients have complied with his request, providing lengthy, detailed accounts of their treatment and expression of their gratitude to Dr. Lauersen. He remains defiant toward the prosecutor and medical board, stating on his website,

> As you all know, I went to prison fighting for the rights of all women to have access to treatment— regardless of their ability to pay. I challenged the insurance companies, but sadly, that fight resulted in a deep personal loss. I am not sorry that I took on the notoriety and attention of my fight, which I believe changed the insurance laws in New York and other parts of the country, which resulted in payment of fertility treatments by insurance companies. I know in my heart I did the right thing by fighting, because today couples who desperately wanted children have them. Today, not just the rich and famous can afford to have fertility treatment. . . . I'm proud that I had a part in making that happen. (Lauersen, n.d.)

1. If you were in Dr. Lauersen's position, would you have conducted yourself similarly? What would you have done differently?

2. What was the strongest aspect of Dr. Lauersen's position? What was the weakest aspect of his position?

3. Do you think there will be fewer or more cases like this in the future? Why?

When faced with ethical conflicts, the coder may fall prey to erosion of agency because he or she is working on behalf of the organization— the medical practice. The coder does not see himself or herself as unethical—it is the organization; the coder is simply a "cog in the wheel." Other justifications that can support the coder's logic against ethical conduct are that "everyone else is doing it" and "if I don't do it, they'll just hire someone who will."

Thinking It Through 4.4

1. In what ways can the objectives of the various parties be better aligned? How might this be accomplished?

2. Explain how health care providers experience increased costs associated with fraud, even if they operate under the most ethical standards possible.

3. Have you personally heard name-calling in association with the health care industry? If so, what were the circumstances? Was there any basis for the comments?

CHAPTER REVIEW

Chapter Summary

Learning Outcomes	Key Concepts/Examples

4.1 Describe the unique elements of the U.S. health care payment system that produce and promote the opportunity for ethical dilemmas. Pages 101–109	• Prior to 1930, health care was a commodity, not unlike other purchased goods and services. Over the years, the introduction of insurance and other economic factors influenced the way in which health care in the United States is financed.
	• A number of different attempts were made to address the issue of dramatically increasing costs, with limited success.
	• The unique economics of health care dramatically influence the way in which health care is financed and managed.
	• The system of health care financing creates the opportunity for ethical dilemmas because:
	  1. Traditional business methods of increasing revenue are not available in the health care field.
	  2. Revenue cycles are considerably longer in health care than in other types of businesses.
	  3. Insurers generally have a greater level of power than providers in determining payment levels.
	  4. The financing system provides a disincentive for the delivery of quality care.

4.2 Identify the stakeholders in business transactions and the medical coding process. Pages 109–111	• Traditional business relationships do have unseen levels of complexity, but the fundamental objectives of each party are usually in line with one another. • In health care transactions, there are usually four separate entities and the objectives are frequently not aligned. This causes the opportunity for conflict and ethical dilemmas.

4.3 Evaluate the role played by each stakeholder in the medical coding process. Pages 112–120	• The four entities involved in most health care transactions are:
	  1. The patient (customer).
	  2. The employer (customer and business).
	  3. The provider (business).
	    • Physician
	    • Administration
	    • Clinical staff
	    • Coder
	  4. The third-party payer (business).

4.4 Analyze the position of stakeholders who face specific ethical dilemmas related to third-party reimbursement. Pages 121–127	• The involvement of a third party in the payment process for health care introduces significant opportunity for ethical dilemmas.
	• Ethical dilemmas are caused in health care because of:
	  1. Conflicting interests that can't be easily reconciled.
	  2. Name-calling.
	  3. Lack of understanding or education.
	  4. Lack of relationship or alignment of objectives.

End-of-Chapter Review

Multiple Choice

Circle the letter that best completes the statement or answers the question.

1. **LO 4.1** Insurance companies first came into being circa
   a. 1880
   b. 1900
   c. 1930
   d. 1952

2. **LO 4.1** Traditionally, when demand increases at the same time that supply decreases, price
   a. Goes up
   b. Goes down
   c. Is unaffected
   d. Is variable, based on the circumstance

3. **LO 4.1** Which of the following was *not* an unintended consequence of health maintenance organizations (HMOs)?
   a. Patients were insulated from the cost of their care.
   b. Health care costs were controlled to a certain degree.
   c. Administrative tasks in the physician office increased dramatically.
   d. Patients resented the attempt to control their behavior and health care expenses.

4. **LO 4.1** In comparison to revenue cycles of most businesses, revenue cycles in health care are generally
   a. Shorter
   b. Longer
   c. Very similar
   d. Better

5. **LO 4.2** Which of the following is *not* a stakeholder in the medical coding process?
   a. Provider
   b. Insurer
   c. Employers
   d. All are stakeholders

6. **LO 4.3** Patient expectations in the provider–patient relationship are increasing because of
   a. Expansion of insurance coverage to a larger number of people
   b. Increasing personal expense and responsibility for the patient
   c. Increasing patient understanding regarding insurance coverage
   d. Improved communication from employers regarding the coverage they provide

7. **LO 4.4** The majority of nongovernmental health care in the United States is purchased by
   a. Individuals
   b. Employers
   c. Large unions
   d. Insurance cooperatives

8. **LO 4.4** Coding accuracy is usually a primary concern of which of the following?
   a. The provider
   b. The patient

c. The coder or billing office staff

d. The employer

9. **LO 4.4** The law that determines which code sets are acceptable for use is the

   a. Correct Coding Act of 1992

   b. Health Insurance Portability and Accountability Act of 1996

   c. Centers for Medicare and Medicaid Services Provider Manual

   d. Omnibus Reconciliation Act of 1995

10. **LO 4.4** Which of the following is *not* a cause of ethical dilemmas in health care coding?

    a. Conflicting interests

    b. Name-calling

    c. Inadequate government regulation

    d. Lack of understanding or education

11. **LO 4.4** *Erosion of agency* refers to

    a. The willingness of people acting on behalf of another to violate their own personal ethical principles

    b. The likelihood of an organization to become more unethical as it grows larger

    c. A personnel selection process by which employers hire "like-minded" personnel who will do what they want

    d. None of the above

12. **LO 4.4** The most significant factor that created ethical challenges in the coding process is the linkage between

    a. Employers and insurance companies

    b. Employers and employees

    c. Providers and insurance companies

    d. Employees and insurance companies

Short Answer

Use your critical thinking skills to answer the following questions.

1. **LO 4.1** Explain why physicians in the 1800s often had second jobs.

2. **LO 4.1** Describe how wage and price controls connected health insurance to a person's employment.

3. **LO 4.1** Explain usual, customary, and reasonable (UCR) reimbursement. Was it a good tool for use in reimbursing health care providers? Why or why not?

4. **LO 4.1** Explain the factors that create the sense of powerlessness that may influence providers' decisions to be unethical in their billing and coding.

5. **LO 4.2** Which is the most significant reason that distrust can exist between customers and businesses? Explain the basis for your opinion.

6. **LO 4.3** Which stakeholder in the medical coding process most influences the ethical behavior of the other parties in the process? Explain why.

7. **LO 4.3** Explain why ICD-10 will improve coding accuracy and reduce unethical coding.

8. **LO 4.3** Explain how payers are the de facto arbiters of coding policies.

9. **LO 4.4** Describe how and why the U.S. health care system facilitates relationships between parties that would not otherwise conduct business together.

10. **LO 4.4** Define how Milgram's sociological experiments in the 1960s relate to health care coding ethics today.

Applying Your Knowledge

Fraud is, unfortunately, an unpleasant fact in the U.S. health care industry, particularly related to billing and coding. Health care billing fraud is considered a much safer way for criminals to commit crimes because the opportunity for "success" is great and "no one is shooting at you" (CBS News-60 Minutes, 2009*).

One common means by which to commit health care fraud is to steal or purchase the names and identification numbers of Medicare patients. In cooperation with other corrupt health care professionals, phony medical corporations are established and huge numbers of claims are submitted for services that never took place. By the time the authorities discover the fraud, the participants in the fraud have disappeared and moved on to their next scheme.

The most common way that the government becomes aware of this fraud is when Medicare patients report that they received an EOB for a service that they did not receive. Today, Medicare and many private insurers instruct patients to call a special hotline if they suspect that billing fraud has occurred.

As mentioned, providers that are engaged in ethical and appropriate billing practices are sometimes accused of fraud by patients and insurers that do not understand the billing process and billing rules. These providers spend a great deal of time and effort defending themselves against charges of fraud when, in fact, they did nothing wrong.

1. In addition to the time and effort associated with the defense of false charges of fraud, what other damages occur to providers?

2. Do you believe that asking patients on EOBs to report suspected fraud is an effective tool in limiting and/or identifying billing fraud?

3. What other options might payers have in controlling health care billing fraud?

4. What effect does the presence of complicated billing rules and widespread fraud have on the health care delivery process?

---

*CBS News-60 Minutes. (2009, October 23). Medicare Fraud: A $60 Billion Crime. **www.cbsnews.com/stories/2009/10/23/60minutes/main5414390.shtml.**

Internet Research

As discussed in this chapter, many of the ethical struggles that exist between providers and payers are related to the issue of coverage; that is, which services are and are not payable under the patient's insurance plan. Moreover, how does a provider correctly designate the difference between covered and noncovered services?

A common historical complaint of providers is that they never knew the provider's rules and, if they did learn them, the rules would change. Payers were hesitant to send out large, bulky provider manuals because of the expense and the fact that they could not control how well the provider office kept the books up-to-date. Providers felt as though they had better things to do than to keep track of new components of a payer's provider manual.

The Internet has changed this because it enables payers and providers to see the most current version of any coding rules and/or guidelines in real time. In addition, providers can obtain detailed information about the patient's particular coverage and benefits. This eliminates much of the variability associated with coverage and clarifies the distinction between covered and noncovered services.

1. What are the advantages of having the payer's provider manual online for a provider? For the payer?

2. Some payers do not allow open access to online provider manuals, requiring the use of a username and password to access the information. What reasons might the payers have for not allowing open access to this information?

3. Using an Internet search engine, locate the website of a payer in your general geographic area that has provider information available online. Identify the website URL and the name of the payer, and provide a brief summary of the information the payer delivers online. If you were a provider contracted with this payer, would you be satisfied with the information that is available? If not, what additional information would you like to have available?

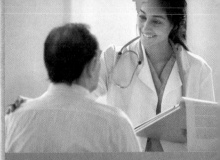

Coding Ethics for Evaluation and Management Services

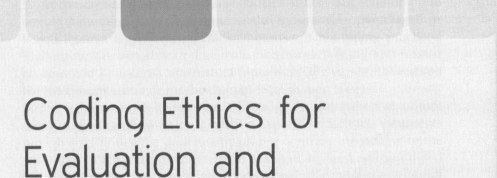

5

Key Terms

Chief complaint

Chronological

Consultation

Documentation
   Guidelines (DG)

History of present
   illness (HPI)

Intuitive

Medical decision
   making

Overcoding

Past, family, and/
   or social history
   (PFSH)

Prognosis

Quantified

Review of systems
   (ROS)

Superbill

Undercoding

Vignette

LEARNING OUTCOMES

After completing this chapter, you will be able to:

5.1   Explain the factors that contribute to the appropriate
       selection and assignment of evaluation and management
       (E/M) codes.

5.2   Distinguish the factors that present ethical challenges in
       association with obtaining and documenting the history
       element of E/M services.

5.3   Differentiate between the 1995 and 1997 Documentation
       Guidelines as they affect the calculation of the physical
       examination component of E/M services, along with the
       ethical ramifications of using each option.

5.4   Explain the factors that contribute to determining a level
       of medical decision making and the ethical difficulties that
       are present in the process.

5.5   Define the circumstances in which time can be used as
       the primary factor in calculating E/M services and list
       occasions in which ethical problems may occur.

5.6   Report the most frequent occasions in which ethical
       lapses may occur in association with E/M service billing.

5.7   Evaluate the ethical problems that can arise during the
       E/M code selection process.

CASE STUDY

Allison Magnuson was excited about her new employment as the administrator with the Franklin Road Medical Clinic. She had a previous career in retail sales, but desired a career change and became interested in the medical field. She initially obtained a position with West End Family Practice as a receptionist. Through hard work, she was promoted to supervisor of the front desk area and, at the same time, she took courses in medical practice management at the local community college. After a number of years of experience and eventually obtaining her degree, she felt ready to be a medical office administrator.

During the afternoon of Allison's first day, an employee from the billing office knocked on her door. The employee indicated that she was very pleased that Allison had joined the practice so that "someone could fix things around here." The employee expressed concern with some of the billing practices in the office and presented Allison with the chart shown in Figure 5.1.

The billing employee indicated that these data reflected one of the physician's billing patterns for office E/M codes for the past six months. The employee felt that this billing pattern was inappropriate and unethical and that the clinic was at great risk for an audit by payers and/or governmental agencies.

Allison examined the chart, but was not particularly familiar with the specifics of CPT coding. The billing office employee seemed to make sense, but Allison wasn't sure if there really was a problem and didn't yet know what to do next—either procedurally or politically.

1. Based on this chart alone, do you believe that this physician has a problem with his billing patterns? Is it an ethical problem?
2. If you were in Allison's position, what step(s), if any, would you take to investigate this matter?

FIGURE 5.1

This chart shows the distribution of E/M codes billed at Franklin Avenue Medical Clinic. It is unusual in that for most practices this chart is in the shape of a bell curve, with the majority of services billed as Level 3 or Level 4, and fewer at each end.

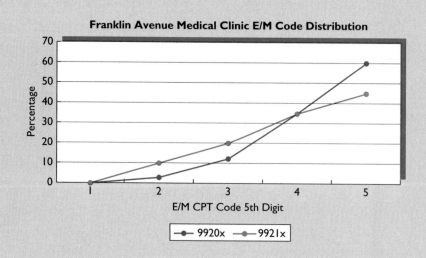

Franklin Avenue Medical Clinic E/M Code Distribution

Introduction

Evaluation and management (E/M) codes are the most commonly used, generally least understood, and most likely source for ethical problems of all the codes that appear in the *Current Procedural Terminology,* Fourth Edition (CPT-4) code book. E/M codes are placed at the front of the CPT-4 manual because of their frequent usage. In fact, of the top 10 codes paid by Medicare in 2008, 7 of the codes are E/M codes, representing 18.1% of Medicare's total outlay for Part B services in that year (Table 5.1). This is particularly remarkable given that the payment levels for individual E/M services are significantly lower than many of the surgical procedures billed by physicians. Physicians must deliver many more E/M services to receive the same amount of money as they would for providing surgical procedures.

The purpose of E/M codes is to facilitate the billing of services provided to patients that are not centered on the performance of medical procedures. The services represented by E/M codes are generally cognitive in nature and are used to recognize the time and effort that it takes to obtain the patient's history, learn about their symptoms, examine the patient, and make a preliminary (or final) diagnosis. E/M services also allow physicians to bill for patient counseling, which can include educating the patient about their condition, patient care instruction, and the answering of patient questions.

5.1 Factors to Consider in Selecting an E/M Code

Correctly selecting E/M codes is generally more difficult than selecting a code for a specific procedure due to the multiple components that must be considered when choosing an E/M code. While selecting procedure codes can be challenging, as discussed at length in Chapter 6, there are few procedure codes whose selection complexity

Table 5.1 Most Frequently Used CPT Codes Billed to Medicare—2008

Rank	Procedure Code	Description	Allowed Charges	Procedures Allowed
1	99214	Office/outpatient visit, est.	$6,031,239,662	68,634,223
2	99213	Office/outpatient visit, est.	5,910,130,389	101,500,558
3	99232	Subsequent hospital care	3,241,808,414	51,027,887
4	66984	Cataract surg w/iol, 1 stage	2,072,478,375	3,097,585
5	99233	Subsequent hospital care	1,885,333,732	20,565,712
6	99285	Emergency dept visit	1,311,734,269	8,078,818
7	88305	Tissue exam by pathologist	1,174,412,562	17,898,126
8	78465	Heart image (3d), multiple	1,097,124,917	3,093,308
9	99244	Office consultation	1,082,579,794	6,141,563
10	99215	Office/outpatient visit, est.	1,017,088,079	8,473,021

Vignette
Brief case study.

Intuitive
Perceived to be true without any particular reasoning process.

compares to the consistent complexity associated with E/M code selection. This complexity is an enormous factor in creating ethical dilemmas for providers and their staff.

WHY E/M CODES ARE IMPORTANT

E/M Code Purpose. E/M codes are important for accurately reporting and billing services to third-party payers. E/M services are delivered by providers in virtually every specialty and in every health care setting. Therefore, every provider's office in the United States must be familiar with these codes and capable of correctly determining and assigning E/M codes.

Prior to 1992, E/M codes by definition did not exist. Previous editions of the CPT code book incorporated all of the office visit and hospital visit codes within 4 pages. In 1992, it took 44 pages to incorporate all of the codes classified as E/M, along with the detailed instructions for code selection. In today's CPT manual, the E/M section remains lengthy and detailed. Appendix C now exists to provide clinical **vignettes** to help coders in selecting the correct code by comparing the situation they are coding with other similar situations.

Perceived effort and time were the two factors that determined code selection prior to 1992 (Cohen, 2002). This was quite acceptable to most providers because of its relative ease to understand and use. However, research at the time revealed that code selection was highly inconsistent with wide variations existing among providers. In fact, when presented with the same clinical vignette, providers from rural areas would usually select a lower code than a provider in a more urban area.

It was the ease and associated inconsistency of code selection prior to 1992 that was actually its downfall. Code selection was relatively arbitrary and "**intuitive**" because there were no specific guidelines or instructions for code selection that were universally recognized. A more scientific approach was needed, particularly for government payers that were attempting to better define the services being delivered and better control runaway health care spending.

The scientific approach selected was the resource-based relative value scale (RBRVS). RBRVS was created over a number of years by Harvard-based researchers who surveyed providers around the nation and carefully calculated the elements that contribute to the delivery of health care services. The vast majority of CPT codes were studied and assigned a "relative value." Services were compared relative to each other, with the primary intent being to more fairly recognize the contribution of cognitive and counseling services to the entirety of health care delivery to each patient. One of the stated purposes of RBRVS was to increase reimbursement for primary care physicians—general practitioners, internists, and so on. Prior to RBRVS, reimbursement was heavily weighted toward compensation for procedures. Primary care physicians frequently complained that they were underpaid compared to their specialist counterparts, because primary care physicians do not perform many procedures or surgeries. Many question whether RBRVS has been successful in this objective because studies show that primary care providers still make substantially less than specialist providers (Grogan, 2011).

Billing for E/M codes is overwhelmingly the largest source of revenue for most primary care providers. While they may be responsible for a lower portion of the specialist's revenue, it is not insignificant for any provider. In addition, correct selection of E/M codes can have a dramatic impact on the practice's financial health—either by inappropriately **undercoding** or by inappropriately **overcoding.** Therefore, a clear understanding of the component elements used to select codes is critically important.

E/M Code Structure.   E/M codes are organized into categories, subcategories, and levels of service. Table 5.2 illustrates the organization of these codes.

Simply based on code structure, the coder cannot be successful in assigning correct codes unless he or she is completely aware of these three factors:

1. The location in which the service was delivered.
2. The status of the patient in relationship to the practice.
3. The nature of the care provided to the patient.

In addition to these fundamentals, the coder must also evaluate a broad range of intraservice factors to select the appropriate code level.

Many frequently asked questions regarding E/M code selection are answered in the CPT instructions provided at the beginning of each section and category. In some cases, code-specific instruction appears in the CPT code book. Careful study of the book and familiarity with the basic fundamentals of E/M code selection are critical in effective and efficient coding.

FACTORS INVOLVED IN SELECTING E/M CODE LEVELS

Seven factors are involved in selecting an E/M code level. They fall within one of three categories: key components, contributing components, and reference factors, as shown in Table 5.3.

History, exam, and medical decision making are the key components that drive code selection. With limited exception, all three of these elements must be present to properly bill for an E/M service. Counseling and coordination of care are frequently significant parts of a face-to-face E/M service, but are not required to be provided at each encounter to bill for an E/M code. The nature of the presenting problem is not a part of the service that can be delivered, but definitely has an impact on the service. Either the presenting problem can be extremely simple and straightforward or it can be highly complex. The nature of that problem will directly affect the level of history, exam, and medical decision making performed during that E/M encounter.

Time is not a primary factor to be used in determining a level of E/M service. This is perhaps the most common misconception about E/M coding, which has its roots in the pre-RBRVS period when there was little but time that differentiated one level of service from another. The issue of time can be one of the major ethical issues associated with E/M coding, which is discussed at greater length beginning on page 157.

Undercoding
Selecting an E/M code that is below the level documented in the medical record.

Overcoding
Selecting an E/M code that is above the level documented in the medical record.

CODING TIP

To select a correct E/M code, the correct location, correct patient status, and nature of the care provided must be documented.

WARNING

Too many providers select E/M codes based on time, when the necessary requirements for using time are not being met.

Table 5.2 Summary of Various E/M Coding Categories

Category	Subcategory	Levels of Service
Office and Other Outpatient Services (99201–99215)	New Patient	5
	Established Patient	5
Hospital Observation Services (99217–99226)	Observation Discharge	1
	Initial Observation Care	3
	Subsequent Observation Care	3
Hospital Inpatient Services (99221–99239)	Initial	3
	Subsequent Hospital Care	5
Consultations (99241–99255)	Office or Outpatient	5
	Inpatient	5
Emergency Department Services (99281–99288)		6
Critical Care Services (99291–99292)		2
Nursing Facility Services (99304–99318)	Initial	3
	Subsequent	4
	Discharge Services	2
	Other Services	1
Domiciliary, Rest Home, or Custodial Care Services (99324–99340)	New Patient	5
	Established Patient	4
	Oversight Services	2
Home Services (99341–99350)	New Patient	5
	Established Patient	5
Prolonged Services (99354–99360)	Direct Contact	4
	Without Contact	2
	Standby Services	1
Case Management Services (99363–99380)	Anticoagulant Management	2
	Medical Team Conference	3
	Care Plan Oversight	6
Preventive Medicine Services (99381–99397)	New Patient	7
	Established Patient	7
Counseling/Risk Factor Reduction (99401–99429)	Preventive Medicine, Individual	4
	Behavior Change, Individual	4
	Group Counseling	2
	Other Services	2
Non-Face-to-Face Services (99441–99444)	Telephone	3
	Online	1
Special E/M Services (99450–99456)	Life/Disability Eval.	1
	Work/Disability Eval.	2
Newborn Care Services (99460–99465)	Basic Newborn Care	4
	Delivery/Birthing Room Services	2
Inpatient Pediatrics and Neonatal Care (99466–99480)	Pediatric Critical Care During Transport	2
	Inpatient Pediatric and Neonatal Critical Care	6
	Inpatient Intensive Care Services	4
Other E/M Services (99499)		1

Table 5.3 The Key Components, Contributing Components, and the Reference Factor Used in Selecting E/M Codes

Key Components	Contributing Components	Reference Factor
History	Counseling	Time
Exam	Coordination of care	
Medical decision making	Nature of the presenting problem	

DEFINING E/M CODE LEVELS: CPT VERSUS MEDICARE

E/M code levels, as defined in the CPT code book, are relatively intuitive in concept but can be open to widely varying interpretation when attempting to define the specific elements. Table 5.4 illustrates the requirements for code selection for a new patient E/M office/outpatient visit.

This would seem to be a fairly easy decision, until you have to answer questions such as:

- What it is the difference between a problem-focused and an expanded problem–focused exam?
- When does medical decision making move from being low to moderate?
- How much history is required to be comprehensive versus detailed?

The problem becomes even more challenging when examining inpatient hospital services. Since there are only three levels of service from which to select, broader ranges of service must be incorporated in each level. Table 5.5 illustrates this issue. Especially in the case of

Table 5.4 CPT Requirements to Be Met or Exceeded for Office or Outpatient Visits—New Patient

Outpatient	History	Exam	Medical Decision Making	Typical Face-to-Face Time
99201	Problem-focused	Problem-focused	Straightforward	10 min.
99202	Expanded problem–focused	Expanded problem–focused	Straightforward	20 min.
99203	Detailed	Detailed	Low	30 min.
99204	Comprehensive	Comprehensive	Moderate	45 min.
99205	Comprehensive	Comprehensive	High	60 min.

Table 5.5 CPT Requirements to Be Met or Exceeded for Inpatient Visits—New Patient

Initial Inpatient	History	Exam	Medical Decision Making	Typical Time
99221	Detailed/Comprehensive	Detailed/Comprehensive	Straightforward/Low	30 min.
99222	Comprehensive	Comprehensive	Moderate	50 min.
99223	Comprehensive	Comprehensive	High	70 min.

Table 5.6 Medicare Documentation Guideline Requirements to Be Met or Exceeded for Office or Outpatient Visits—New Patient

New Patient	99201	99202	99203	99204	99205
History					
Chief Complaint	Required	Required	Required	Required	Required
History of Present Illness	1–3 elements	1–3 elements	4+ elements	4+ elements	4+ elements
Review of Systems	N/A	Pertinent	2–9 systems	10–14 systems	10–14 systems
Past, Family, Social History	N/A	N/A	1 of 3 elements	3 of 3 elements	3 of 3 elements
Physical Examination					
1997	1–5 elements	6–11 elements	12 or > elements	Comprehensive	Comprehensive
1995	System of complaint	2–4 systems	5–7 systems	8 or > systems	8 or > systems
Medical Decision Making					
	Straightforward	Straightforward	Low	Moderate	High
Time					
Face-to-face	10 min.	20 min.	30 min.	45 min.	60 min.

Documentation Guidelines (DG)
A document created by CMS to provide direction as to the documentation requirements necessary for the use of a particular E/M code.

initial inpatient visits, medical decision making is the driving factor in determining the code level because the levels of history and exam are fundamentally the same. However, how do you determine the difference between low and moderate decision making?

To address the issue of medical decision making, Medicare established **Documentation Guidelines (DG).** The purpose of the guidelines was, in part, to remove the variability of interpretation and to establish more quantifiable criteria in making code selections. To that end, Medicare established specific guidelines for each element of code selection, as illustrated in Table 5.6.

The Medicare Documentation Guidelines added a degree of clarity by specifically defining the requirements needed to bill a given level of service. However, they also added a significant level of complexity to the coding and auditing process. Many complained that it would take longer to code for a service than it would take to actually deliver the service, because of all the factors that had to be considered when selecting a code. Others complained that the complexity of the process would only create a disincentive for providers to try to code correctly because it was just "too hard." Therefore, providers would just go back to their default mode for code selection—time.

Since the Medicare Documentation Guidelines were introduced, most providers have adapted their practice and have made a good-faith effort to select the correct codes for the services they provide. Most of the "doomsday" predictions made in the early 1990s about inaccuracy in code selection did not come to pass. On the other hand, this does not mean that there are not significant opportunities for ethical dilemmas related to E/M code selection.

1. What do you believe are the possible reasons that cognitive services are not reimbursed as highly as procedural services?

2. Do you agree with the assertion that the selection of E/M codes is more difficult than selecting procedural codes? Why or why not?

3. Which do you believe occurs more frequently—undercoding or overcoding? On what do you base your belief?

5.2 Elements of History Documentation and the Occurrence of Ethical Problems in Relationship to History

A medical history is the relevant facts concerning the patient's past medical conditions and treatment. Within the context of medical coding, four elements are involved in the history, of which three are differing types of history. A history is not necessarily a *complete* history and, in fact, it would be exceptionally rare for a history to be complete for the patient's entire life or to cover every symptom the patient has historically experienced. However, the level of history is an important facet of choosing an appropriate E/M code level.

CHIEF COMPLAINT

To bill for an E/M service, except for preventive medicine or counseling services, a provider must document a **chief complaint.** The chief complaint is a brief summary that describes *why* the patient presents for treatment during that encounter. In most cases, the complaint is documented in terms used by the patient and involves a description of symptoms or problems the patient may be experiencing. If it is a chronic condition, the patient may be familiar with the definitive diagnosis. If it is new problem, he or she may not know the cause of the symptoms—the patient just knows that something is not right and attention is required.

This seems to be a straightforward issue—why did the patient schedule an appointment to visit the provider that day? However, even an issue that is this basic can be the source of ethical dilemmas. The following example demonstrates this issue.

Chief complaint
A brief summary that describes *why* the patient presents for treatment during that encounter.

WARNING

Many medical records for E/M services do not specifically state a meaningful chief complaint. This is a minimal standard that must be met.

Example

Jane Clark presented on December 21, 2011, for her annual well-woman exam. She stated that the reason for her visit was to have a Pap smear and complete well-woman exam. During the review of systems (ROS) portion of the visit, she mentioned that she had occasional headaches, which she attributed to stress. The physician made some lifestyle recommendations regarding stress relief, but no further medical intervention or treatment occurred for this issue.

Jane's insurer denied the claim because they pay for one well-woman exam each year. Jane forgot that she had a well-woman exam on January 14, 2011. However, the insurance company representative told Jane that the service would be covered if the doctor used a "problem" visit code. Jane called the provider's billing office and asked that the codes on the claim be changed to indicate that she had the visit due to her headaches.

In this case, the provider's decision seems fairly simple—the medical record clearly indicated that she scheduled the appointment for a well-woman exam. She had a Pap smear, pelvic exam, and counseling generally associated with a well-woman exam. Yet, in a situation this straightforward, the provider is still faced with the ethical decision about changing the chief complaint—the reason the patient was seen—for the purpose of obtaining insurance benefits for the service on behalf of the patient. The provider must decide which is more important: accurately reporting the nature of the service (in this case, through the chief complaint) or keeping a long-time patient satisfied?

HISTORY OF PRESENT ILLNESS

History of present illness (HPI)
A chronological description of the development of the patient's present illness from the first sign and/or symptom to the present.

Chronological
Time-based; usually presented in order from first to last.

Quantified
Defined; concretely measured.

The CPT manual defines the **history of present illness (HPI)** as a **chronological** description of the development of the patient's present illness from the first sign and/or symptom to the present (American Medical Association [AMA], 2010). The HPI is **quantified** in the following terms:

- Location
- Quality
- Severity
- Timing
- Context
- Modifying factors
- Associated signs and symptoms affecting the present problem

The recording of the HPI is illustrated as follows for a 63-year-old man brought to a hospital emergency department:

Example

Patient complains of chest pain (location), which began 45 minutes ago (duration). Pain has been continuous since that time with several periodic episodes of more intense pain, lasting two to three minutes each (timing). The pain is described as "crushing" (quality) and at times is rated as a 10 on a scale of 1 to 10 (severity). The pain occurs with or without exertion (context) and is associated with shortness of breath (associated signs and symptoms). The pain was somewhat relieved with sublingual nitroglycerin in the ambulance (modifying factors).

Ethical dilemmas can exist, even in the reporting of the HPI, in two primary areas. First, Medicare rules are very explicit that the provider must participate in the recording or documentation of the HPI for the patient. The review of systems (ROS) and past, family, and/or social history (PFSH) may be recorded by ancillary personnel and acknowledged by the provider. However, this is not an option for the recording of the chief complaint or HPI (CMS, 1999). Therefore, even if the chief complaint or HPI is properly recorded in the medical record, it is not proper if the provider does not record this information.

COMPLIANCE TIP

Compliance programs must ensure that the history of present illness (HPI) is recorded by the provider *and* all *relevant* history is included in the medical record.

Example

Dr. Smith works within the ambulatory care department of an academic medical center. It is her practice to have the medical students actively participate in the care of the patients by having the student take the history of the patient, including the history of present illness, review of systems, and past, family, and/or social history. Dr. Smith then reviews the student's notes and initials them.

Arlene, who is a coder in the university's billing office, is assigned the task of coding Dr. Smith's E/M services. After reviewing the chart, she notes that the physician did not participate in the recording of the HPI. According to her training, the HPI recorded by a student cannot be credited when calculating the E/M service level. Arlene talks to her supervisor about this problem, showing her the documentation. The supervisor advises Arlene that the fundamental information is there and, therefore, "don't stir things up." Arlene is quite uncomfortable with this advice.

The second area of opportunity for ethical dilemmas in the documentation of the HPI is the temptation to electively ignore certain elements of the HPI because inclusion of that information could result in the denial of payment by the patient's insurer due to specific policy exclusions. In this situation, the provider and coder must face the challenge of determining what is relevant to the care of the patient without providing an unnecessarily long, and potentially irrelevant, medical history.

Example

Dr. Elliott, a reproductive endocrinologist, sees a couple who have concerns about infertility. He records the HPI as follows:

The patient, a 34-year-old G2P2, complains of secondary infertility (chief complaint). They have had unprotected intercourse for two years (duration). She reports that both fallopian tubes are blocked (location). She describes periodic dyspareunia with sharp, stabbing pain (quality) which is rated as a 7 on a scale of 1 to 10 (severity). The pain occurs more frequently before her period (context). The husband's semen analysis is normal and he has a child from a previous relationship (context).

Dr. Elliott's note would qualify as an extended HPI, as at least five different elements are noted. However, key information regarding this patient is missing from the HPI because it does not report that the fallopian tube blockage is the result of an elective sterilization (tubal ligation) that was done five years ago while the patient was in a previous marriage. The patient's insurer specifically excludes any infertility treatment that follows an elective sterilization.

If Dr. Elliott's coder reviewed the records from the patient's previous physician and noted the elective sterilization, he or she would have an ethical dilemma because the HPI excluded pertinent information. The physician's intent was to enable the patient to have coverage for the treatment they desired, but to which they are not contractually entitled.

In summary, ethical dilemmas can exist in relationship to the HPI based on two questions:

1. Who did the recording of the information in the medical record?
2. Is *all* pertinent information included in the HPI?

REVIEW OF SYSTEMS

Review of systems (ROS)
An inventory of body systems obtained through a series of questions, seeking to identify signs and/or symptoms that the patient may be experiencing or has experienced.

In addition to the chief complaint and history of present illness, the third major component of "history" required to fulfill the CPT and Medicare Documentation Guidelines for E/M code assignment is **review of systems (ROS).** CPT defines the review of systems as "An inventory of body systems obtained through a series of questions, seeking to identify signs and/or symptoms that the patient may be experiencing or has experienced" (AMA, 2009). In essence, the purpose of reviewing systems is to help the provider better understand the patient's condition, gain insight into the potential causes of the condition, and/or discover clues about the patient's health that may or may not be directly related to the patient's present chief complaint (Tables 5.7 and 5.8).

For the lower levels of E/M office/outpatient services an ROS is not necessary. For the higher levels, however, a rather thorough ROS is required. The CPT book defines the systems that are to be considered for review. The Medicare Documentation Guidelines specify how many of these systems must be evaluated to qualify for a given level of service.

Table 5.7 Medicare Documentation Guideline Requirements to Be Met or Exceeded for the Review of Systems Component of Office or Outpatient Visits—New Patient

New Patient	99201	99202	99203	99204	99205
History					
Review of Systems	N/A	Pertinent	2–9 systems	10–14 systems	10–14 systems

Table 5.8 Medicare Documentation Guideline Requirements to Be Met or Exceeded for the Review of Systems Component of Office or Outpatient Visits—Established Patient

Established Patient	99211	99212	99213	99214	99215
History					
Review of Systems	N/A	N/A	Pertinent	2–9 systems	10–14 systems

The 14 systems available for consideration are:

- Constitutional
- Eyes
- Ear, nose, throat, mouth
- Cardiovascular
- Respiratory
- Gastrointestinal
- Genitourinary
- Musculoskeletal
- Integumentary (skin and/or breasts)
- Neurological
- Psychiatric
- Endocrine
- Hematologic/lymphatic
- Allergic/immunologic

CODING TIP

A major problem with the review of systems is that it is too easy to say, "All other systems negative" and thereby take credit for a complete ROS when it was not necessary for the treatment of the patient's condition.

The ROS element can be captured in a number of ways:

- The patient can complete a written or online questionnaire that addresses the possible symptoms that may exist in connection with each of the systems. The provider can then review the questionnaire and expand on any specific issues that the patient notes.
- A member of the provider's staff, such as a nurse or medical assistant, can review the systems with the patient, making note of any relevant findings.
- The provider can personally review the systems with the patient.

Most medical practices elect either option 1 or 2 to make best use of the provider's time. This is completely acceptable, according to the Medicare Documentation Guidelines, provided that there is a notation by the provider confirming or supplementing the information recorded by the patient or staff member (CMS, 2010b).

When counting systems to establish an ROS level, it is acceptable to include those systems specifically noted, as well as all other systems if the provider notes "all other systems negative." At this point, ethical dilemmas can arise because by using this standard, it is very easy to provide a "complete" ROS for every patient. The question then becomes, "Was a complete review of systems necessary to provide appropriate treatment to the patient?"

FYI

The patient and/or the provider's medical staff can complete forms that serve as the documentation for the ROS and PFSH.

Example

Peter, a 13-year-old boy, had visited Dr. McGregor in August for his annual "back-to-school" physical. Dr. McGregor billed 99394 for the exam, as well as for a number of vaccines, including tetanus (90718). In mid-September, Peter sustained a 3-cm laceration on his arm. His mother brought him to Dr. McGregor to determine if stitches were necessary to close the wound. The physician determined that the laceration was not deep and did not require stitches. The wound was closed with Steri-Strips and Peter was given instructions regarding care of the wound.

Dr. McGregor, when calculating the level for the E/M visit associated with this service, took credit for a comprehensive review of systems. He did this because he referred to the comprehensive ROS that was done the previous month in the history section of his note for this service.

While the physician in this case study was technically correct in referencing a previous ROS, the ethical dilemma remains: Was a complete review of systems required and/or necessary for the appropriate assessment and treatment of this minor arm laceration? Was the fact that Peter had no gastrointestinal symptoms relevant to the care that was delivered? Was the physician's medical care better because of the notation of the comprehensive review of systems than it was if he had not noted the comprehensive ROS?

PAST, FAMILY, AND/OR SOCIAL HISTORY

Past, family, and/or social history (PFSH)
The recording of components of the patient's past used in helping the physician diagnose and properly treat the patient.

Relevant components of the patient's past can be very important in helping the physician diagnose and properly treat the patient. In coding terminology, these three components are called the **past, family, and/or social history (PFSH)**. The patient's history could be very extensive and relevant or it may be noncontributory to the patient's current health status or condition. Either way, the physician will generally obtain some sort of history to properly evaluate the patient (Tables 5.9 and 5.10).

Past History.   The past history can include a number of specific items from the patient's distant past, including prior major illnesses and injuries, prior operations, and prior hospitalizations. It also can include current issues such as medications, allergies, and immunization status, as well as the specific cause that is prompting the current encounter.

The issue of third-party payers and preexisting conditions can create significant ethical problems for providers in relationship to reporting all relevant historical information. The provider may not be aware of the ethical issue if the patient is not forthcoming with a complete history. However, the provider can be directly involved in an ethical issue if the patient requests that the provider not record information that was reported.

Table 5.9 Medicare Documentation Guideline Requirements to Be Met or Exceeded for the Past, Family, and/or Social History Component of Office or Outpatient Visits—New Patient

New Patient	99201	99202	99203	99204	99205
Past, Family, Social History	N/A	N/A	1 of 3 elements	3 of 3 elements	3 of 3 elements

Table 5.10 Medicare Documentation Guideline Requirements to Be Met or Exceeded for the Past, Family, and/or Social History Component of Office or Outpatient Visits—Established Patient

Established Patient	99211	99212	99213	99214	99215
Past, Family, Social History	N/A	N/A	N/A	1 of 3 elements	2 of 3 elements

Example

Frank Elmont, a 53-year-old male, desired to get additional life insurance. As part of the underwriting process, Mr. Elmont had to have a physical exam to check on his general health status. Two years previously, he was told by another physician that his blood glucose levels were high and that he should seek further treatment from an endocrinologist. However, he did not do so.

The provider performing the insurance exam asked Mr. Elmont about his past health status. The patient mentioned his previous high-glucose test to the provider. When the provider began to ask more questions about the tests to determine its significance, the patient realized that mention of the possible diabetes could result in denial of coverage or significantly higher premiums. He asked the provider, "Could you just not write that down?"

Family History. The importance of family history is directly related to the risk or susceptibility of a patient to contract a particular illness or disease. This is becoming increasingly important as greater understanding of genetic processes provide the ability to identify and quantify a patient's risk for experiencing a disease in the future.

As noted previously, one of the elements in calculating the appropriate level of history is counting how many different types of history are obtained. Ethical dilemmas related to the patient's history occur when history elements are recorded that are not particularly relevant to the patient's care, strictly for the purpose of upgrading the level of coding. This is complicated by the fact that history that is unnecessary in one case is absolutely essential in another. Consider the following two examples:

Example

1. Dr. McGregor, the physician treating Peter, the 13-year-old boy with the laceration, included information about his family history that reflected that his grandfather passed away from lung cancer and that his aunt has a history of mental illness. Was this family history relevant to Peter's laceration?

2. Dr. McGregor reported that several of Peter's family members, including two siblings, have a serious blood clotting disorder. Could this family history be relevant to Peter's laceration?

In one case, the recording of information related to the family history was critical in the treatment process—in the other case, it was completely irrelevant. In both cases, the documentation of the family history alone would support the billing of a 99214 service. However, the ethics and integrity of doing so in the case where it was not relevant to the treatment is certainly questionable.

> **COMPLIANCE TIP**
>
> The critical element of the PFSH is, "Is it relevant to the patient's current condition?"

Social History. The purpose of the social history is to reflect age-appropriate information that can impact treatment and the decision-making process supporting that treatment. This includes items such as:

- Marital status and/or living arrangements.
- Current employment.
- Occupational history.

- Use of drugs, alcohol, and tobacco.
- Level of education.
- Sexual history.
- Other relevant social factors.

Recording the social history can be completely irrelevant to the care of the patient, or it may be highly relevant. The following case illustrates the importance of social history:

Example

Marjorie Ellis, a 63-year-old female, presented to Dr. Mixon's office with complaints of severe fatigue and depression. The social history portion of Dr. Mixon's notes stated:

SH: Patient was recently widowed (18 months ago). The factory at which she worked was recently closed and she was laid off from her job. She reports that she is under extreme financial stress.

The physician in this case could not have made an appropriate diagnosis without this relevant social history information.

Summary of History for E/M Services.   When calculating the level of history taken for a given E/M encounter, it is vital to note that to select a given level of service, *all three criteria for that level must be met or exceeded.* Therefore, it may be tempting for the provider to document an additional element of the history to facilitate the billing of a higher level of service than he or she might otherwise be entitled (Table 5.11).

Example

Dr. McGregor's history for his patient Peter is documented as follows:

HPI: Peter reports that he ran into a chain-link fence about two hours ago, resulting in a laceration on his right arm, just above his wrist. Initially there was heavy bleeding (as reported by the patient), but pressure on the wound stopped the bleeding in less than five minutes. Patient reports moderate pain associated with the injury. Patient's mother provided him with acetaminophen before deciding to bring him to the office for evaluation.

ROS: Integumentary: Simple 3-cm laceration on lower part of patient's right arm. No loss of consciousness during collision with fence. All other systems negative.

PFSH: Peter sustained a 5-cm cut on his foot last year while fishing. Tetanus vaccine was provided at that time. Grandfather has stage 4 lung cancer.

Table 5.11 CPT Categorization of the Requirements for Each Level of History

Type	HPI	ROS	PFSH
Problem-focused	Brief (1–3)	None	None
Expanded problem–focused	Brief (1–3)	Problem pertinent	None
Detailed	Extended (4+)	Extended (2–9)	Pertinent (1 of 3)
Comprehensive	Extended (4+)	Complete (10+)	Complete (2 of 3 or 3 of 3)

Table 5.12 Elements Documented by Dr. McGregor in the First Case of Peter

Type	HPI	ROS	PFSH
Problem-focused	Brief (1–3)	None	None
Expanded problem–focused	Brief (1–3)	Problem pertinent	None
Detailed	Extended (4+)	Extended (2–9)	Pertinent (1 of 3)
Comprehensive	Extended (4+)	Complete (10+)	Complete (2 of 3 or 3 of 3)

Based on the example provided, Peter received a comprehensive history because more than four items were reported in connection with the HPI, all systems were reviewed in the ROS, and two of the three (past and family) history elements were described (PFSH). However, which of these were truly significant in the patient's treatment (Table 5.12)?

Example

HPI: Peter reports that he ran into a chain-link fence about two hours ago, resulting in a laceration on his right arm, just above his wrist. Initially, there was heavy bleeding (as reported by the patient), but pressure on the wound stopped the bleeding in less than five minutes. Patient reports moderate pain associated with the injury. Patient's mother provided him with acetaminophen before deciding to bring him to the office for evaluation.

ROS: Integumentary: Simple 3-cm laceration on lower part of patient's right arm. No loss of consciousness during collision with fence. ~~All other systems negative.~~

PFSH: Peter sustained a 5-cm cut on his foot last year while fishing. Tetanus vaccine was provided at that time. ~~Grandfather has stage 4 lung cancer.~~

If the two struck-out lines are removed from the history, the decision-making chart now looks as shown in Table 5.13.

The type of history that can be billed is, at best, detailed, which could reduce the level of E/M service that is billable for this encounter.

E/M coding is not strictly an exercise in counting elements in a history. It involves both counting and evaluation of significance. Throughout the instructional materials of the E/M section of the CPT

Table 5.13 Elements Documented by Dr. McGregor in the Second Case of Peter

Type	HPI	ROS	PFSH
Problem-focused	Brief (1–3)	None	None
Expanded problem–focused	Brief (1–3)	Problem Pertinent	None
Detailed	Extended (4+)	Extended (2–9)	Pertinent (1 of 3)
Comprehensive	Extended (4+)	Complete (10+)	Complete (2 of 3 or 3 of 3)

code book, the word *significant* appears in multiple locations. For example:

- HPI: "... signs and symptoms significantly related to the presenting problem(s)."
- Past History: "A review ... that includes significant information about...."
- Social History: "An age-appropriate review ... that includes significant information ..." (AMA, 2010).

Provider participation in the selection of E/M codes is critical because the provider is the person in the best position to determine significance. A skilled coder may be able to surmise the provider's thought process, based on the context of the information provided. However, given that the provider is ultimately responsible for the codes selected and is the only person who legitimately knows what he or she was thinking, it is incumbent on the provider to both understand the coding process and to actively participate in code selection—particularly E/M codes.

Thinking It Through 5.2

1. Why is it incorrect to state, "As much history as possible should be documented for all E/M services provided"?

2. Which of the four elements of the patient's history is most frequently associated with unethical practices? On what do you base your opinion?

3. To select a given level of E/M service, all four elements for that level must be met or exceeded. Does this create potential ethical challenges? Why or why not?

5.3 Examination Documentation Guidelines and the Opportunity for Ethical Problems

Providers often claim that understanding the rules and guidelines associated with the examination portion of the E/M service documentation are the most complex and difficult to grasp. This can't be denied because Medicare has produced two different sets of guidelines for the examination (1995 guidelines and 1997 guidelines). These guidelines differ significantly from each other and are not easily explained, particularly when considering the comprehensive exam under the 1997 guidelines. This difficulty in understanding and interpreting exam guidelines creates the opportunity for ethical challenges in selecting exam levels—some of them unintentional or occurring out of ignorance.

1995 EXAMINATION GUIDELINES

Since the creation of the E/M codes in 1992, four types of examinations have existed: problem-focused, expanded problem–focused,

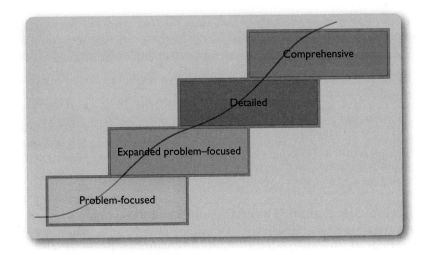

FIGURE 5.2
The problem with defining the level of exam was that initially, there was not a clear distinction as to the difference between the various levels. Instead of clear steps between one level and the next, the definitions were more blurred and ill-defined.

detailed, and comprehensive (Figure 5.2). The difficulty with this terminology was that there was significant disagreement over the placement of the line between the various types of exam. What constituted an expanded problem–focused exam? How was it different than a problem-focused exam? What did you have to do to have a "detailed" exam?

In an attempt to clarify the definitions, the Health Care Financing Administration (HCFA—now CMS) issued the *1995 Examination Documentation Guidelines.* This supplied providers with very clear-cut rules as to what constituted each type of exam.

The 1995 guidelines featured "organ systems" or "body areas." The organ systems that were "counted" in the guidelines were as follows:

COMPLIANCE TIP

Both the 1995 and 1997 Documentation Guidelines are acceptable for use for Medicare and most third-party payers. Providers can use whichever one provides them the greatest advantage.

Organ Systems

- Constitutional
- Eyes
- Ear, nose, throat, mouth
- Cardiovascular
- Respiratory
- Gastrointestinal
- Genitourinary
- Musculoskeletal
- Skin
- Neurological
- Psychiatric
- Hematologic/lymphatic/immunologic

Body Areas

- Head (including face)
- Neck
- Chest (breasts)
- Abdomen
- Genitalia/groin
- Back (including spine)
- Each extremity

Table 5.14 1995 Examination Requirements from the Medicare Documentation Guidelines

Type of Exam	1995 Requirements
Problem-focused	1 body area or organ system
Expanded problem–focused	2–4 organ systems (including affected area)
Detailed	5–7 organ systems (including affected area)
Comprehensive	8 or more organ systems

If a provider examined a certain number of these organ systems or body areas, it was counted as an element of the exam. The different types of exams were classified as shown in Table 5.14.

This was fairly straightforward, easy to comprehend, and easy to calculate. The problem with this guideline is that it did not recognize the work involved in the detailed single-organ-system exams often performed by specialists. For example, the 1995 guidelines essentially did not give ophthalmologists the opportunity to bill for anything above a "problem-focused" exam because the eyes were defined as only one organ system, regardless of how detailed the exam, how expensive and specialized the equipment required to perform the exam, and so on.

For the provider in 1995, the temptation was to do one of two things:

1. Very briefly examine parts of the body that were not relevant to the patient's chief complaint.
2. Count the individual portions of the single-system exam and report that as the number of organ systems, to "pump up" the examination level.

Both of these options are ethically challenged because the first option challenges the principle of examining only things that were "significant" and the second option was specifically prohibited in the 1995 Documentation Guidelines. No opportunity was provided to count a single-organ exam as anything more than "one" organ system.

1997 EXAMINATION GUIDELINES

To address the outcry, primarily from specialist providers and their professional organizations, HCFA issued the *1997 Examination Documentation Guidelines*. These were intended to allow specialists to be recognized for the work they did that was limited to a single-organ system. Therefore, specialists could legitimately perform a comprehensive examination without going through the unnecessary steps of examining organ systems that were not truly relevant to the exam or part of their specialty.

The 1997 guidelines were based on the same organ systems as the 1995 guidelines. The primary difference is that the 1997 guidelines also supplied detailed single-organ-system examinations. Those exams are as follows:

General Multisystem

- Skin
- Eyes

- Ear, nose, throat, mouth
- Cardiovascular
- Respiratory
- Gastrointestinal
- Genitourinary
- Musculoskeletal
- Hematologic/lymphatic/immunologic
- Neurological
- Psychiatric

Each of these exams has numerous components, all much more specific than simply identifying an organ system. For example, the female genitourinary system exam is shown in Table 5.15.

Table 5.15 1997 Examination Requirements from the Medicare Documentation Guidelines for the Female Genitourinary Exam	
System/Body Area	**Elements of Examination**
Constitutional	• Measurement of *any 3 of the 7* vital signs: BP___ (sitting or standing), BP___ (supine), P___, R___, T___, Ht___, Wt___ • General appearance of patient
Neck	• Examination of neck • Examination of thyroid
Respiratory	• Assessment of respiratory efforts • Auscultation of lungs
Cardiovascular	• Auscultation of heart, with notation of abnormal sounds and murmurs • Examination of peripheral vascular system by observation and palpation
Chest (breasts)	(See genitourinary female)
Lymphatic	• Palpation of lymph nodes in neck, axillae, groin and/or other location
Skin	• Inspection and/or palpation of skin and subcutaneous tissues
Neurological/psychiatric	Brief assessment of mental status including: • Orientation • Mood and affect
Gastrointestinal (abdomen)	• Examination of abdomen with notation of masses or tenderness • Examination for presence or absence of hernia • Examination of liver and spleen • Obtain stool sample for occult blood test when indicated
Genitourinary	Includes at least 7 of the following 11 bulleted elements: • Inspection and palpation of breasts • Digital rectal examination including sphincter tone, presence of hemorrhoids, rectal masses Pelvic examination including: • External genitalia • Urethral meatus • Urethra • Bladder • Vagina • Cervix • Uterus • Adnexa/parametria • Anus and perineum

Table 5.16 1997 Examination Requirements from the Medicare Documentation Guidelines

Type of Exam	1997 Requirements
Problem-focused	1–5 elements
Expanded problem–focused	6–11 elements
Detailed	12 or more elements
Comprehensive multisystem	2 elements from at least 9 areas/systems
Comprehensive single system	All elements in the shaded boxes
	At least 1 element in all unshaded boxes

The 1997 guidelines classify the various types of exams ranging from problem-focused to comprehensive single system, as shown in Table 5.16.

The single-system exams provide specialists with more realistic requirements for the completion of a comprehensive exam. In the case of the female genitourinary system, the physician is not required to examine anything from the head and face, eyes, ear, nose, and throat, musculoskeletal system, or the extremities. In the case of the eye single-system comprehensive examination the provider is not required to examine any body system, other than the eyes, and must perform only a general neurological/psychiatric assessment.

For the first three levels of examination, the process is uncomplicated—bullet points are counted, regardless of the category in which they fall. However, when it comes to the comprehensive exam, providers must pay attention to "shaded" and "unshaded" boxes. This distinction introduces complexity and confusion to the process. The added complexity is evidenced by the fact that the 1995 Documentation Guidelines are 15 pages in length. The 1997 guidelines are 53 pages in length, with the majority of the additional content addressing the examination requirements (Centers for Medicare and Medicaid Services [CMS], 2010b).

Example

Dr. Peters, an OB/GYN, sees his established patient, Marilyn, who complains of irregular and painful vaginal bleeding, diffuse abdominal pain, as well as fatigue and depression. During the course of the visit, Dr. Peters performs and documents an examination that includes all of the components of the 1997 exam guidelines, except he does not document the presence or absence of a hernia and he does not document any findings related to the spleen or liver. When calculating the level of E/M service, Dr. Peters assumes credit for a comprehensive female genitourinary exam.

Dr. Peters's coder, while reviewing the record, sees that all of the requirements for the 1997 examination were not met because he did not document all of the required elements of the gastrointestinal system (a shaded box). This contributes to the lowering of the E/M code level for the entire encounter. Dr. Peters and his coder engage in a heated exchange over the particulars of the 1997 Documentation Guidelines. Dr. Peters claims that he did perform the hernia, liver, and spleen exams—he just didn't document it. The coder claims that "if it wasn't documented, it wasn't done." Who is right?

The interpretation of the documentation guidelines provide many opportunities for challenging ethical principles. Is it sufficient to be "close enough" in completing the majority of the requirements for a given level? The guidelines are detailed and complex—can providers take refuge in the claim that they were doing their best and any error was inadvertent? Many providers are dissatisfied with the reimbursement levels paid by many insurers—doesn't the inadvertent overcrediting of a particular area of an exam simply level the playing field?

In this example, there truly is no ethical dilemma and the crediting of a comprehensive exam is appropriate. The reason that it is appropriate is that the exam did meet the standards required for the 1995 comprehensive exam (Dr. Peters examined nine systems—only eight are required). The Medicare rules indicate that the physician can use either the 1995 or 1997 Documentation Guidelines—whichever is most advantageous to them (CMS, 2010b). However, it is not appropriate to bill a comprehensive examination using the 1997 guidelines because the required documentation was not supplied.

Some may argue that the documentation of a hernia or spleen and liver exams, or lack thereof, does not substantially change the nature of the service provided and therefore should not change the billing level. Others would argue that Medicare has provided very specific guidelines that, if studied carefully and fully grasped, can be followed appropriately. The following observations are important related to this matter:

- If an exam element is performed, it makes no sense not to document it. Systems should be established within the practice to make the documentation process easier. In fact, documentation processes can be created that will prompt the physician to perform certain exam elements, which may improve the quality of patient care.

- Given this patient's symptoms, reviewing the spleen and liver and the presence or absence of a hernia is only good medicine. Examining these elements is not simply adding to "the score" for E/M code level calculation—these are legitimate exam components.

- Often, ethical dilemmas can be avoided simply by being fully aware of the coding and documentation rules. The argument between the doctor and the coder over the specifics of the 1997 guidelines was unnecessary because the 1995 guidelines were easily met for a comprehensive examination.

Thinking It Through 5.3

1. Does the fact that providers can choose either the 1995 or 1997 examination guidelines create ethical dilemmas or does it solve them? Explain.

2. If you were an orthopedic surgeon, would you be more likely to use the 1995 or 1997 examination guidelines? Why?

3. In your opinion, what is the biggest ethical challenge associated with selecting an E/M examination level? Why?

5.4 The Role of Medical Decision Making in Code Assignment and Ethical Problems

Medical decision making
The selection of the best possible course of action to treat a particular patient's condition.

Determining the level of **medical decision making** for a given encounter is the least complex element of the process, yet also the one most open to interpretation by the provider. There are four specific levels of medical decision making: (1) straightforward, (2) low, (3) moderate, and (4) high.

Some coders would argue that medical decision making is the element that has the most influence over ultimate code selection because the decision-making process is what drives the medical necessity of obtaining a given level of history or performing a certain level of examination. For example, when selecting codes for E/M in the hospital inpatient or observation setting, the primary differentiation between the three levels of codes is the medical decision-making component (Table 5.17).

In other words, if medical decision making is easy with regard to a case (e.g., a common cold in an otherwise healthy adult with no chronic illnesses or disease), is a comprehensive physical examination required to adequately treat the patient? However, if the same patient presents with several known chronic conditions, a more detailed history related to this episode of care may be required to make the appropriate decision concerning the appropriate treatment.

The American Medical Association (AMA) provides a significant number of clinical vignettes in Appendix C of the Current Procedural Terminology (CPT) book to help providers and coders identify various types of conditions that would meet the criteria for various levels of medical decision making. The key differentiator between these examples is the relative difficulty of the medical decision making, in light of the presenting problem. The intent is that providers would compare their patient's presenting symptoms with those illustrated in the examples provided.

In the Medicare Documentation Guidelines there is no counting of bullet points, although some recommended systems have been established that incorporate counting into the decision-making selection process. The guidelines do break down the process into several components to help establish a level of decision making. Those components are:

- Number of diagnosis/management options.
- Amount and complexity of data that must be considered.

Table 5.17 CPT Guidelines for Code Selection for Initial Inpatient Services

Inpt./Observ./ Same Date Admit & Discharge	History	Exam	Medical Decision Making
Level 1	Detailed/ Comprehensive	Detailed/ Comprehensive	SF/Low
Level 2	Comprehensive	Comprehensive	Moderate
Level 3	Comprehensive	Comprehensive	High

- Risk of:
  - Various management options.
  - Morbidity and mortality to the patient.
  - The presenting problem.

Compared to the potential ethical problems associated with selecting the appropriate levels of history and exam, there are fewer ethical issues associated with choosing the level of medical decision making. The primary ethical challenges associated with medical decision making are correctly identifying the provider's thought process within the medical record (as there does not necessarily have to be a medical decision-making section in the notes) and ensuring that the provider doesn't exaggerate the complexity of the medical decision making to justify a higher coding level. The lack of a specific counting protocol for code selection does introduce an element of variability to the process. On the other hand, selecting a level of medical decision making is the most intuitive of the three primary elements that ultimately contribute to overall code selection.

Thinking It Through 5.4

1. Do you agree that selecting a level of medical decision making is the least complex element of the E/M code selection process? Why or why not?

2. How could the use of clinical vignettes *create* ethical dilemmas if not used properly?

3. Why do you believe bullet points are not used to determine levels of medical decision making? Explain your position.

5.5 Time as the Determining Factor in E/M Code Selection

Many providers like to use the element of time in their code selection process because it is relatively simple, compared to considering the three key components—history, exam, and medical decision making—that are ordinarily required to make a code selection. If a patient is in the room with the provider for 30 minutes, it is easy to go to the chart, identify the code that has a recommended time of 30 minutes, select that code, and move on to the next patient. Unfortunately, this is not an appropriate method of code selection.

According to the *1997 Medicare Documentation Guidelines* (CMS, 2010b):

In the case where counseling and/or coordination of care dominates (more than 50%) of the physician/patient and/or family encounter (face-to-face time in the office or other or outpatient setting, floor/unit time in the hospital or nursing facility), time is considered the key or controlling factor to qualify for a particular level of E/M services. (p. 5)

Therefore, when applying the instructions provided earlier, time can be a factor only when counseling and/or coordination of care *dominates* an encounter (Table 5.18). If counseling does not constitute more than 50% of the encounter, then the use of time in code selection is not an option. In fact, some code categories—such as Preventive

Table 5.18 Average Times for Various E/M Services

Outpatient—New

Codes	99201	99202	99203	99204	99205
Times	10 min.	20 min.	30 min.	45 min.	60 min.

Outpatient—Established

Codes	99211	99212	99213	99214	99215
Times	5 min.	10 min.	15 min.	25 min.	40 min.

Outpatient—Consultations

Codes	99241	99242	99243	99244	99245
Times	15 min.	30 min.	40 min.	60 min.	80 min.

Medicine, Emergency Department, Admission/Discharge from Inpatient or Observation Status on the same day, and Admission to Observation Status/Observation Discharge—explicitly do not supply time as an option in code selection. On the other hand, there are certain code categories in which time is the only factor that can be used in code selection. Examples include 99401–99412 and hospital discharge (99238 for less than 30 minutes and 99239 for more than 30 minutes).

When using time as a tool for code selection, several issues must be considered. The first consideration is the definition of *counseling*. For E/M code selection, *counseling* does not necessarily refer to psychotherapy or any type of mental health service. Rather, *counseling* includes talking with the patient and/or family members about issues such as:

- Test results.
- **Prognosis.**
- Risks and benefits of management options.
- Instructions.
- Compliance issues.
- Risk factor reduction.
- Education.

The use of time as a tool in code selection is designed to compensate providers appropriately for the time involved in supplying cognitive services, such as education regarding illness and disease, treatment options for a patient's condition, and communication regarding the patient's prognosis. If time was not supplied as an option, a provider could be discouraged from providing these services, which have great value in improving the health and well-being of patients.

Although time is a valuable option available to providers, there are specific prohibitions to using time as a factor for code selection. Time cannot be used as a factor in code selection if the visit was extended because the

- History was extensive.
- Patient was a poor historian.
- Physical exam was lengthy.

None of these items meet the definition of *counseling* or *coordination of care* and are instead part of the other elements used in code selection (history, examination, and medical decision making). Simply because the patient

Prognosis
Likelihood of a particular outcome.

WARNING

The fact that an encounter with a patient lasted a specific period of time does not *automatically* mean that the corresponding level of E/M code can be billed. The guidelines for billing using time must be met to bill based solely on time.

had an extensive medical history that required detailed review or the patient was not sure of the important dates in his or her medical history, the physician is not entitled to use time as a tool in code selection.

Ethical dilemmas associated with the use of time in code selection occur when the physician is inclined to calculate the time improperly or overstate the amount of time involved in counseling and care coordination. Sometimes this erroneous calculation occurs as the result of a lack of awareness of guidelines and rules. On other occasions it occurs because of an intentional decision to mislead the third-party payer concerning the intensity of the service provided and thereby receive payment to which the provider is not entitled.

Example

Dr. Elmets's practice is primarily consultative in nature and therefore it is fairly rare that he performs a physical exam in connection with the majority of his patient encounters. He advised his billing staff that he is basing all of his E/M coding decisions on the time spent with the patient. All of Dr. Elmets's charts are prepopulated with the statement, "Counseling and coordination of care constituted more than 50% of today's encounter."

Susan, Dr. Elmets's new billing coordinator, did not feel that this was an appropriate methodology by which to assign codes for E/M services. To investigate her suspicions, she selected a particular day to examine Dr. Elmets's billing pattern. On the day in question, Dr. Elmets's first patient was scheduled for 9:00 A.M. Patients were scheduled to be seen until 12:00 P.M. Following a break for lunch, patients were seen again beginning at 1:00 P.M. and Susan noted that the last patient left that day at 5:15 P.M. Although she did not observe Dr. Elmets all day she assumed that he began seeing patients at the appointed times and stopped seeing patients around noon, as the support staff did not complain about not having their full lunch break.

The next day, Susan reviewed the **superbills** that had been completed for the previous day. The code distribution recorded on the documents is shown in Table 5.19.

Superbill
A tool (often paper) on which the provider marks the services provided and diagnoses associated with the visit.

The billing pattern in the example, on the surface, does not appear to be outrageous as it is not uncommon for many health care providers to see 30 or more patients per day. However, Susan became very

Table 5.19 Summary of Dr. Elmets's Billing Pattern for Services Provided			
E/M CPT Code Billed	# Billed	Standard Time for Code	Cumulative Time per Code
99203	2	30	60
99204	2	45	90
99205	2	60	120
99213	10	15	150
99214	10	25	250
99215	5	40	200
Total	31		870

Compliance and E/M Service Coding

As indicated throughout this chapter, many opportunities exist for ethical dilemmas in relationship to coding for E/M services. The existence of an effective compliance program is a vital element of a provider's long-term success, as it ensures that the provider is:

1. Aware of the dilemmas, both before and after they are a problem.

2. Constantly defining and refining methodologies to address and correct shortcomings that are identified.

3. Protective of its staff members who are committed to doing the "right" or "ethical" thing.

All providers should have a compliance program in place, whether or not they provide and bill for E/M services. However, compliance and E/M are particularly important and require three separate, yet interwoven components: education, documentation, and auditing (Figure 5.3). The parties involved in the process must be educated about what is required for documentation. Then the documentation must be consistently produced. Finally, the documentation must be audited to confirm that it is appropriate and correct. The results of the audit must be communicated back to the parties to ensure that continuous improvement in the process occurs.

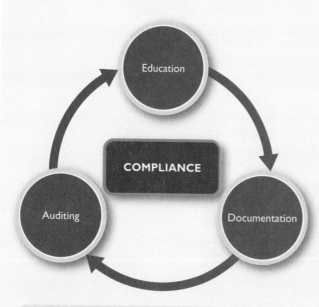

FIGURE 5.3

The three components of an effective compliance program for E/M services: education, documentation, and auditing.

Education

Because of the sheer volume of information to be considered when selecting an E/M code, the compliance program must have a significant education component. An organization can't be in compliance with Medicare and other payer rules if the end users (e.g., physicians, nurses, coders, etc.) are not aware of how E/M codes are properly selected and what elements are included in determining service levels.

Repetitive educational opportunities are essential for all parties involved to be effective in E/M code selection and, in turn, compliance with billing rules and guidelines. These educational opportunities can take a number of forms, including formal classroom education, one-on-one coaching and counseling, informal discussions of coding rules, and case study review. Repetition is essential to cement the concepts in the minds of the learners. Also, case studies are particularly effective because they provide a practical feel to what could be considered an otherwise sterile academic exercise. Case studies also draw in the learner and promote creative thinking around the code selection process.

Documentation

The most important element of ensuring compliance in relationship to E/M coding is complete and accurate documentation. Whereas the documentation of a particular procedure could be fairly brief or very detailed, successful E/M documentation requires detail proportionate to the level of service being reported and billed. A new patient office/outpatient service could be billed as a Level 5 (99205), but the billing could be noncompliant if Level 5 history, examination, and medical decision making are not documented—even if they actually occurred.

Compliant documentation for E/M services does not have to be a long, intensive free-form note dictated by the provider. Extra credit is not available for making the process more difficult or time-consuming than it needs to be. Documentation can be obtained from patient questionnaires, past medical records, and many other sources, provided that they are adequately referenced in the current note. However, providers must be aware of how to effectively document those sources of information in the record for a given service so that it can be appropriately credited for compliance purposes. Various provider-created forms and checklists are also quite acceptable for documentation purposes. Approval of these forms and checklists prior to their usage, as part of the overall compliance program, is critical in ensuring that all the information needed to be compliant is recorded properly.

Auditing

The auditing of the medical record associated with E/M services is the third element critical to a successful compliance program. To be consistently satisfied that the documentation meets the criteria for compliance, the records must be reviewed on a regular basis.

The amount of auditing required for a compliance program varies widely from setting to setting. The past track record of a particular provider's documentation should have an enormous impact on how much or little auditing is required on a continuous basis. Providers who consistently demonstrate high-quality documentation that is consistent with the level of service billed can likely

be placed on a reduced schedule of auditing. Providers that have had problems in the past in relationship to their E/M coding may undergo a more intensive auditing process. The number of encounters reviewed is going to vary based on the type, size, and nature of a specific practice.

There is no "right" or "wrong" amount of auditing that must occur to have an effective compliance program. The minimum standards of auditing should be:

- The sample selected should be done on a random basis.

- The sample should be of sufficient size to be representative of the provider's documentation.

- The results of the audit should be reported to the designated parties responsible for the compliance program and should be reported back to the provider, coder, and any other persons involved in the process.

concerned when she realized that there were only 435 minutes available in that day to see patients (7 hours, 15 minutes of clinic time). How could Dr. Elmets bill, based on time, nearly twice as many minutes as there were available?

The problem becomes worse when you consider that these assumptions do not allow for *any* time between patients—100% efficiency, and there was no social time involved in any patient encounter, which can't be counted when calculating code levels either by time or by meeting key elements (history, exam, and medical decision making). Susan determined that she had a problem with the level of service being billed because the documentation that she had indicated that the services being billed were literally impossible to accomplish in the timeframe observed.

The use of time in selecting codes is not intended as a quick and simple bypass of the more complicated and difficult to understand guidelines for key element selection. Nor is it intended as a panacea for the provider who does not move quickly from patient to patient. It is a tool to be used by physicians when the code calculated by using the key elements is not equitable relative to the quantity of time spent counseling the patient.

Thinking It Through 5.5

1. Do you believe that it is fair that time cannot be used as a factor in selecting an E/M code when the patient's condition causes the examination to take extended time?

2. Explain why compliance programs must have a special focus on E/M services.

3. Explain the factors that may cause a particular provider undergo more intense internal audits than other providers within the same practice do.

5.6 Common Opportunities for Ethical Dilemmas in Billing and Coding for E/M Services

This chapter presented a number of examples of ethical dilemmas associated with E/M coding. These were real-life examples that could occur in a number of settings. However, a number of specific circumstances exist in which E/M coding can be ethically challenging on a regular or routine basis.

BILLING FOR AN E/M SERVICE ON THE SAME DATE AS A PROCEDURE

The CPT manual indicates that all surgical procedure codes include "Subsequent to the decision for surgery, one related Evaluation and Management (E/M) encounter on the date immediately prior to or on the date of procedure" (AMA, 2010). This means that, ordinarily, E/M services provided on the date of a procedure are assumed to be part of the procedure and are not separately billable.

However, the CPT manual also allows for the billing of E/M services on the same day as a procedure by affixing a −25 modifier to the E/M service. This is appropriate when, "the patient's condition required a significant, separately identifiable E/M service above and beyond the other service provided or beyond the usual preoperative and postoperative care associated with the procedure that was performed" (AMA, 2010).

The use of the −25 modifier is somewhat controversial because it has been deemed to be frequently overused. A 2004 Office of Inspector General (OIG) report indicated that in 2002, Medicare paid $1.96 billion for approximately 29 million claims that were submitted with a -25 modifier attached. As part of the study, the OIG analyzed the medical records associated with 431 of these claims and found that the modifier was attached improperly in 35% of the submissions. When extrapolated, this resulted in an overpayment to physicians estimated at $538 million in 2002 alone (Office of Inspector General, 2005).

The most common overuse of this modifier occurs when the medical record does not provide documentation of a service that is significant and separately identifiable from the procedure performed. Many providers automatically attach a −25 modifier to the E/M service because it is often reimbursed by third-party payers without any prospective medical record review. Some justify this additional billing because they believe that the payers do not adequately compensate them for the procedures performed. The additional reimbursement for the E/M service helps "level the playing field."

> **STOP**
>
> **WARNING**
>
> It is not acceptable to simply attach a −25 modifier to an E/M service when performed on the same day as a procedure. Separately identifiable E/M services must be provided and documented to bill using a −25 modifier.

Example

Marie, a 28-year-old established patient of Dr. Marston, was seen with complaints of vulvar pain and swelling occurring over the last three days. She denied discharge, bleeding, urgency, and frequency. Following a brief history and an examination of the affected area, Dr. Marston determined it was a Bartholin's gland abscess and recommended an I&D (incision and drainage) be performed the same day. Marie agreed and Dr. Marston performed the procedure.

In this situation, it is appropriate to bill an E/M service with a -25 modifier, in addition to the procedure, because separately identifiable and significant E/M services were required before Dr. Marston arrived at a definitive diagnosis and made a recommendation for treatment. Now, consider the following similar circumstances.

Example

Marie, a 28-year-old established patient of Dr. Marston, was seen with complaints of vulvar pain and swelling occurring over the last three days. She denied discharge, bleeding, urgency, and frequency. Following a brief history and an examination of the affected area, Dr. Marston determined it was a Bartholin's gland abscess and recommended an I&D be performed the same day. Marie did not want to undergo the procedure at that time. Dr. Marston instead recommended conservative management and scheduled her for a follow-up visit in three days to assess the condition and perform the procedure, if necessary. Dr. Marston billed for an E/M visit for this service.

Three days later, Marie returned and Dr. Marston quickly determined that her condition was not improved. He then performed the I&D. Dr. Marston billed for the procedure and a Level 2 established patient E/M service (attached a -25 modifier to the E/M service).

In the second circumstance, the billing of an E/M service is not appropriate because significant and separately identifiable work was not provided by Dr. Marston at the time of the procedure. As a net result, Dr. Marston overbilled for the services provided. Table 5.20 illustrates the overbilling, revealing that Dr. Marston provided essentially the same service to the patient in both cases, but received additional revenue from inappropriate billing.

Physicians and coders must accurately report services that occur in connection with procedures (particularly those that occur in the physician office setting) with great care because there is a significant ethical risk of overbilling when E/M services are reported with procedures in the absence of documentation of significant and separately identifiable services.

Table 5.20 Various Billing Options Available to Dr. Marston		
Example	**Visit**	**Service Billed**
1	First	9921x–25
		56420
2 (incorrect)	First	9921x
	Second	9921x–25
		56420
2 (correct)	First	9921x
	Second	56420

APPROPRIATELY CLASSIFYING NEW AND ESTABLISHED PATIENTS

E/M services are often classified based on whether the patient is "new" or "established." The CPT manual states, "A new patient is one who has not received any professional services from the physician or another physician of the same specialty who belongs to the same group practice, within the past three years" (AMA, 2010). This can become an ethical issue because of the ways in which medical practices are splitting and merging in today's health care environment.

For example, a physician may leave a group practice to open her own private practice. Some of that physician's patients may follow her to the new practice. It is not uncommon for this physician at the new practice to bill all of her patients as "new" patients, even though she may have seen these patients dozens of times before at the previous group practice.

Some argue that the fact that the patient is seen in a different practice with a different federal tax identification number is sufficient to warrant the billing of a "new" patient service. The argument is further supported by the fact that the new practice has to incur the costs associated with registering the patient, preparing a chart, and, in many cases, receiving transferred records from the previous practice. Many feel this practice is acceptable because of its frequency of occurrence and the low likelihood that payers will recognize the provider as the same physician who saw the patient at the previous practice—although the use of National Provider Identifier (NPI) numbers increases this risk.

The same issue of inappropriate code selection can occur when the opposite situation occurs—a solo practitioner nearing retirement joins another group practice in the same geographic area, with a reduced schedule. The patients of the solo practitioner follow him to the new practice. Because of the reduced schedule, his patients are not able to see him when desired and, as a result, choose to see one of the other physicians in the group practice. The physician in the group practice who sees the patient has never seen the patient before, nor has the patient ever physically been in the building. However, according to CPT guidelines, the patient is an established patient for any one of the physicians in the group because the patient does not meet the definition of a new patient. The guidelines state, "A new patient is one who has not received any professional services from the physician or another physician of the same specialty who belongs to the same group practice, within the past three years." In this case, the physician seeing the patient belongs to same group practice as a physician who has seen the patient within the last three years (the solo practitioner). This means that the patient is, by definition, an established patient.

This is a particularly difficult ethical struggle because it is easy for the staff of the group practice to not recognize this patient as an established patient. In addition, it is even easier for the practice not to be noticed by payers because only a highly sophisticated system would be able to identify the association between the current physician and the previous physician. If the practice is aware of this potential occurrence, but does nothing to address the issue, then a serious ethical dilemma exists.

This can be significant because of the comparative relative value units (RVUs) assigned to E/M codes based on a new versus an established patient. Table 5.21 illustrates the 2011 total nonfacility-based

Table 5.21 Relative Value Units for Outpatient E/M Codes 2011

CPT Code	RVUs	CPT Code	RVUs	CPT Code	RVUs
99201	1.25	99211	.56	99241	1.37
99202	2.16	99212	1.24	99242	2.58
99203	3.13	99213	2.09	99243	3.52
99204	4.80	99214	3.08	99244	5.20
99205	5.95	99215	4.15	99245	6.36

RVUs for each of these commonly used E/M codes. For example, the new practice bills a "medium" code of 99203 instead of 99213; its reimbursement is inappropriately increased by nearly 50%.

Regardless of the justification and/or risk associated with this practice, it is in violation of CPT coding guidelines and may result in an overpayment to the provider because of the higher reimbursement associated with new patient visits versus established patient visits.

INAPPROPRIATE BILLING OF CONSULTATIONS

A **consultation** is a type of E/M service provided by a physician at the request of another physician or other appropriate source to either recommend care for a specific condition or problem *or* to determine whether to accept responsibility for entire care or care of a specific condition or problem. To bill for a consultation, both of these criteria must be met:

- A written or verbal request may be documented by either or both the consulting or requesting physician (or other appropriate source).
- The consultant must supply a written report of findings to the requesting party, which can take the form of:
  - A copy of the consultant's note.
  - A separate letter.
  - An entry in a shared medical record.

A common ethical lapse can occur when a consultation is billed when these criteria are not *both* met. If a consultation is billed when a request is made, but no letter is sent from the consultant to the requesting provider, the billing is inappropriate. Conversely, just because the provider sends a letter to another physician does not constitute a consultation.

Consultations are frequently billed inappropriately because of the additional reimbursement that ordinarily accompanies the billing of this service (Table 5.21). The reason behind the additional reimbursement is the additional time, effort, and work involved in providing consultative services. If a consultation is billed without provision of all the required services, the consultant is being overpaid.

The problem became so prevalent that, in 2010, the Centers for Medicare and Medicaid Services (CMS) eliminated the use of consultation codes (99241–99245; 99251–99255) because they were used improperly so frequently. The reason provided by CMS was that there was a great deal of confusion regarding the use of the codes and improper coding

Consultation
A type of E/M service provided by a physician at the request of another physician or other appropriate source to either recommend care for a specific condition or problem *or* to determine whether to accept responsibility for entire care or care of a specific condition or problem.

FYI

The primary reason that Medicare stopped paying for consultation services was excessive use and abuse of these codes.

resulted in overpayments and excessive resources dedicated to auditing consultation claims (American College of Rheumatology, 2010).

Medicare's elimination of consultation codes does not affect the use of consultation codes for claims submitted to all commercial third-party payers. Therefore, the opportunity for the unethical use of consultation codes still remains. However, if improper consultation coding continues to occur, third-party payers may also join Medicare in eliminating their availability for usage.

Thinking It Through 5.6

1. Do you believe it is fair to providers to presume that any E/M service provided on the same day as a procedure is related to that procedure? Why or why not?

2. Explain the ethical dilemma that occurs when a patient is billed as a new patient when, in fact, he or she is an established patient—especially when the third-party payer does not catch the error and pays the claim as a new patient.

3. What is the primary reason that consultation codes are billed inappropriately? Why do you believe this occurs?

5.7 Summarizing the E/M Coding Process

When selecting a code for a procedure, the process is relatively straightforward. First, the procedure performed must be identified. Next, a determination is made as to whether a code describing the procedure exists—ensuring that the code accurately describes both the procedure and the approach or method used by the provider. Finally, a code is selected and assigned.

The process of code selection for E/M codes is significantly more complex than selecting a procedure because more variable factors are involved. Where did the service take place? What type of service was provided? Was the patient a new or established patient? Was a procedure performed on the same day as the proposed E/M service? Is the E/M service part of a larger procedure and therefore not separately billable (e.g., within a global surgical period)?

Once these questions are answered, then the various elements of the service must be quantified. What was the level of history provided? What was the level of examination provided, and are the 1995 or 1997 guidelines more appropriate for code determination? What type of medical decision making was required for code establishment (Figure 5.4)?

The E/M code selection process is ripe for ethical shortcuts and dilemmas because there are so many "moving parts" in the process. In addition to defining the appropriate classification and place of service criteria, selecting the correct level of service is often misunderstood and abused. For providers and coders to be successful in maintaining ethical standards when using E/M codes, the primary requirement is thorough education regarding the process. Providers face a nearly impossible challenge in correctly selecting E/M codes if they don't understand the criteria and guidelines. Ignorance of the coding rules is

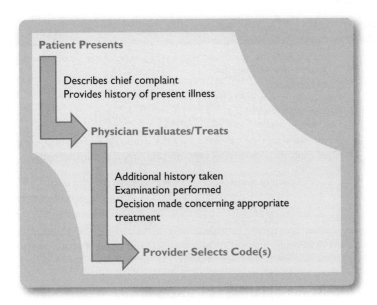

not an appropriate defense for incorrect coding and intentionally disregarding education regarding code usage is, in itself, a possible ethical breach. Coders and providers must choose, in advance, to adhere to the specific coding guidelines that are unique to E/M codes in order to successfully bill for the services in an ethical manner.

CHAPTER REVIEW

Chapter Summary

Learning Outcomes	Key Concepts/Examples

5.1 Explain the factors that contribute to the appropriate selection and assignment of evaluation and management (E/M) codes. Pages 135–141	• E/M codes are used by virtually every health care provider in the United States, across every specialty, to describe services that are not focused on procedures. Instead, they are used to report cognitive services required by doctors to make diagnostic decisions.
	• E/M codes are the most frequently billed codes and were introduced in 1992, in conjunction with the implementation of the resource-based relative value scale (RBRVS).
	• E/M services are divided into categories, subcategories, and levels of service
	• The key components in selecting E/M codes levels are:
	  1. History.
	  2. Exam.
	  3. Medical decision making.
	• Other contributing factors used in determining E/M code levels are:
	  1. Counseling.
	  2. Coordination of care.
	  3. Nature of the presenting problem.
	• Time can be a factor in selecting an E/M code when more than 50% of the encounter is dedicated to the provision of counseling.
	• The CPT guidelines for code selection are far less specific than the Medicare Documentation Guidelines published by CMS.

Learning Outcomes	Key Concepts/Examples
5.2 Distinguish the factors that present ethical challenges in association with obtaining and documenting the history element of E/M services. Pages 141–150	• Four components are associated with the reporting of the history element for E/M documentation. They are: 1. Chief complaint. 2. History of present illness (HPI). 3. Review of systems (ROS). 4. Past, family, and/or social history (PFSH). • The most significant ethical challenge associated with each component is: 1. Chief complaint—accurately capturing the nature or purpose of the encounter. 2. History of present illness—documenting sufficient relevant detail. 3. Review of systems—overstating the number of systems actually reviewed; determining if the review is medically necessary. 4. PFSH—including only elements that are relevant.
5.3 Differentiate between the 1995 and 1997 Documentation Guidelines as they affect the calculation of the physical examination component of E/M services, along with the ethical ramifications of using each option. Pages 150–155	• The 1995 Documentation Guidelines were based on number of body/organ systems examined. They were most conducive to primary care physicians and were not suitable for specialists. • The 1997 Documentation Guidelines were more appropriate for specialist services by creating defined single-organ-system examinations. This allowed specialists to bill for comprehensive examinations. • The most significant ethical issue regarding the examination is overstating the number of systems examined and/or examining systems that are not pertinent to the patient's condition to bill a higher level of service.

5.4 Explain the factors that contribute to determining a level of medical decision making and the ethical difficulties that are present in the process. Pages 156–157	• Determining the level of medical decision making for a given encounter is the least complex element of the process, yet is also the one most open to interpretation by the provider.
	• There are four possible levels of medical decision making:
	1. Straightforward
	2. Low
	3. Moderate
	4. High
	• The components used to calculate the decision-making level are:
	1. Number of diagnosis or management options.
	2. Amount and complexity of data that must be considered.
	3. Risk of:
	  • Morbidity and mortality to the patient.
	  • The presenting problem.
	  • The various management options.
	• The ethical challenge of medical decision making is accurately assessing the components that contribute to the decision and not overstating the level.

5.5 Define the circumstances in which time can be used as the primary factor in calculating E/M services and list occasions in which ethical problems may occur. Pages 157–161	• In the case where counseling and/or coordination of care dominates (more than 50%) of the physician–patient and/or family encounter (face-to-face time in the office or other or outpatient setting, floor/unit time in the hospital or nursing facility), time is considered the key or controlling factor to qualify for a particular level of E/M services. • Ethical problems may occur when time is used, regardless of whether counseling actually dominated the encounter. • Counseling encompasses discussing: 1. Test results. 2. Prognosis. 3. Risks and benefits of management options. 4. Instructions. 5. Compliance issues. 6. Risk factor reduction. 7. Education.
5.6 Report the most frequent occasions in which ethical lapses may occur in association with E/M service billing. Pages 162–166	• The most common incidents of ethical lapses in conjunction with E/M service billings are: 1. Billing for an E/M service on the same date as a procedure. 2. Inappropriately classifying new and established patients. 3. Inappropriately billing consultations.

Learning Outcomes	Key Concepts/Examples
5.7 Evaluate the ethical problems that can arise during the E/M code selection process. Page 166–167	• The process of properly selecting an E/M code is more complex than selecting a correct procedure code because the following questions must be asked and answered: 　1. Where did the service take place? 　2. What type of service was provided? 　3. Was the patient a new or established patient? 　4. Was a procedure performed on the same day as the proposed E/M service? 　5. Is the E/M service part of a larger procedure and therefore not separately billable (e.g., within a global surgical period)? • Once these questions are answered, the various elements of the service must be quantified and then a code selected.

End-of-Chapter Questions

Multiple Choice

Circle the letter that best completes the statement or answers the question.

1. **LO 5.1** E/M codes can be best described as all of the following *except*

    a. Codes used most commonly

    b. Codes that are most/best understood

    c. Codes that are the most likely source of ethical problems

    d. Codes used in any/all service settings

2. **LO 5.1** When presented with the same vignettes, providers from which areas selected lower E/M code levels?

    a. Urban areas.

    b. Rural areas.

    c. Suburban areas.

    d. There was no significant variance between providers from different areas.

3. **LO 5.1** Which of the following is a *category* of E/M codes?

    a. Office and outpatient services

    b. New patient

    c. Level 3

    d. Discharge services

4. **LO 5.1** Which key component has 1995 and 1997 versions that can be used in the selection of E/M code levels?

    a. History

    b. Exam

    c. Medical decision making

    d. All three

5. **LO 5.2** A history of present illness (HPI) is a _____ description of the development of a patient's illness.

    a. Detailed

    b. Comprehensive

    c. Chronological

    d. Technical

6. **LO 5.2** Which of the following *must* be recorded by the provider?

    a. History of present illness
    b. Review of systems
    c. Past, family, and/or social history (PFSH)
    d. All of the above

7. **LO 5.2** Which of the following is *not* an acceptable way to collect the information for the review of systems?

    a. Written or online questionnaire completed by the patient
    b. Collected by the provider's staff (e.g., nurse, medical assistant, etc.)
    c. Collected directly by the provider
    d. All are acceptable

8. **LO 5.2** When recording information related to the patient's history, it is most important that the information is

    a. Comprehensive
    b. Significant
    c. Brief
    d. Personal

9. **LO 5.3** Which of the following is true about the 1995 examination guidelines?

    a. They are generally preferred and used by specialist physicians.
    b. They are generally preferred and used by primary care physicians.
    c. It is more difficult to document a comprehensive exam using the 1995 guidelines than the 1997 guidelines.
    d. There are specialty-specific exams provided as part of the guidelines.

10. **LO 5.3** Which of the following statements is true regarding the 1995 and 1997 examination guidelines?

    a. Providers must choose one set of guidelines and apply it to all patients in their practice.
    b. Medicare has indicated that the 1995 guidelines can be used as a reference, but all providers are audited according to the 1997 guidelines.
    c. Providers may apply either 1995 or the 1997 guidelines and it can vary from patient to patient.
    d. The 1995 guidelines are considered by most to be more complex than the 1997 guidelines.

11. **LO 5.4** The clinical vignettes that assist coders in selecting levels of medical decision making can be found in the CPT manual in

    a. Appendix A
    b. Appendix B
    c. Appendix C
    d. Appendix M

12. **LO 5.4** Which of the following is *not* a factor in determining the level of medical decision making?

    a. Number of diagnosis or management options
    b. Length of time required to determine a diagnosis
    c. Amount or complexity of data that must be considered
    d. Risk to the patient (morbidity/mortality, various management options)

13. **LO 5.5** The purpose of allowing time as a factor in selecting E/M codes is to

    a. Compensate physicians when the patient takes a long time to provide his or her history
    b. Compensate physicians for the time involved when counseling dominates the encounter
    c. Compensate physicians who work with patients that are not fluent in the physician's language
    d. Simplify the process of code selection

14. **LO 5.6** To bill for an E/M service on the same day as a procedure, all of the following may occur *except*

    a. A -25 modifier must be added to the E/M code.

    b. A significant, separately identifiable service must be provided and documented.

    c. Decision making regarding the need to perform the procedure is necessary.

    d. Basic education regarding the procedure is provided.

15. **LO 5.6** Which of the following is an acceptable circumstance for a patient to be classified as a new patient for billing purposes?

    a. The patient is being seen after having not been seen by anyone in the practice for more than three years.

    b. The patient's regular physician leaves a group practice and sees another physician in the same group, whom he or she has not seen previously.

    c. The patient follows the physician who leaves one group and moves to another practice.

    d. The patient sees another physician of the same specialty within the same group because the regular physician is on a leave of absence.

Short Answer

Use your critical thinking skills to answer the following questions.

1. **LO 5.1** Why are E/M codes more difficult to select correctly than procedure codes?

2. **LO 5.1** Discuss the various ways in which using the CPT guidelines for E/M code selection can be challenging.

3. **LO 5.2** Certain elements of the history must be recorded by the provider. List the elements that must be recorded by the provider and describe the possible reasons these elements must be recorded by the provider.

4. **LO 5.2** Discuss the possible ethical ramifications of stating "all other systems negative" on a review of systems, regardless of the patient's condition.

5. **LO 5.3** Discuss the pros and cons of using the 1995 versus the 1997 Documentation Guidelines.

6. **LO 5.4** Explain why you believe there are not bullet points or elements to count in the Documentation Guidelines when assigning a level of medical decision making.

7. **LO 5.5** List the various categories of E/M codes for which time is not an option when selecting codes. Why is time not a factor for these codes?

8. **LO 5.6** What are the factors that determine whether or not an E/M code can be billed on the same day as a procedure? How should these be documented in the medical record?

9. **LO 5.6** Outline Medicare's reasoning for discontinuing the use of consultation codes for reimbursement. Do you agree with the decision? Why or why not? As a payer, how would you address the problem related to consultations that caused the elimination of these codes?

Applying Your Knowledge

At the beginning of this chapter you were introduced to Allison Magnuson, who just received a great opportunity to become a clinic administrator. Although she was not an expert coder, she had received training in management and research processes and felt that she had the skill set necessary to solve the problem with which she was presented by a member of her office's billing department.

   Allison knows that making assumptions and jumping to conclusions is not the appropriate way to investigate and, if necessary, address a problem. If she acted solely on the information she was presented, Allison may have a brief career at the Franklin Avenue Clinic. While the information she received was certainly disturbing, there was a significant amount of important information that was missing. Some of the missing information included:

1. Does the documentation support the level of service reflected on the chart she was presented?

2. Is this pattern of billing for E/M services unique to this physician or is it consistent throughout the practice?

3. Are there contributing factors that might explain the billing pattern demonstrated?

4. Has there been any change in the billing patterns compared to a similar period in the past?

5. What is the process at this clinic for E/M code selection? What is the process, if any, for auditing E/M service billing?

These questions must be investigated and answered as the first stage of the process—long before any conclusions can be reached. To determine how you might proceed in this process, consider the following questions:

1. What role might a practice's culture play in the investigative process for Allison? Why would culture have an impact and what type of impact might it have?

2. Outline, in order, the steps that Allison should take to look into this matter. What data should she gather and to whom should she speak during each step?

3. If the investigation shows that incorrect E/M coding exists, what are some possible reasons this could be occurring? Would the reason it is occurring affect the manner or steps that you choose to correct the problem? Why?

4. If the practice is not very large, there may not be a compliance officer (or Allison may be the compliance officer). What can Allison do to address the issues she finds while controlling the risk she may experience if the results anger her new employer?

5. If it is learned that incorrect coding is taking place, what should Allison do to prepare for the future to address or avoid this problem?

6. What are some options that Allison has available in communicating her findings to the providers who may be coding incorrectly?

Internet Research

Since its introduction in 1992, RBRVS has become the standard in determining provider reimbursement in the United States. Initially a complex and mysterious formula, availability of RBRVS data on the Internet has increased the understanding of providers and coders. RBRVS tables assist providers in calculating their reimbursement from Medicare and from third-party payers that adapted the RBRVS methodology, and provide a tool for calculating costs and establishing fees.

The Centers for Medicare and Medicaid Services (CMS) publishes the full RBRVS database several times each year on the CMS website (www.cms.hhs.gov). The tables, which are published using Excel spreadsheets, can be downloaded and manipulated for the particular needs of the provider (Figure 5.5). They are massive because they include every CPT code and are not particularly user-friendly. Many publishers, including specialty medical societies, publish redacted versions of the RBRVS database. These smaller versions include only the codes relevant to providers in a particular specialty or codes in a particular section. The advantage of the CMS website publication is that it is free of cost.

Three components comprise the RVU:

- Work RVU.

- Practice Expense RVU.

- Malpractice RVU.

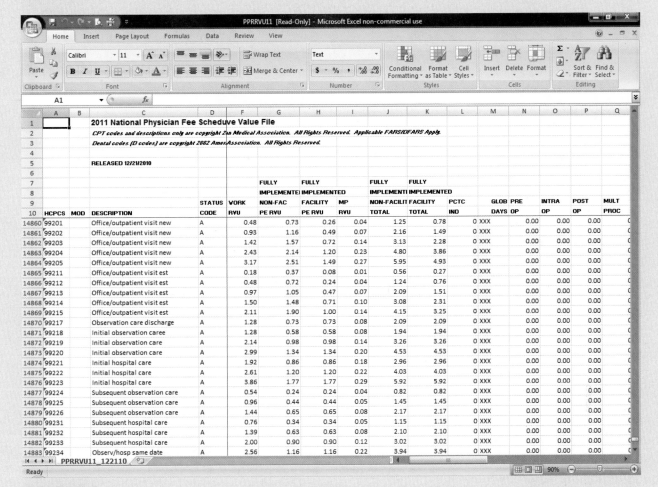

FIGURE 5.5

This portion of an Excel spreadsheet illustrates the relative value units (RVUs) assigned to the office and outpatient-based E/M codes. The spreadsheet can be downloaded from the Medicare section of the Health and Human Services website (www.cms.gov).

Each of the three components is added together to arrive at the total RVUs. The allocation varies by CPT code, but on average, Work RVUs represent 55% of the total, Practice Expense, 42%, and Malpractice, 3%. The amount that a provider receives in reimbursement for each CPT code is calculated by multiplying the RVUs by the conversion factor—a dollar amount determined each year. Adjustments are made using the Geographic Practice Cost Indices (GPCI), which are multiplied with the individual RVU components to recognize the differences (both higher and lower) in the economics of different areas of the country.

1. Locate the latest RVU table from the Medicare website. Find CPT code 99213 in the Excel spreadsheet and report the total Fully Implemented Non-Facility Total RVU for that code.

2. Why do you believe there are two different columns for practice expense (facility and nonfacility)? When there is a difference between the two columns, which is higher? Why?

3. Examine the other columns in the table. Which information do you believe would be most helpful to a coder? Why?

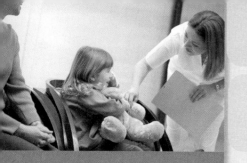

6

Coding Ethics for Surgical and Procedural Services

LEARNING OUTCOMES

After completing this chapter, you will be able to:

6.1   Detail the components that are ethically billed in conjunction with global surgical procedure codes.

6.2   Ethically apply the principles of bundling and unbundling to surgical CPT codes.

6.3   List the modifiers used to facilitate ethical billing for services that are normally bundled with another procedure.

6.4   Explain the ethical risk of improper code selection and the incorrect usage of "unlisted" procedure codes.

6.5   Evaluate the circumstances in which the separate billing of supplies is and is not ethical.

CASE STUDY

Margaret performs all of the billing services for Dr. Smitkins, a general surgeon. The majority of Dr. Smitkins's services are provided in the operating room setting, but he also has office hours, during which consultative services and surgical postoperative are provided. Margaret is responsible for billing all of Dr. Smitkins's services, based on operative reports and office charge tickets supplied by the physician.

Margaret begins to notice that the frequency of office-based evaluation and management (E/M) services for established patients increased in the recent past. At the same time, the number of postoperative visits (CPT code 99024), which are usually billed as a $0.00 charge, has decreased. Margaret is particularly concerned, given that the total number of surgical procedures performed has increased approximately 15% compared to the same period in the previous year.

In an attempt to understand the changes in the billing pattern, Margaret looks at the billing records for the patients who had surgical procedures and compares to them to the patients' medical records. Margaret cannot find any substantive difference in the way in which services were provided and billed for patients who had major surgical procedures. However, she does note that CPT code 99024 (no charge postoperative visit) is rarely used in conjunction with patients who had "minor" surgical procedures, such as diagnostic laparoscopies (CPT code 49320) and percutaneous needle biopsies (CPT code 49180). Instead of seeing the patient one week following the procedure, Dr. Smitkins saw the patient 12 to 14 days following the procedure and billed an E/M service.

Pursuing the matter further, Margaret checks the medical records for these postoperative visits and compares them to the notes for similar postoperative visits for the same surgical procedure in the previous year. Although not a physician, Margaret's 20 years of medical coding experience lead her to believe that there is not a substantive difference in the services that were provided, even though there was a difference in the CPT code billed for the postoperative services, and a difference in the reimbursement collected by the practice for these services.

1. Is there a problem with Dr. Smitkins's billing pattern? If so, is it a problem with usage of E/M codes or is it a problem with procedure code usage?

2. After Margaret discusses the matter with Dr. Smitkins, he indicates to her that it is acceptable for him to bill for E/M services that occur outside the global surgical period. Is he correct? How should Margaret respond?

Introduction

Compared to code selection for E/M services, the selection of procedural service codes is significantly less complex. However, this does not mean that care is not required when selecting these codes, or that there is not significant opportunity for ethical dilemmas in association with billing for procedures. For procedure codes, the opportunity for dilemmas exists more in the application of specific coding rules associated with using the codes than with the actual code selection process.

6.1 Services Included in the Global Surgical Package

The Surgery section of the CPT code book is by far the largest in the book, with 5,566 codes in 2011. It is divided into 15 chapters, based on organ system. They are organized as shown in Table 6.1.

Although the organ systems described are vastly different and the individual procedures are even more varied and unique, the CPT manual has provided some general direction that is applicable to any of these codes. The remainder of this chapter will focus on coding issues that are consistent throughout this portion of the CPT book. After the fundamentals of coding from this section are reviewed, the possible ethical issues specific to surgical codes will be explored in detail.

THE CPT DEFINITION OF THE GLOBAL SURGICAL PACKAGE

Even though the services are, by their nature, variable, CPT codes that represent a surgical procedure include a consistent set of services. Services that are "included" are as follows:

- The operation (procedure) itself.
- Local infiltration, metacarpal/digital block, and/or topical anesthesia.

Table 6.1 Chapters of the Surgery Section of the CPT Code Book

Chapter	CPT Codes
Integumentary (Skin)	10021–19499
Musculoskeletal	20005–29999
Respiratory	30000–32999
Cardiovascular	33010–37799
Hemic and Lymphatic	38100–38999
Mediastinum and Diaphragm	39000–39599
Digestive	40490–49999
Urinary	50010–53899
Male Genital System	54000–55899
Female Genital System	56405–58999
Maternity Care and Delivery	59000–59899
Endocrine System	60000–60699
Nervous System	61000–64999
Eye and Ocular Adnexa	65091–68899
Auditory System	69000–69990

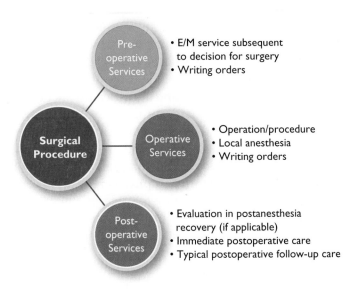

• E/M service subsequent to decision for surgery
• Writing orders

Pre-operative Services

Surgical Procedure

Operative Services

• Operation/procedure
• Local anesthesia
• Writing orders

Post-operative Services

• Evaluation in postanesthesia recovery (if applicable)
• Immediate postoperative care
• Typical postoperative follow-up care

FIGURE 6.1

Various components are included as part of a standard global surgical procedure. Any CPT code that has a global period includes the preoperative, intraoperative, and postoperative services.

• One related E/M encounter on the date immediately prior to or on the date of the procedure if the decision for surgery was previously made (includes H&P [history and physical]).

• Writing orders.

• Evaluation in the postanesthesia recovery area.

• Supplies and materials usually used as part of the procedure.

• Immediate postoperative care, including dictating operative notes and talking with family and physicians.

• Typical postoperative care.

The concept of **global procedure** coding is illustrated by Figure 6.1. Note that procedural coding spans a variety of services, from preoperative services such as E/M consultation to postoperative evaluation and follow-up care.

The opportunity for ethical struggles, as they relate to the billing of global procedures, exists primarily in defining and applying the **preoperative** and **postoperative periods.** The coding process allows for some variability because of the wide variety of procedures that are defined through the process. This variability also allows for some confusion and, for those so inclined, allows the opportunity to circumvent the billing guidelines meant to be followed when billing for a global procedure.

THE PREOPERATIVE PERIOD

The purpose of the global concept is to discourage providers from individually billing extra services that are not medically necessary, simply to generate additional revenue. It standardizes the billing process around the country so that providers receive similar reimbursement (adjusted for local cost of living factors) for similar services. There are occasions in which separately billing services related to the procedure are allowed—but these are intended to be exceptions to the general rule.

The Standard Preoperative Period. The CPT manual states that the global surgical period, in part, includes "One related E/M

CODING TIP

All codes in the Surgery section of the CPT code book include eight separate components, which cannot be billed separately.

Global procedure
The concept that the reimbursement for a particular procedure includes the services before and after the procedure, as well as all of the individual components required to complete the procedure.

Preoperative period
The period prior to a surgical procedure during which any services related to that procedure are provided.

Postoperative period
The period following a surgical procedure during which any services related to that procedure are provided.

encounter *on the date immediately prior to or on the date of the procedure* if decision for surgery previously made (includes H&P)" (italics added) (American Medical Association [AMA], 2010b). The intent of the italicized language is to indicate that the standard preoperative services that are provided every time the procedure is performed are included in the surgical code and are therefore not separately billable. Examples of services that are provided for every procedure are (1) education of the patient about the procedure and obtaining informed consent (including the completion of consent forms), (2) performance of a basic history and physical (H&P) to confirm that the patient is in satisfactory condition to undergo the procedure, and (3) completion of other paperwork and documentation necessary to fulfill the requirements of the facility at which the procedure is being performed.

For the E/M service to be included as part of the global procedure (and not separately billable), three assumptions must exist:

1. The decision for surgery must have been made at some previous time or encounter.
2. The services provided are "routine" and are provided to every patient.
3. All services provided during the encounter are directly linked to the procedure itself.

Some providers avoid the issue of whether or not a service is directly linked to the procedure or if it is separately billable by simply moving the E/M service to a point outside the window defined by the CPT manual.

Example

Dr. Collins ordinarily performs all of her scheduled surgeries on Friday. It is her practice that all of the patients who are having surgery on Friday come in on Thursday to have the standard preoperative services (signing of consents, performance of a basic history and physical, etc.). These services clearly were preoperative services that are part of the global surgery package and therefore were not separately billed.

Dr. Collins attended a meeting at which the issue of underreimbursement for surgical procedures was discussed. One recommended solution for obtaining additional reimbursement was to ensure that the preoperative services occurred more than one day in advance of the surgery. The presenter argued that it was acceptable for providers to do this because they clearly were within the "letter of the law."

Upon return to the office, Dr. Collins instructed her nursing and scheduling staff to have Tuesday mornings dedicated to providing preoperative services to patients who were going to have surgery on Friday. Dr. Collins billed these services as 9921x and saw that she was receiving reimbursement for these services, in addition to the fact that her reimbursement for the procedure was unaffected. Dr. Collins felt that the information received at the conference was well worth the travel expenditure because of the increased reimbursement that she realized.

WARNING

Just because preoperative services are provided more than one day in advance of a surgical procedure does not mean that the services are automatically separately billable.

In the case study featuring Dr. Collins, the conference speaker and Dr. Collins are correct in that they comply with the specific language of the CPT code book. However, this does raise the question as to whether the actions are a violation of the "spirit" of the guidelines. Regardless of whether the surgeon feels that the reimbursement from a payer for a specific CPT code is adequate relative to the services provided, the intent of the code is to include compensation for the basic preoperative services described. In addition, some commercial payers have elected to expand the preoperative period to one week or more before the surgery because of the belief that these guidelines are being abused to obtain additional, undeserved reimbursement. Expanding the preoperative period in effect eliminates the opportunity to have these routine services billed separately—primarily because of the documentation timing requirements instituted by the hospitals and/or facilities at which the services are provided.

Outliers.   In medical coding there are always legitimate exceptions to the rules, called **outliers.** The primary exception to the prohibition against separately billing for preoperative services occurs when significant services that are "over and above" the standard preoperative services are provided.

Outlier
Something that occurs outside the expected or normal range.

Urgent or Emergent Services.   One instance in which outliers occur with relative frequency is when surgery is performed on an **urgent** or **emergent** basis. If the performance of the surgery is delayed by any significant period of time, significant risk to the patient may occur and his or her well-being may be adversely affected.

Urgent
Requiring action or attention in the very near future to prevent permanent physical harm.

Emergent
Requiring immediate action or attention to prevent permanent physical harm.

Example

Ms. Deming is a 22-year-old who presents to the emergency room (ER) with complaints of a severe headache and a brief loss of consciousness. The emergency department physician, Dr. Charles, checks her vital signs, orders a brain CT scan, and immediately calls Dr. Gardiner, a neurosurgeon, to come in and evaluate the patient. Dr. Gardiner reviews the CT results and finds an aneurysm of blood vessel in the brain.

Based on these findings, Dr. Gardiner discusses the various treatment options with the patient, but recommends immediate surgery. Ms. Deming wants to wait until her parents arrive tomorrow from out-of-town to make a decision, but Dr. Gardiner emphasizes the urgent nature of the treatment required. Ms. Deming is taken to the operating room (OR) the same day for surgery to treat the aneurysm.

In the case of Ms. Deming, Dr. Gardiner is entitled to bill for an E/M service because her evaluation of the patient's condition and the decision to perform surgery was far in excess of the standard preoperative services that are provided in connection with this procedure. A modifier must be attached to the E/M service to signify that unusual services were provided at the time, over and above those usually provided. The level of E/M service provided would be determined based on the levels of history, examination, and medical decision making that were performed.

BILLING TIP

To receive payment for a preoperative service on the day of or prior to a surgical procedure, a modifier must be added to support the reason the service was medically necessary.

In situations like that of Ms. Deming, it was never intended that the E/M service provided was part of the global procedure code. Not all aneurysms are necessarily as emergent as the scenario described here and therefore several days could pass between the time the condition is diagnosed and the time that the surgical procedure is performed. In that case, both services would be billed separately and would be separately payable.

Additional Education or Counseling. A separate situation that is not as clear as occasions that are urgent or emergent occurs when additional education or counseling of the patient is required prior to the performance of a surgical procedure. If significant, separately identifiable services are provided, over and above the normal preoperative services, these are not included in the global procedure package and are separately billable.

Example

Mr. Evans visited Dr. Kotler, a general surgeon, because his primary care physician noted some abnormal laboratory values during a recent physical exam. Dr. Kotler reviewed the results and ordered additional tests, the results of which suggested that Mr. Evans had pancreatic cancer. Dr. Kotler felt that the best course of action would be to perform an open wedge biopsy of the pancreas to define more specifically the patient's condition. Dr. Kotler advised Mr. Evans of his medical opinion and his recommended course of treatment. The procedure would be scheduled for one week later.

The day prior to the surgery, Mr. Evans and his wife came to the office for the preoperative examination, the signing of consents for the procedure, and so on. Over the course of the week he had done some research on the Internet and this produced a significant number of questions. In addition, his anxiety level about his potentially serious condition had increased significantly.

Mr. Evans expressed doubt about the need for the procedure, as he had received advice that a more natural or holistic approach could be used to address the condition. Dr. Kotler acknowledged the benefits of certain holistic approaches, but still strongly recommended that Mr. Evans undergo the procedure. The physician documented a total of 50 minutes with the patient, discussing the possible diagnoses, prognoses, and treatment options, in addition to the 15 minutes spent performing the physical exam and obtaining informed consent. Eventually, he convinced Mr. Evans that the biopsy procedure was in his best interest.

Discussion of the risks, benefits, and options associated with a procedure are a fundamental part of the preoperative process, during which consents are signed and education is provided. However, the E/M services provided during the preoperative visit in Mr. Evans's case significantly exceed those routinely provided in conjunction with this procedure. Therefore, it is not part of the global service and is separately billable.

Because of the quantity of time and the fact that the selection of the E/M code was based on time as the controlling factor (see Chapter 5), the decision to bill this service was not difficult. However, circumstances may occur in which the decision is not as easy because

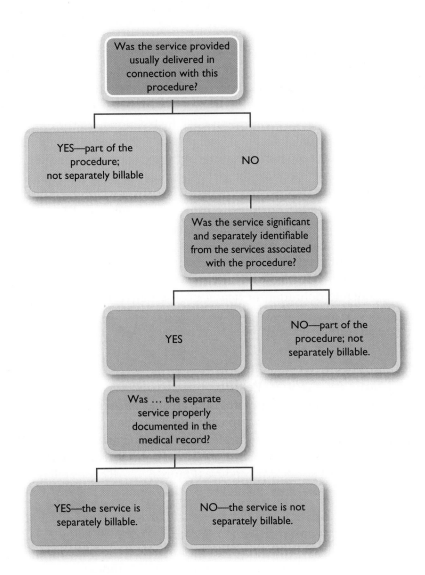

FIGURE 6.2
Some preoperative and postoperative services are separately billable; some are not. This decision tree illustrates the process by which the coder can determine whether a service can be billed.

the additional services required were slightly greater than those normally provided, as opposed to significantly greater.

There is no simple guideline that precisely defines when a preoperative E/M service is separately billable and when it is not. The decision tree in Figure 6.2 can help in the decision-making process.

THE POSTOPERATIVE PERIOD

The CPT manual indicates that "immediate postoperative care" and "typical postoperative follow-up care" are included in the global procedure code. Although not explicitly detailed, most interpret immediate postoperative care to mean services on the same day as the procedure or, in the case of major surgical procedures, the services that are provided until the patient is discharged from the hospital. Typical postoperative follow-up care is generally considered services that are provided after a period of time has passed, usually in an outpatient setting.

The challenge with the definition of "typical postoperative follow-up care" is specifying the definition of "typical." Typical follow-up care following an anterior cruciate ligament repair (CPT code 27407) for one physician may not be typical for another physician who performed the same procedure. One physician may routinely see a patient twice on an outpatient basis following this surgery, whereas another physician may routinely see a patient four times following the surgery. Both are typical for the respective physicians, but the physician who sees the patient for additional visits is not able to bill for these follow-up services, based on CPT instructions for the Surgery section of the manual.

Because of the nonspecific nature of "typical," substantial ethical dilemmas can exist because the provider may be financially encouraged to provide additional postoperative services by claiming that the additional services are not typical. Does the patient need to be routinely seen two times following a minor surgical procedure? Is a physician who does not see a patient following a minor surgical procedure meeting the standard of care for the procedure? To help resolve this issue, the Centers for Medicare and Medicaid Services (CMS) adopted a more concrete definition of *typical* postoperative follow-up care in conjunction with the implementation of the resource-based relative value scale (RBRVS). Many other third-party payers have adopted the same or a similar system.

The Medicare Global Period.   CMS, which is responsible for the operation of the Medicare program, created its own definitions for "typical postoperative follow-up care" because the lack of specificity in the CPT definition made accurate claim tracking and payment difficult. To that end, it assigned a postoperative period to every CPT code that represented a surgical procedure (Figure 6.3). All codes fell within one of three classes—each defined by a time period.

- *0-day postoperative period.* These procedures are generally minor and relatively noninvasive. All services associated with the procedure provided on the day of the procedure are included in the reimbursement for the procedure code. If additional care related to the procedure is required on the next day or any other day, the service is separately billable because it would be considered an outlier. In the ordinary course of events, additional follow-up care associated with the procedure is not necessary.

- *10-day postoperative period.* These are commonly known as "minor" surgical procedures. Examples could include needle biopsies, various types of endoscopy, and certain laparoscopy codes. Any services provided within 10 days following the procedure are presumed to be connected with that procedure and are not separately reimbursable. The Relative Value Update Committee (RUC), which is responsible for making recommendations to CMS concerning the relative values of surgical procedures, builds one postoperative visit into the reimbursement value for all codes with a 10-day postoperative period.

- *90-day postoperative period.* These are commonly considered to be "major" surgical procedures, which require significant recovery time and follow-up care. Virtually any "open" procedure has a 90-day postoperative period, as well as many of the more complex laparoscopic codes. It is assumed that any procedure that has a 90-day postoperative period will require at least two outpatient postoperative visits, which is built into the value of these codes.

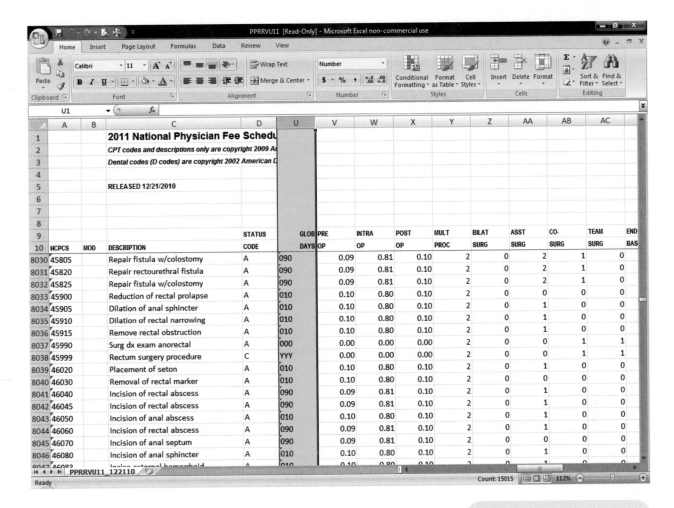

Spreadsheet (Microsoft Excel — PPRRVU11 [Read-Only]):

	HCPCS	MOD	DESCRIPTION	STATUS CODE	GLOB DAYS	PRE OP	INTRA OP	POST OP	MULT PROC	BILAT SURG	ASST SURG	CO-SURG	TEAM SURG	END BAS
8030	45805		Repair fistula w/colostomy	A	090	0.09	0.81	0.10	2	0	2	1	0	
8031	45820		Repair rectourethral fistula	A	090	0.09	0.81	0.10	2	0	2	1	0	
8032	45825		Repair fistula w/colostomy	A	090	0.09	0.81	0.10	2	0	2	1	0	
8033	45900		Reduction of rectal prolapse	A	010	0.10	0.80	0.10	2	0	0	0	0	
8034	45905		Dilation of anal sphincter	A	010	0.10	0.80	0.10	2	0	1	0	0	
8035	45910		Dilation of rectal narrowing	A	010	0.10	0.80	0.10	2	0	1	0	0	
8036	45915		Remove rectal obstruction	A	010	0.10	0.80	0.10	2	0	1	0	0	
8037	45990		Surg dx exam anorectal	A	000	0.00	0.00	0.00	2	0	0	1	1	
8038	45999		Rectum surgery procedure	C	YYY	0.00	0.00	0.00	2	0	0	1	1	
8039	46020		Placement of seton	A	010	0.10	0.80	0.10	2	0	1	0	0	
8040	46030		Removal of rectal marker	A	010	0.10	0.80	0.10	2	0	0	0	0	
8041	46040		Incision of rectal abscess	A	090	0.09	0.81	0.10	2	0	1	0	0	
8042	46045		Incision of rectal abscess	A	090	0.09	0.81	0.10	2	0	1	0	0	
8043	46050		Incision of anal abscess	A	010	0.10	0.80	0.10	2	0	1	0	0	
8044	46060		Incision of rectal abscess	A	090	0.09	0.81	0.10	2	0	1	0	0	
8045	46070		Incision of anal septum	A	090	0.09	0.81	0.10	2	0	0	0	0	
8046	46080		Incision of anal sphincter	A	010	0.10	0.80	0.10	2	0	1	0	0	

Billing for Complications. The services included in the global surgical postoperative period are those that are *normally* provided to the typical patient. Therefore, any surgery that required sutures that subsequently have to be removed would include the removal of those sutures as part of the postoperative services, making suture removal not a separately billable service.

However, even if the service is not typical, it does have to be of sufficient intensity to warrant independent or separate billing. Consider the following scenarios related to the issue of intensity with respect to separate billing:

- Mary underwent a diagnostic laparoscopy (CPT code 49320). She had a postoperative visit one week following the surgery, which was unremarkable. Two days later, she felt a "pulling sensation" near one of her incisions and was concerned. She called the physician office and he advised her to come in to have it checked. The nurse examined it and did not identify any specific problem. The physician briefly looked at the incision and did not find any sign of infection or wound separation. He advised the patient that it was simply part of the healing process and there was no reason for concern.

- Walker underwent a gastric bypass procedure (CPT code 43846). At the follow-up visit 10 days after surgery, the physician noted a slight separation in one of the incision repairs. The physician documented the following: "Soft abdomen with well healing incisions, with the exception of a 1-cm opening at the right apex of his incision, draining clear fluid. Probing the incision with a sterile swab reveals underlying tissue to be intact with approximately 10 cc of clear fluid drainage. This caused another 3–4 cm of the incision to open spontaneously. This was packed with wet to dry gauze, followed by a sterile dressing." Walker was advised to return in one week for a further check and to call sooner if any problems were noted.

- Evelyn underwent the placement of a pacemaker (CPT code 33208). At her follow-up visit one week following surgery, she complained of lightheadedness and a general sense of not feeling well. The physician ordered some blood tests and found that her hemoglobin and hematocrit results were highly abnormal. He suspected that the patient was bleeding internally and had her immediately go to the hospital for monitoring.

Each of these cases reflects a potential complication associated with the surgery. Now, the provider and coder must review the same decision tree that was supplied earlier in this chapter. In light of this decision tree, are any of these services separately billable outside the global postoperative period?

Because different observers can arrive at different results when examining these cases, CMS simplified the decision-making process by eliminating the ability of the provider to bill any services provided to Medicare patients that are related to the procedure in the postoperative period, unless a return to the operating room is necessary. This created a separate and distinct decision tree, as shown in Figure 6.4, for billing for postoperative complications for Medicare patients.

In general, commercial third-party payers will compensate providers for the treatment of complications associated with a procedure, provided that the circumstances are justified. Justification can be demonstrated by completing the decision tree in Figure 6.2 on page 181, which indicates that the service was not typical, was significant, and was properly documented.

On the other hand, Medicare will not pay for a postoperative service unless a return to the operating room is required (Figure 6.4). In the three scenarios provided, the surgeon is not able to bill for any postoperative services described if these patients are covered by Medicare. The only case that could possibly be payable by Medicare would be

> **BILLING TIP**
>
> Postoperative services that occur in the global period cannot be billed to Medicare unless a return to the operating room is necessary to treat the condition.

FIGURE 6.4

The decision tree for determining separately billable postoperative services is simple when the patient is covered by Medicare.

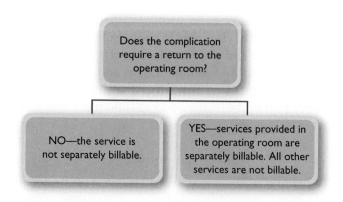

the third case (Evelyn) and that would require that the physician take her to the OR to identify and/or stop her internal bleeding.

BILLING ABUSE WITHIN THE GLOBAL POSTOPERATIVE PERIOD

The case study at the beginning of this chapter provides a prime example of improper billing of services within the postoperative period. Specific actions were being taken to achieve additional billings and additional reimbursement. However, there may be cases in which the ethical ramifications are not as clearly defined, such as the case of Mr. Jameson.

Example

Mr. Jameson underwent a vasectomy (CPT code 55450), which has a 10-day global postoperative period. He was scheduled one week following the procedure (Friday) for a follow-up visit. However, he realized on Thursday that his son's school program was the same time as his appointment. He called the physician office and rescheduled the appointment for Tuesday.

In the case of Mr. Jameson, there was no intent on the part of the physician to provide the service outside the global period. In a strict, literal interpretation of the coding rules, the physician would be able to bill separately for the service provided. However, the service provided on Tuesday was identical to the service that would have been provided on Friday, when the service was originally scheduled. In addition, the procedure includes reimbursement for postoperative services (Figure 6.5). If the physician billed separately for the postoperative services, in effect she would be collecting twice for the same service, as reflected in Figure 6.5.

Application of strict ethical guidelines is required when considering the billing of services done in conjunction with a global surgical procedure—both preoperatively and postoperatively. Following the "letter of the law" will likely result in the receipt of additional payment and has a very low risk of being detected by auditors. However, this is done at the cost of sacrificing ethical principles, by disregarding the intent of the coding guidelines.

WARNING

If a service is being billed primarily to obtain additional revenue, the chances of it being unethical are very high.

Thinking It Through 6.1

1. Do you agree that defining and applying pre- and postoperative periods is the greatest ethical challenge associated with surgical procedure coding? Why or why not?

2. State your opinion of the CPT definition for "global surgical package." Is it adequate or not? If not, how should it be changed to minimize unethical billing?

3. Explain the primary differences between CPT and Medicare rules for billing for postoperative complications. Is there an ethical component associated with the differences? Explain your response.

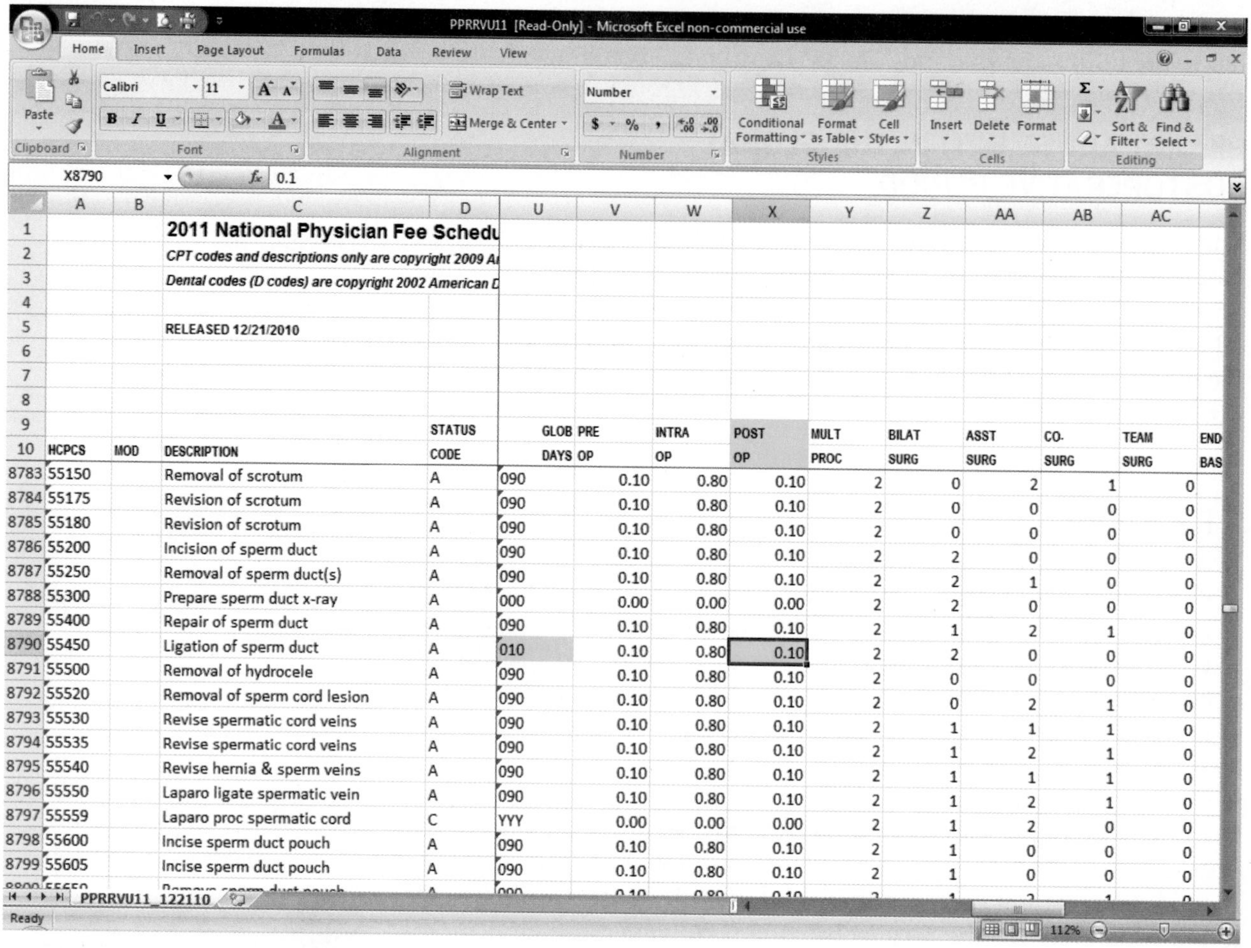

	HCPCS	MOD	DESCRIPTION	STATUS CODE	GLOB DAYS	PRE OP	INTRA OP	POST OP	MULT PROC	BILAT SURG	ASST SURG	CO-SURG	TEAM SURG	END BAS
8783	55150		Removal of scrotum	A	090	0.10	0.80	0.10	2	0	2	1	0	
8784	55175		Revision of scrotum	A	090	0.10	0.80	0.10	2	0	0	0	0	
8785	55180		Revision of scrotum	A	090	0.10	0.80	0.10	2	0	0	0	0	
8786	55200		Incision of sperm duct	A	090	0.10	0.80	0.10	2	2	0	0	0	
8787	55250		Removal of sperm duct(s)	A	090	0.10	0.80	0.10	2	2	1	0	0	
8788	55300		Prepare sperm duct x-ray	A	000	0.00	0.00	0.00	2	2	0	0	0	
8789	55400		Repair of sperm duct	A	090	0.10	0.80	0.10	2	1	2	1	0	
8790	55450		Ligation of sperm duct	A	010	0.10	0.80	0.10	2	2	0	0	0	
8791	55500		Removal of hydrocele	A	090	0.10	0.80	0.10	2	0	0	0	0	
8792	55520		Removal of sperm cord lesion	A	090	0.10	0.80	0.10	2	0	2	1	0	
8793	55530		Revise spermatic cord veins	A	090	0.10	0.80	0.10	2	1	1	1	0	
8794	55535		Revise spermatic cord veins	A	090	0.10	0.80	0.10	2	1	2	1	0	
8795	55540		Revise hernia & sperm veins	A	090	0.10	0.80	0.10	2	1	1	1	0	
8796	55550		Laparo ligate spermatic vein	A	090	0.10	0.80	0.10	2	1	2	1	0	
8797	55559		Laparo proc spermatic cord	C	YYY	0.00	0.00	0.00	2	1	2	0	0	
8798	55600		Incise sperm duct pouch	A	090	0.10	0.80	0.10	2	1	0	0	0	
8799	55605		Incise sperm duct pouch	A	090	0.10	0.80	0.10	2	1	0	0	0	

2011 National Physician Fee Schedu
CPT codes and descriptions only are copyright 2009 A
Dental codes (D codes) are copyright 2002 American D

RELEASED 12/21/2010

FIGURE 6.5

Each CPT code has a defined preop, intraop, and postop valuation. In the case of a vasectomy (CPT code 55450), 10% of the reimbursement for the procedure is allocated to the preoperative services, 80% is allocated to the intraoperative services, and 10% is allocated to the postoperative services. If the global surgical concept is not applicable to a code, all three categories reflect 0.00 as their percentage allocation.

Bundling
Billing for a package of related services, instead of billing for every element provided in the course of a procedure.

Unbundling
The improper practice of billing separately for every service element provided in the course of a procedure.

6.2 Bundling and Unbundling

One of the elements of coding that many providers and coders find confusing is the concept of **bundling**. The principle of bundling is based on the fact that it is not appropriate to bill for every element provided in the course of a procedure. Unlike the specific line-by-line detail that must be supplied in a cooking recipe, accurate coding does not require a line-by-line detail of every service provided in the course of the encounter. There are several ways in which the principle of bundling is applied. Each must be understood to properly report the services provided.

In some cases, the focus of an activity is the individual procedures. The failure to perform even one aspect of the individual procedures will produce an undesirable result. Figure 6.6, which illustrates the relationship of the ingredients to the formation of a pumpkin pie, shows that if one or more of the ingredients is incorrect or missing, the entire pie will be "wrong."

In other cases, such as procedural coding, each individual component is important and those that are necessary to complete the procedure should be provided. However, when the time comes to describe and report the procedure for billing purposes, it is not necessary or appropriate to individually detail each line item or element provided. In fact, doing so would be **unbundling** a bundled procedure. Figure 6.7, which reflects all of the elements provided, demonstrates that

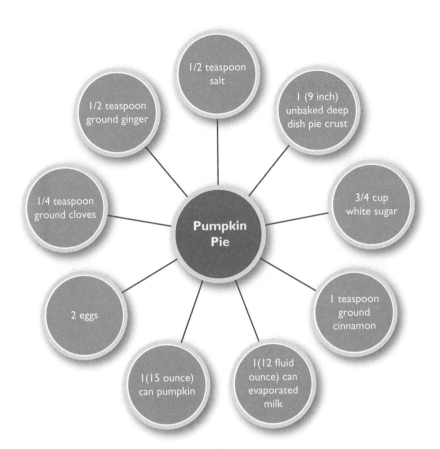

FIGURE 6.6
Examining the ingredients of a pumpkin pie is somewhat similar to looking at the ingredients of a global surgical service. Most people don't think about the individual components of a pie—they think about the end result.

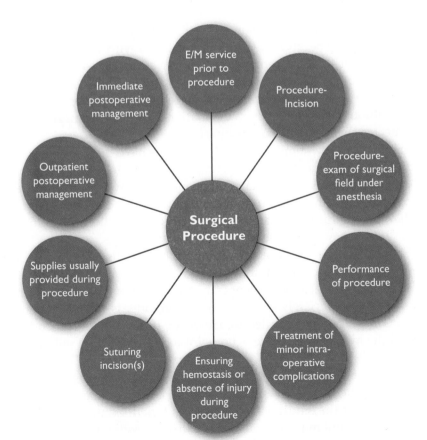

FIGURE 6.7
There are many different parts of a global surgical procedure. All of the parts are provided and necessary, but they are not separately billed.

> ### FYI
>
> Bundling is the principle that not every service associated with a particular surgical procedure should be billed separately.

> ### CODING TIP
>
> Whenever a code is designated as a separate procedure it generally means that it can't be billed separately, unless it is the only procedure performed during the encounter.

the key element is the reporting of the totality of the procedure—not the individual pieces.

SEPARATE PROCEDURE

Throughout the CPT manual there are many codes that have a designation indicating "separate procedure." For example:

- 49000 Exploratory laparotomy, exploratory celiotomy with or without biopsy(s) (separate procedure)
- 49320 Laparoscopy, abdomen, peritoneum, and omentum, diagnostic, with or without collection of specimen(s) by brushing or washing (separate procedure)
- 52000 Cystourethroscopy (separate procedure)
- 58700 Salpingectomy, complete or partial, unilateral or bilateral (separate procedure)

The purpose of this designation is to indicate that these procedures are commonly carried out as an integral part of a larger service or procedure. These occur most commonly with procedures that involve the abdomen or pelvis, where a wide variety of procedures could theoretically occur via the same incision.

The most easily understood circumstance is that of the exploratory (diagnostic) laparotomy or diagnostic laparoscopy. Initially, the provider may begin the procedure not knowing exactly the cause of the patient's symptoms. A diagnostic laparoscopy (CPT code 49320) is scheduled to diagnose the patient's condition. While performing the diagnostic laparoscopy, the provider, for example, discovers a severely inflamed appendix and makes the decision to remove it (CPT code 44970).

Under the principles of bundling, it is inappropriate to bill both 49320 and 44970 because the services associated with 49320 are a component part of 44970. When relative values were assigned to 44970, the work associated with 49320 was calculated as part of the value. This is logical, in that it is improbable that a surgeon would perform a procedure without doing a thorough evaluation of the entire surgical field (in effect, a diagnostic laparoscopy).

While the overwhelming majority of payers have their systems configured to allow the reimbursement of 44970 and to deny 49320, it is possible that some payers may inappropriately pay both procedures. Some providers may adhere to the philosophy that they are going to "bill out everything" and let the payer "decide what they are going to pay." This policy is problematic on a number of levels.

First, the only reason a provider might bill in this fashion is to attempt to collect for services that the provider *knows* are not separately billable. This is ethically challenged because, unless the intent is to return the inappropriately paid money, the provider is receiving money that it knows it is not entitled to. However, if the provider intends to return the money, then there is no point to the individual unbundled billing.

The second problem is that if the individual services are billed separately, the total price of the procedure is going to be higher than it would be if the single bundled code is billed. Some might argue that this does not matter because if the insurer denies the unbundled

Table 6.2 The Potential Difference in Charges in Global Billing Versus Individual Billing

Bundled Accounting		Unbundled Accounting	
Global surgical procedure	$1,000.00	Preoperative service	$ 100.00
		Unbundled intraoperative service	200.00
			800.00
			300.00
		Postoperative service	150.00
Accounts receivable amount	1,000.00	Accounts receivable amount	1,550.00
Allowed by insurer	600.00	Allowed by insurer	600.00
Adjusted receivable	600.00	Adjusted receivable	600.00
Gross vs. adjust receivable		**Gross vs. adjust receivable**	
Variance	**$ 400.00**	**Variance**	**$ 950.00**

service, the provider will simply write off the charges and the net effect to the patient will be the same. Yet, if the patient does not have insurance or the service provided is noncovered, there will not be a writeoff or price adjustment, unless the provider makes a specific effort to do so. If this, in fact, is what is going to be done, then you have to ask the question, "What is the objective of the individual billing?"

The third problem is that the billing of individual services, which likely are not separately payable, will unnecessarily inflate the accounts receivable of the provider. Unless the provider adjusts the accounts receivable at the time of the charge entry, the assets of the practice will be overstated. Table 6.2 illustrates the overstated receivables, which if not properly considered, could cause inappropriate decision making on the part of practice administration.

Finally, if the provider organization is interested in the internal division of work for the proper allocation of the reimbursement to providers, the RBRVS does provide tools by which to assign values to the individual components of a bundled procedure. If one provider in a group supplies the preoperative service and another provider does the procedure itself, and another provider provides the postoperative services, each provider's contribution to the global service can be calculated and distributed, even if only a single global payment is received. Individual line-item billing is not necessary to determine work levels and allocate payments accordingly.

> **BILLING TIP**
>
> Unbundling almost always results in unethical billing, with charges inflated beyond what is appropriate.

PARENT–CHILD CODES

A common **convention** within the CPT code manual is the use of parent–child codes. To save space and be more concise, CPT has grouped codes that have common components and do not repeat all of the code description for each individual code. For example:

Convention
Rule or method of conducting a task.

51725	Simple cystometrogram
51726	Complex cystometrogram;
51727	with urethral pressure profile studies, any technique
51728	with voiding pressure studies, any technique

CODING TIP

Parent–child coding relationships are a feature in the CPT code book, primarily to save space. If codes that appear in this type of relationship are performed at the same encounter, it may or may not be appropriate to bill them separately.

51729   with voiding pressure studies and urethral pressure profile studies

When codes are indented beneath another code, the primary code is assumed to be a part of the indented codes. In this case, it would be inappropriate unbundling to bill 51726 and 51727 together because 51726 is, by definition, included in 51727. The full definition of 51727 would be "Complex cystometrogram; with urethral pressure profile studies, any technique." Similarly, it would be inappropriate to bill 51727 and 51728 individually when performed at the same time because 51729 includes both procedures.

Just because codes are in a parent–child relationship, it does not mean that multiple codes cannot be billed. For example, see the following abbreviated set of codes:

58660   Laparoscopy, surgical; with lysis of adhesions (separate procedure)
58661   with removal of adnexal structures
58662   with fulguration or excision of lesions of the ovary, pelvic viscera, or peritoneal surface by any method
58670   with fulguration of oviducts

For each of these codes, the common language within each code is "Laparoscopy, surgical." In the case of 58660, any language to the right of the semicolon (;) is not part of the primary "shared" code language. Therefore, if a physician removes the fallopian tube(s) (58661) and also removes endometriosis (58662) during the same operative session, they can ethically be billed separately because the CPT coding conventions allow it. Some private payers may establish their own bundling rules that may prevent this type of billing, however.

MULTIPLE PROCEDURE BUNDLING AND UNBUNDLING

To this point, the discussion has focused on the unbundling of the internal components of a single procedure—that is, separating individual procedural elements. Unbundling can also occur when multiple procedures are performed at the same operative session. These procedure may appear to be independent and, therefore, separately billable. However, specific CPT rules and/or specialized payer or Medicare rules may indicate that one procedure is bundled with another and separate billing would be inappropriate and unethical.

Using the previous code set, it is not appropriate to bill both 58660 and 58661 because 58660 has the separate procedure designation. This means that if the physician is removing the fallopian tube(s) (58661), the removal of any adhesions necessary to accomplish the procedure is considered to be a part of the primary procedure. It is inappropriate and unethical to bill these separately. (There are occasions in which adhesion removal is substantial and requires significant time and effort, which may be entitled to additional reimbursement. However, separate billing of each code is not the appropriate manner in which to obtain this reimbursement.)

There are several reasons why it is not ethical to bill multiple procedures performed at the same operative session, even if they are not explicitly bundled by CPT definition. The first reason is that some of the procedures performed are not substantial in light of the totality of the procedures provided. There is a separate code for the lesser procedure, but given the circumstances, it does not justify additional reimbursement.

One example could include the billing of an ovarian cyst drainage (58805) at the same time as a total abdominal hysterectomy (58150), which may or may not include removal of the ovaries. It would generally be unethical to bill for an ovarian cyst drainage that is immediately followed by the removal of the ovary during the same operative session. However, it may also be inappropriate to bill for a minor cyst drainage in this circumstance even if the ovaries are left intact. It may be inappropriate for three reasons:

1. The reimbursement for an ovarian cyst drainage includes the necessary abdominal incision to perform the procedure. In this case, no additional incision is needed because the hysterectomy incision can be used to access the cyst.

2. The amount of work performed in the cyst drainage may not justify a separate billing. An important question to ask is, "Would the cyst have been drained if no other surgical procedure were being performed?" In other words, "Would the cyst or the symptoms it caused have required a separate surgical procedure?" If the answer to this question is no, then it is highly likely that separate billing is not appropriate.

Third-Party Payers and Ethics for Procedure Codes

In the last two decades, many providers and patients have complained that insurance companies and other third-party payers have gained an unfair advantage in their relationship with providers. Although not a monopoly, some payers have dominant market share that makes it difficult, if not impossible, for providers to survive without contracting with the payer as a participating provider.

Unfortunately, because of their relative size and strength, the third-party payer has a disproportionate share of the power in the negotiation process. Providers are, at times, forced to accept terms that they find unacceptable and must live with rules that they perceive are unfair. When complaints are made to payers about these rules, they are sometimes found to be unresponsive or simply refuse to address the complaints of the providers.

A common area in which this occurs is related to bundling and unbundling of multiple procedural services. Although the expanded usage of Correct Coding Initiative (CCI) edits has standardized the process and made payer processing more consistent, some payers still maintain their own set of bundling edits, which are not consistent with the CCI edits or any other recognized coding organization guidelines.

Dozens of lawsuits have been filed against payers in recent years by providers that allege that the payers are engaging in unfair coding and payment processes. Many of the providers have been successful in filing class action lawsuits and there have been multimillion-dollar settlements with providers to compensate them for unfair and unethical practices that resulted in underpaid and improperly paid claims (Physician Advocacy Institute, 2010).

Although the focus of this text is ethical behavior on the part of the provider and coder, equal emphasis should be placed on the conduct of third-party payers in their coding and payment rules and guidelines. Although inappropriate, many providers attempt to justify their unethical behavior toward payers because they feel that they have been treated unfairly or unethically by the payer. If all parties in the process conduct themselves in an ethical manner, the likelihood of ethical behavior increases in a dramatic fashion.

3. Even minor or lesser procedures have a preoperative and postoperative period associated with them. If a major procedure is occurring, it is not appropriate to be compensated for both the global period for the major procedure and the global period for the minor procedures. This is often managed by the use of the −51 modifier and decreased reimbursement for the lesser procedures. However, in some cases the procedures are so minor that independent billing would not be justified.

CORRECT CODING INITIATIVE (CCI) EDITS

Beyond the bundling rules that explicitly exist within the CPT code book through general coding instruction and code-specific guidelines, a major source of bundling information is the **National Correct Coding Initiative (NCCI) edits.** The purpose of the NCCI edits is to create a system that was developed to nationally standardize correct coding methodologies and eliminate improper coding. These edits are based on fundamental principles of CPT coding, current standards of medical and surgical coding practice, input from specialty societies, and analysis of current coding practices (Centers for Medicare and Medicaid Services [CMS], 2006).

Prior to the creation of the CCI edits, there were no universal rules regarding what codes could and could not be billed when performed during the same encounter. Many third-party payers developed their own set of guidelines or purchased commercially available "coding edit" sets. Unfortunately, these coding edit guidelines were often viewed as proprietary and the information was not available to providers. Only after denials were received from the payer did the provider know that services were mutually exclusive. Because providers did not know and could not know the guidelines, they were often called "black box" edits because it was as if the rules were hidden inside a black box.

Partially in response to provider complaints and partially in an effort to increase provider compliance with standardized coding rules, the CCI edits were initially created and implemented on January 1, 1996. Initially, the CCI codes had to be purchased from third-party publishers that obtained the rights to the code sets. However, after several years these edits were available online at the Medicare website (www.cms.hhs.gov) at no cost to providers.

Three types of CCI edits govern bundling and unbundling rules: medically unlikely edits, Column 1/Column 2 edits, and mutually exclusive edits.

Medically Unlikely Edits. Medically unlikely edits (MUEs) are the most recently added component of the CCI system. Implemented in January 2007, CMS developed MUEs to reduce the number of erroneous paid claims for physician services. Not all codes have an MUE, but those that do indicate the maximum number of units that a single provider would ordinarily report for a single patient on a single date of service (CMS, 2010). The purpose of MUEs is to prevent providers from recklessly or erroneously stating that they had provided multiple services in the same day, and be paid multiple times.

National Correct Coding Initiative (NCCI) edits
A publication of guidelines that detail what codes can and cannot be billed during the same encounter. It serves, in part, as the definition of what services are bundled.

CODING TIP

One of the biggest challenges for coders is knowing when multiple procedures performed at the same encounter are separately billable. Medicare uses the NCCI edits to make this determination, but many private payers may have their own guidelines.

FYI

NCCI edits are available on the Medicare website at no cost to providers. The edits are updated on a quarterly basis.

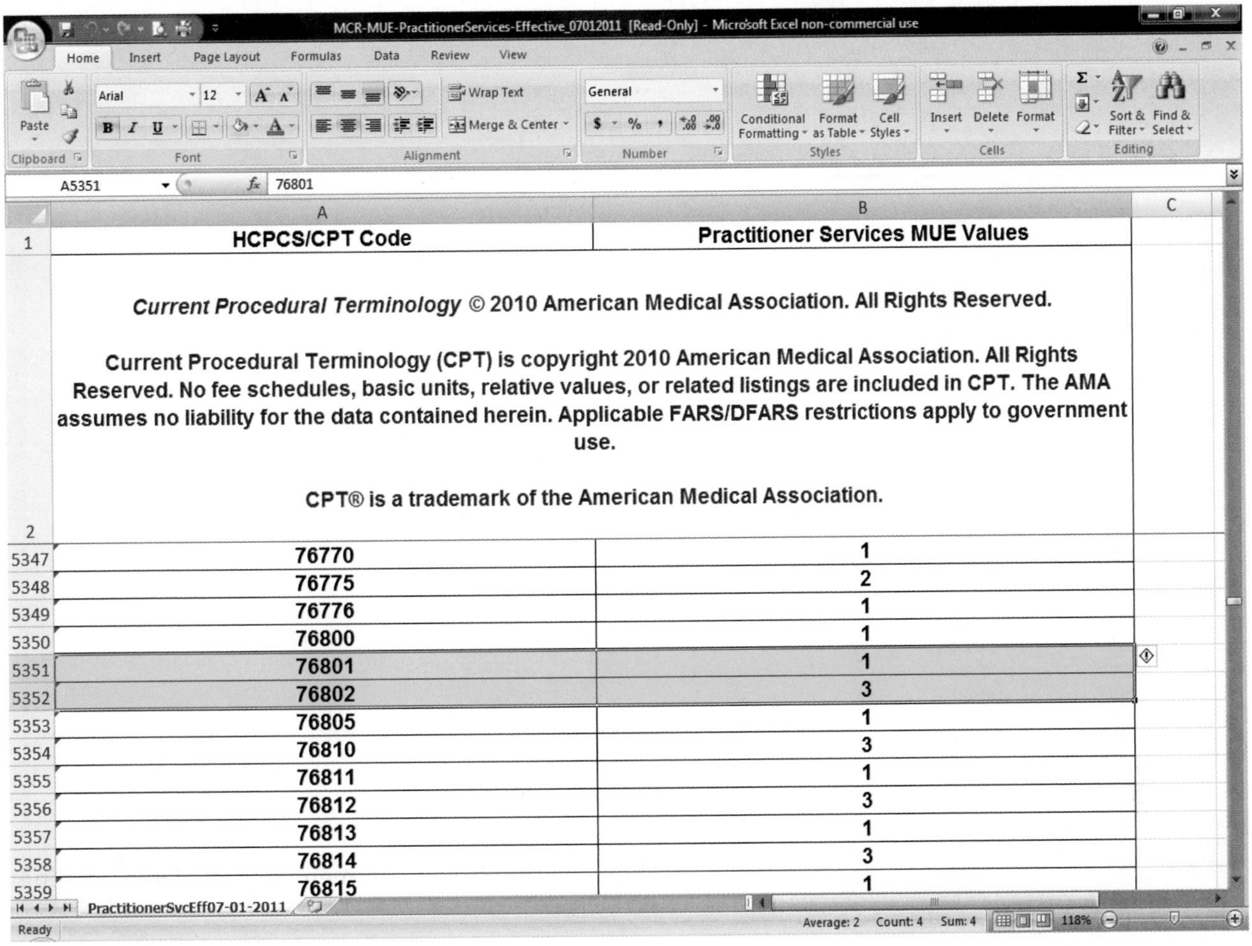

	A	B	C
1	**HCPCS/CPT Code**	**Practitioner Services MUE Values**	
2	*Current Procedural Terminology* © 2010 American Medical Association. All Rights Reserved. Current Procedural Terminology (CPT) is copyright 2010 American Medical Association. All Rights Reserved. No fee schedules, basic units, relative values, or related listings are included in CPT. The AMA assumes no liability for the data contained herein. Applicable FARS/DFARS restrictions apply to government use. CPT® is a trademark of the American Medical Association.		
5347	76770	1	
5348	76775	2	
5349	76776	1	
5350	76800	1	
5351	76801	1	
5352	76802	3	
5353	76805	1	
5354	76810	3	
5355	76811	1	
5356	76812	3	
5357	76813	1	
5358	76814	3	
5359	76815	1	

FIGURE 6.8

This partial sample of an MUE table shows that certain ultrasound codes have maximum limits as to the number of times a service can be billed on any given day for a single patient. For example, obstetric ultrasound code 76801 can be billed only once (by definition) and ultrasound code 76802 (which is an add-on code to 76801) can be billed only three times. This means that if a patient is carrying more than quadruplets, the claim will be denied because the MUE has been exceeded. After submitting supporting documentation, additional units may be payable.

There are occasions in which a provider may provide a given service an unusually significant number of times to the same patient on the same day. However, the provider needs to supply documentation to justify these additional services and explain what prompted a quantity of services that would not be expected (Figure 6.8).

Column 1/Column 2 Edits. Column 1/Column 2 edits are self-explanatory (Figure 6.9). There are two columns. The first column (Column 1) lists codes that are comprehensive in nature. These tend to be more complex services that have a number of different components. The second column (Column 2) lists codes that are often an integral part of a major procedure. If a particular code appears in Column 2, it means that the service cannot be billed during the same encounter as the corresponding code in Column 1. Therefore, any code that appears in Column 1 by definition also includes any associated procedures that appear in Column 2.

The CCI edits are printed by a wide variety of specialty societies and publishers, focusing on the codes that are specific to a given subset of physicians. They are usually organized in a user-friendly format that is easier to view and interpret than the extraordinarily large Microsoft Excel spreadsheets that appear on the Medicare website (e.g., in 2010 the Column 1/Column 2 edits for CPT codes 50000–59999 alone had 85,801 rows in the spreadsheet).

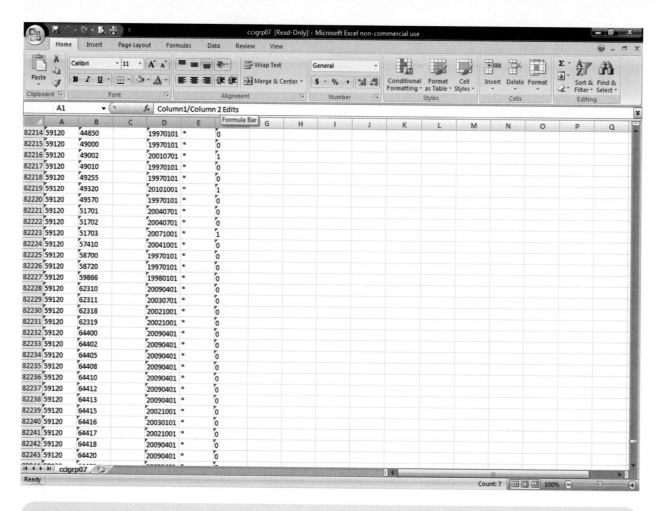

	A	B	C	D	E	F	G	H	I	J	K	L	M	N	O	P	Q
82214	59120	44850		19970101	*	0											
82215	59120	49000		19970101	*	0											
82216	59120	49002		20010701	*	1											
82217	59120	49010		19970101	*	0											
82218	59120	49255		19970101	*	0											
82219	59120	49320		20101001	*	1											
82220	59120	49570		19970101	*	0											
82221	59120	51701		20040701	*	0											
82222	59120	51702		20040701	*	0											
82223	59120	51703		20071001	*	1											
82224	59120	57410		20041001	*	0											
82225	59120	58700		19970101	*	0											
82226	59120	58720		19970101	*	0											
82227	59120	59866		19980101	*	0											
82228	59120	62310		20090401	*	0											
82229	59120	62311		20030701	*	0											
82230	59120	62318		20021001	*	0											
82231	59120	62319		20021001	*	0											
82232	59120	64400		20090401	*	0											
82233	59120	64402		20090401	*	0											
82234	59120	64405		20090401	*	0											
82235	59120	64408		20090401	*	0											
82236	59120	64410		20090401	*	0											
82237	59120	64412		20090401	*	0											
82238	59120	64413		20090401	*	0											
82239	59120	64415		20021001	*	0											
82240	59120	64416		20030101	*	0											
82241	59120	64417		20021001	*	0											
82242	59120	64418		20090401	*	0											
82243	59120	64420		20090401	*	0											

FIGURE 6.9

This section of the Column 1/Column 2 table shows that when billing CPT code 59120—Surgical treatment of an ectopic pregnancy, abdominal or vaginal approach (Column 1 or Column A), none of the codes in Column 2 (Column B) can be billed at the same time. Some of the examples include 58720—Salpingo-oophorectomy (because it can be, by definition, part of 59120), 62310—Injection, single . . . of diagnostic or therapeutic substance(s) (because anesthesia provided by the surgeon is included in the primary procedure and is not separately billable), and so on.

Mutually Exclusive Edits. These edits identify code pairs that Medicare has determined, for clinical reasons, are unlikely to be performed on the same patient on the same day (Figure 6.10). For example, a mutually exclusive edit might identify two different types of testing that yield equivalent results or are by definition impossible to accomplish simultaneously. When two mutually exclusive services are submitted on a claim, only the service of lesser value will be reimbursed (American College of Emergency Physicians, 2008).

The CCI edits exist to make very clear the rules by which Medicare governs service bundling and unbundling. CCI edits are an important tool as they pertain to ethical coding because much of the speculation that existed previously in association with coding for multiple services during the same encounter has been removed. It not only draws clear distinctions between correct and incorrect coding for those that might be tempted to push boundaries, but it also helps the diligent coder confidently follow the rules.

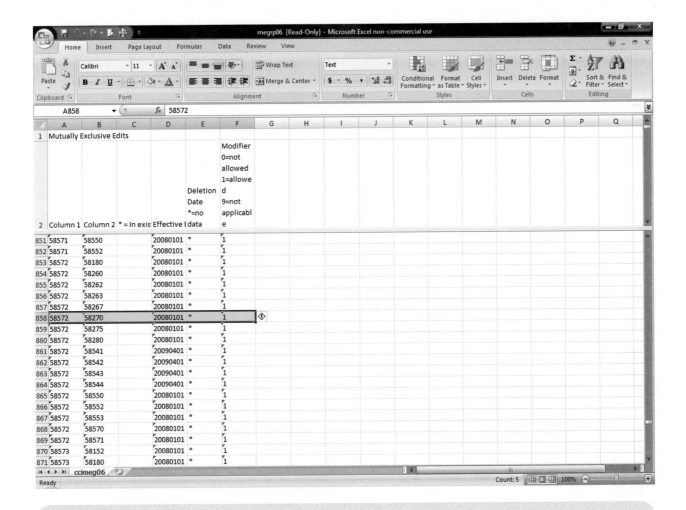

FIGURE 6.10

This small section of the Mutually Exclusive table shows that 58572 and 58570 cannot be billed during the same operative session. This makes sense in that it is impossible to perform a hysterectomy on a uterus greater than 250 grams at the same time that a hysterectomy is performed on a uterus of less than 250 grams.

Thinking It Through 6.2

1. Do you agree that bundling is beneficial for both payers and providers? Why or why not? What are the ethical considerations if every service was billed separately?

2. Should all payers be required to use the CCI edits, as opposed to creating their own edits? Support your position. What are the ethical ramifications of this type of requirement?

3. How could the concept of separate procedure be better explained to minimize ethical issues?

6.3 The Use of Modifiers and Ethical Procedural Coding

In general, whenever there are rules, there are also exceptions. This is also the case as it pertains to billing for global or bundled procedural services. Although a procedure may generally not be payable in a given circumstance, an unusual situation may make that payment

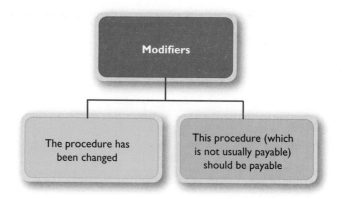

FIGURE 6.11
Modifiers have two uses: to communicate either that the procedure has been changed in some fashion, or to indicate that a procedure is payable that ordinarily would not be payable.

Modifiers

The procedure has been changed

This procedure (which is not usually payable) should be payable

Modifier
A two-digit numeric code indicating that a service or procedure that has been performed has been altered by some specific circumstance, but not changed in its definition or code.

CODING TIP

The purpose of modifiers is to indicate that a service has been altered in some way. The primary purpose is not to obtain additional reimbursement.

not only appropriate, but also fully justified. In coding, these special circumstances are identified using **modifiers.**

GENERAL PRINCIPLES REGARDING MODIFIERS

The purpose of modifiers is to provide a method to indicate that a service or procedure that was performed was altered by some specific circumstance, but not changed in its fundamental definition or code. In many cases, the use of modifiers is required by payer policies to indicate circumstances in which an otherwise nonpayable service is payable. Modifiers address unusual circumstances and situations, which may or may not directly influence reimbursement (Figure 6.11).

A major contributor to the unethical use of modifiers is the erroneous notion that the primary purpose of modifiers is to obtain additional reimbursement. While additional reimbursement can certainly result from the proper use of modifiers, it is not the primary purpose. The primary purpose of modifiers is to facilitate the accurate reporting of a service that does not precisely match the CPT code descriptions of the services provided.

ETHICAL STRUGGLES AND THE MODIFIERS THAT CONTRIBUTE TO THEM

The purpose of all modifiers is the same—to show that a service has been altered in some way. However, there are some modifiers that by their nature more easily contribute to ethical dilemmas.

Modifier –59. When the National Correct Coding Initiative (NCCI or CCI) was introduced in 1996, it formalized the concept of bundling and unbundling procedures that were not necessarily explicitly or implicitly bundled in the CPT code definition. This created a great deal of controversy because providers demonstrated occasions in which two procedures that normally are done in conjunction with each other could and should be billed separately. Therefore, in 1997 the –59 modifier was introduced to allow providers the opportunity to properly report legitimately unbundled services (Andrews, 2009).

Unfortunately, many uninformed coders and physicians felt that modifier –59 was essentially a license to unbundle. This is not the case. Over time, the definition of the modifier and the accompanying instructions were changed to more specifically clarify the conditions

COMPLIANCE TIP

The use of the –59 modifier should be a primary focus of any compliance program. This modifier is one of the more frequently abused modifiers.

that had to exist to properly use the modifier. The purpose of modifier −59 is to indicate that a service was provided during a different session, as part of a different procedure or surgery, a different site or organ system, a separate incision or excision, a separate lesion, or a separate injury that doesn't usually occur for the same individual on the same day. The documentation must adequately explain and support the code usage. Consider the example of Grace's visit to her gynecologist.

Example

Grace was seen by her gynecologist, Dr. Grimaldi, for menorrhagia with resulting anemia. After an appropriate evaluation and discussion, Dr. Grimaldi scheduled Grace for a supracervical hysterectomy the following week. Grace elected not to have her tubes and ovaries removed. On February 8, Dr. Grimaldi took Grace to surgery. An exploratory laparotomy revealed an enlarged fibroid uterus extending to the umbilicus. The left ovary had an approximately 4-cm cyst that appeared simple. The ovaries were freed and a supracervical hysterectomy was performed. Clear straw-colored fluid was drained from the left ovarian cyst and a biopsy of the cyst wall was sent to pathology. The cyst capsule was removed from the ovary.

In Grace's case, three procedures for which CPT codes exist were performed:

58180	Supracervical abdominal hysterectomy, with or without removal of tube(s), with or without removal of ovary(ies)
58805	Drainage of ovarian cyst(s), unilateral or bilateral (separate procedure); abdominal approach
58925	Ovarian cystectomy, unilateral or bilateral

Without a modifier, the only procedure that could be paid is 58180 because the other two procedures are bundled into it. It would be unreasonable and perhaps unnecessary to perform ovarian cyst drainage and a cystectomy when the ovaries are removed anyway, as a component part of the hysterectomy. (Note that in the description, 58180 includes the removal of ovary[ies], if it is performed. In this case, it was not.)

Since an oophorectomy (removal of ovaries) was not performed in this case, then the cystectomy becomes a separate procedure that may be separately reimbursable. The only way this can be done is by attaching the −59 modifier. This states, "This situation is very unusual—it needs special consideration when the claim is adjudicated." Therefore, the claim should be reported as follows:

58180

58925-59

Note that CPT code 58805 was not billed separately because it is bundled as part of the ovarian cystectomy (58925). It is not reasonable to bill for a cyst drainage and a cyst removal on the same cyst, as in the case here. However, if there were two cysts—one on each ovary— and one was drained and the other completely removed, it could be

ICD-10-CM and Procedure Codes

As indicated earlier, no direct relationship exists between diagnosis codes and procedure codes. Therefore, the change from ICD-9-CM to ICD-10-CM does not have an obvious effect on how procedure codes are reported.

However, the greater specificity that ICD-10-CM supplies may make the reporting of unusual circumstances related to procedure codes much easier to communicate. In fact, if payers are alert to the details of the new ICD-10 codes that are reported, special reports may not be necessary to obtain payment for unusual situations. The biggest factor that may assist in this process is the location-specific characteristics of ICD-10 codes.

There are occasions in which multiple services are provided during the same operative session that are normally bundled and therefore are not separately payable. An example might be the repair of an elbow deformity and the amputation of an arm above the elbow. Most payers would look at this as a bundled service because there would be no need to repair the deformity if the arm was going to be amputated anyway. However, if the left arm was going to be repaired and the right arm was going to be amputated, the only way to obtain payment for this service is to submit the left arm repair with a −59 modifier and an operative report that explains the unusual circumstance.

ICD-10 allows greater specificity and allows the full circumstances to be communicated without submission of additional supporting paperwork. Using ICD-10, the diagnosis codes would be reported as shown in Table 6.3. The reporting mechanisms of ICD-10 diagnosis codes will help clarify unique situations in which services that are normally bundled are billed separately. The last characters of A and B designate services provided on different arms.

The ability of the provider to report services in this way will provide cost savings to both payer and provider because there will be less expense in claim preparation and processing and faster receipt of payment by the provider.

separately reimbursable. This would be done using HCPCS Level II modifiers RT and LT, which designated "right side" and "left side," respectively. Coding for this service would appear as follows:

> 58180
>
> 58925-59-RT
>
> 58805-59-LT

It is not ethical to attempt to receive separate reimbursement for a procedure when the circumstances do not warrant the use of the modifier and are not deserving of extra reimbursement. The −59 modifier is not an automatic route to additional payments. In fact, the use of the −59 modifier may require the submission of medical records, which could delay payment. It should be used only when the circumstances call for it.

Modifier −24. Although modifier −24 is attached to E/M codes, it is addressed here because it can be used only when a procedure with an associated global period is performed. The improper or unethical usage of this modifier can occur when a service not directly related to the procedure is performed, but it is not significant or separately

Table 6.3 CPT Codes with Possible Accompanying ICD-10-Codes	
CPT Code	**ICD-10 Code**
24920	S48.911A
24665-59	S52.122B

identifiable, and/or it is not properly documented in the medical record. Consider the case of Holly's broken ankle and follow-up.

Example

Holly was mountain climbing and in the process broke her ankle. Her ankle was treated surgically by an orthopedic surgeon, Dr. Hammer. At a surgical follow-up visit, Holly mentioned to Dr. Hammer that she was experiencing some knee pain on the opposite leg. After doing a brief examination and taking a brief history, Dr. Hammer determined that the cause of her discomfort was the improper use of her crutches. He showed her how to maneuver the crutches properly and gave her instruction to let him know if the problem persisted. In the medical record Dr. Hammer recorded, "Knee pain—caused by crutches."

In this circumstance, the medical record documentation does not support the billing of an E/M service with a −24 modifier attached. Even if the record was more complete, the question remains as to whether this was significant enough to warrant the separate billing of a service. In addition, the proper use of crutches could easily be considered part of the follow-up to the ankle surgery.

On the other hand, there are circumstances in which is it perfectly legitimate to use the −24 modifier, as in the case of Mikaela's accident.

Example

Mikaela had been in an automobile accident, resulting in a significant scar to her face. The plastic surgeon, Dr. Fisher, performed a repair of the wound. At the surgical follow-up visit, Mikaela wanted to discuss her interest in having breast reduction surgery. Dr. Fisher documented in the record, "A 25-minute discussion was held concerning the patient's desire to have breast reduction surgery. The discussion included the back pain experienced by the patient, the risks associated with the surgery, and alternatives to the surgery. The patient will talk about these items with her husband and call the office next week to let us know what treatment option she would like to pursue."

In this example, a documented 25-minute discussion is far in excess of what normally is provided during a follow-up visit after a wound repair. Therefore, billing 99214-24 (based on time) is an appropriate coding option.

Modifier −26. The occurrence of unethical usage of modifier −26 professional component is not dependent on when it is used, but rather when it is *not used*. Many procedures in the CPT code book have two separate components—a **professional component (PC)** and a **technical component (TC).** The professional component encompasses the *professional* services delivered in conjunction with a procedure, including the performance of the procedure, the interpretation of the results, and the preparation of a report. The technical component includes the *technical* aspects of delivering the procedure, including the purchase, maintenance, and operation of the required equipment; compensation for the staff that performs or assists in the exam; and the general overhead associated with the care delivery (Figure 6.12).

Professional component (PC)
The services delivered in conjunction with a procedure by the provider, including the performance of the procedure, the interpretation of the results, and the preparation of a report.

Technical component (TC)
The technical aspects of delivering a procedure, including the purchase, maintenance, and operation of the required equipment; compensation for the staff that performs or assists in the exam; and the general overhead associated with the care delivery.

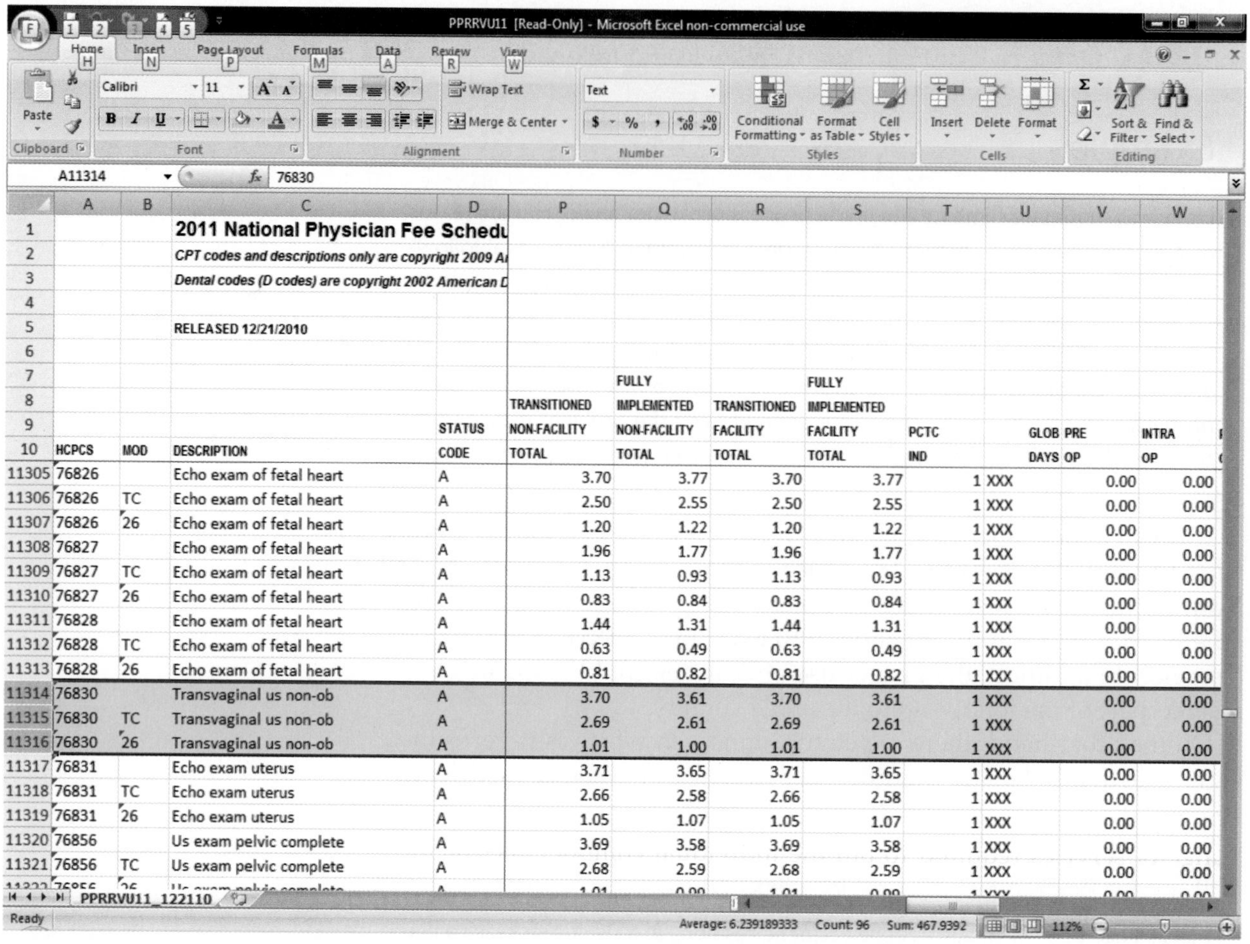

2011 National Physician Fee Schedu
CPT codes and descriptions only are copyright 2009 A
Dental codes (D codes) are copyright 2002 American D
RELEASED 12/21/2010

	HCPCS	MOD	DESCRIPTION	STATUS CODE	TRANSITIONED NON-FACILITY TOTAL	FULLY IMPLEMENTED NON-FACILITY TOTAL	TRANSITIONED FACILITY TOTAL	FULLY IMPLEMENTED FACILITY TOTAL	PCTC IND	GLOB DAYS	PRE OP	INTRA OP
11305	76826		Echo exam of fetal heart	A	3.70	3.77	3.70	3.77	1	XXX	0.00	0.00
11306	76826	TC	Echo exam of fetal heart	A	2.50	2.55	2.50	2.55	1	XXX	0.00	0.00
11307	76826	26	Echo exam of fetal heart	A	1.20	1.22	1.20	1.22	1	XXX	0.00	0.00
11308	76827		Echo exam of fetal heart	A	1.96	1.77	1.96	1.77	1	XXX	0.00	0.00
11309	76827	TC	Echo exam of fetal heart	A	1.13	0.93	1.13	0.93	1	XXX	0.00	0.00
11310	76827	26	Echo exam of fetal heart	A	0.83	0.84	0.83	0.84	1	XXX	0.00	0.00
11311	76828		Echo exam of fetal heart	A	1.44	1.31	1.44	1.31	1	XXX	0.00	0.00
11312	76828	TC	Echo exam of fetal heart	A	0.63	0.49	0.63	0.49	1	XXX	0.00	0.00
11313	76828	26	Echo exam of fetal heart	A	0.81	0.82	0.81	0.82	1	XXX	0.00	0.00
11314	76830		Transvaginal us non-ob	A	3.70	3.61	3.70	3.61	1	XXX	0.00	0.00
11315	76830	TC	Transvaginal us non-ob	A	2.69	2.61	2.69	2.61	1	XXX	0.00	0.00
11316	76830	26	Transvaginal us non-ob	A	1.01	1.00	1.01	1.00	1	XXX	0.00	0.00
11317	76831		Echo exam uterus	A	3.71	3.65	3.71	3.65	1	XXX	0.00	0.00
11318	76831	TC	Echo exam uterus	A	2.66	2.58	2.66	2.58	1	XXX	0.00	0.00
11319	76831	26	Echo exam uterus	A	1.05	1.07	1.05	1.07	1	XXX	0.00	0.00
11320	76856		Us exam pelvic complete	A	3.69	3.58	3.69	3.58	1	XXX	0.00	0.00
11321	76856	TC	Us exam pelvic complete	A	2.68	2.59	2.68	2.59	1	XXX	0.00	0.00

FIGURE 6.12
This portion of the RBRVS table shows the RVUs for CPT code 76830 and demonstrates the value of the total code, the amount attributable to the technical component (TC) and the amount attributable to the professional component (PC). In this and every case the technical component RVUs added to the professional component RVUs equals the total service RVUs.

When a provider bills a service that has both technical and professional components without a modifier, the implication is that the provider delivered both elements of the service. However, if the service is delivered in a facility that is not owned by the provider (e.g., services delivered in the hospital radiology department, ultrasounds performed in an inpatient hospital setting, etc.) it is not possible for the provider to have supplied 100% of the service because he or she does not contribute to the cost of delivering the technical component of the service. Consider the billing practices of Dr. Monserat in the following case.

Example

Dr. Monserat is an OB/GYN who frequently meets her patients in the hospital radiology department to perform hysterosalpingograms (HSGs; CPT code 58340). In this procedure, dye is injected into the patient's uterus to determine whether or not the fallopian tubes are clear and functional. While the dye is being injected, a radiological exam is done to watch the dye flow through uterus, into the fallopian tubes, and ideally out into the pelvis. If the dye does not leave the tubes, this means that the tubes are not open and the opportunity for a successful pregnancy is very unlikely, if not impossible, without some sort of medical intervention. In addition to the CPT code for the injection of the dye, there is also a code to report the radiological component (CPT code 74740) of the exam.

Dr. Monserat bills 58340 and 74740-26 because she interpreted the exam while it was being performed and he discussed the results with the patient at the time of the exam. However, hospital policy requires that a radiologist in the radiology department view the radiology results and write the final report. Traditionally, Dr. Monserat does not write a report concerning the HSG, other than a very brief note in her medical record.

In this case, if Dr. Monserat bills 58340 and 74740-26 and the radiologist bills 74740, it is likely that there will be a problem with one or both claims when they are considered by the third-party payer. Dr. Monserat has had numerous conversations with hospital administration and the chair of the radiology department, vigorously defending her right to bill the professional component of the service. The hospital defends with equal vigor its right to bill for the full radiological component for this service because the hospital employs the radiologists.

The key to the ethical usage (or nonusage) of modifier −26 is a clear understanding of the difference between the professional and the technical component and ensuring that the provider is supplying the full range of services required to bill the individual components—or the full service that entitles the provider to bill the entire procedure, without a modifier.

Modifier −52. The purpose of modifier −52 is to report occasions in which the provider did not provide the full service described by the CPT code used to report the service. The specific reason for not providing the full service is unimportant in determining whether or not to use the modifier, but the medical record should clearly reflect the reason why the full service was not reported. The key is that the fundamental procedure or service must remain the same and undisturbed.

Again, like modifier −26, the ethical risk is *not* using modifier −52 when in fact it should be used. If a reduced service is provided, but modifier −52 is not used, the implication is that the full procedure was performed. This supplies the opportunity for the provider to receive a reimbursement level that is higher than that to which they are entitled. Consider the case of Serena's surgical procedure.

FYI

The most frequent misuse of the professional and technical component modifiers (−26 and −TC) is *not* using them when they should be used.

Example

Serena, a 37-year-old who has had three children, desires permanent sterilization. She had a left salpingectomy as the result of an ectopic pregnancy. After consultation with Dr. Garnett, Serena elects to have a hysteroscopic approach, which was scheduled for two weeks later.

Following assessment of the uterine cavity and fallopian tubes immediately prior to performing the procedure, Dr. Garnett successfully places the micro-insert in the right tube. Dr. Garnett billed CPT code 58565—Hysteroscopy, surgical; with bilateral fallopian tube cannulation to induce occlusion by placement of permanent implants.

Unfortunately, the approach followed by Dr. Garnett in Serena's case is not an ethical coding methodology for this service. In this case the patient had one tube removed on a previous occasion. Therefore, the insert was placed in only one tube, when the code explicitly states that the procedure is to be done bilaterally. The failure to add a −52 modifier (58565-52) in this case could result in more payment than Dr. Garnett is entitled to.

The ethical challenge that some providers face is that the odds of this improper billing being detected by a third-party payer or government entity is very low. The payer would have to have record of the initial procedure (CPT code 59120, which it may not have available if the patient was covered by another payer at the time of that procedure) and it would need to have the software programmed to note that the performance of the first procedure would preclude complete performance of the second procedure (58565). It may be unlikely that any payer would be capable of this type of data management.

The second factor that may create a challenge for providers is the feeling or opinion that the payers are not reimbursing them adequately for the procedure. If a procedure is reported as a "reduced service," it is likely that the reimbursement will be reduced further. By simply failing to report this modifier (which probably will not be caught anyway), they will be simply "leveling the playing field" in the "competition" with the payers.

Modifier −53. In certain situations, the physician may elect to terminate a surgical or diagnostic procedure due to unusual circumstances or if the well-being of the patient is threatened. It can be necessary to indicate that a surgical or diagnostic procedure was started, but discontinued. In addition, the CPT manual specifically excludes the use of this modifier when a procedure is electively canceled (either by the patient or by the physician) prior to the administration of anesthesia or before the patient is brought in to the procedure room or operating suite.

It is ethically appropriate to use this modifier in two instances:

1. When the patient's condition deteriorates to the point that it is no longer safe to continue the procedure.
2. When the patient's condition is stable but the physician, for whatever reason, is not able to complete the procedure.

Example

Gladys, a 68-year-old woman, was scheduled to undergo a cardiovascular stress test (CPT code 93015) with her cardiologist, Dr. Lemon. Approximately two minutes into the procedure, Gladys complained of intense chest pain and the procedure was stopped. Dr. Lemon determined that her heart rate and rhythm were highly abnormal and arrangements were made to transport Gladys to the nearest emergency room for further evaluation and treatment. Dr. Lemon billed this service as 93015-53.

In Gladys's case, the patient's condition prevented the physician from completing the procedure. The physician did incur expense associated with providing the procedure such as supplies, staff time, and other administrative expense. Yet, the procedure was not fully completed and it would be inappropriate and unethical to report that it was completed.

Example

Rebecca is a 25-year-old patient who came to Dr. Emerson, a dermatologist, with numerous premalignant lesions. After obtaining additional history and performing a limited examination, Dr. Emerson decided that the lesions should be removed on the same day. As part of the procedure, she prepped the surgical area and injected local anesthetic. However, the patient's blood pressure dropped dramatically and she passed out due to her anxiety level. The physician did not feel that it was appropriate to continue the procedure and so the procedure was rescheduled for the next day at a facility where an anesthesiologist would be available to provide services.

In Rebecca's case, the patient's emotional condition made the intended procedure (CPT code 17004) impossible to perform. This could not be known until the procedure was attempted. In this case, billing the service as 17004-53 accurately reflects the service provided and explains why additional services the next day were necessary.

The ethical dilemma in this case is, again, the temptation to not report the −53 modifier because the use of this modifier can result in reduced payment. In some cases, this is entirely appropriate because the quantity of services provided was substantially less than that normally delivered in conjunction with the service (e.g., a surgery that normally takes 90 minutes is stopped after 10 minutes because of the patient's systemic condition). However, in other cases the work involved is actually more intense than if the procedure had been completed without complication.

Different payers respond to the submission of modifier −53 in different ways. Even different Medicare carriers have different policies as to how the procedure is reimbursed. For example, one carrier instructs providers to submit a charge proportionate to the amount of work provided (Noridian Administrative Services, 2009), whereas others indicate that each case will be reviewed on an individual basis (WPS Insurance Corporation, 2007).

Regardless of how the payer responds, the provider is discouraged from using the modifier because payment will either be reduced or, at best, will be delayed while the case is individually reviewed. It is easier for the provider to disregard or "forget" the modifier, especially if the billing of the procedure that was not completed will not affect the billing of a procedure for the patient in the near future. This is the true source of the ethical dilemma associated with this modifier use.

Modifier −22. Modifier −22 is probably the most well-known modifier among physicians because it is perceived as the modifier that will provide additional reimbursement for difficult procedures. Over the years, the definition of this modifier was adjusted from focusing on "unusual" procedural services to "increased" procedural services. The reason for the change was that defining "unusual" was more open to interpretation and ill-defined than identifying "increased" services.

Compliance and Procedure Coding

Compliance efforts, as they relate to procedural coding, should focus primarily on ensuring that the documentation of a procedure is consistent with the codes billed for the procedures. It is a severe compliance problem if a provider bills for a procedure and the chart does not have a corresponding procedure note that supplies the details of the procedure.

Specifically within physician practices, the biggest compliance risk is the failure to ensure that the procedures or diagnostic tests marked on the superbill by the provider have a corresponding procedure note. When developing a compliance program, it should include random audits of surgical procedures to ensure that the billing and the documentation match. However, special attention should be given in these circumstances:

1. When the frequency of a certain procedure suddenly increases.
2. When the frequency of a certain procedure performed by a particular physician is significantly different than that performed by other physicians of the same specialty within the same practice.
3. When an unusual number of multiprocedure surgical encounters are billed.

In addition, special care should be taken to ensure that surgical procedures are billed correctly, based on the type of procedure, location of procedure, and method of procedure performance. Without a compliance program that checks the correctness of code selection, providers are exposed when payer audits are conducted and incorrect coding is identified.

BILLING TIP

Ethical issues may arise in the use of the −22 modifer in two ways: Payers may not provide additional reimbursement that is legitimately documented, and coders may not want to deal with the hassle associated with attempting to receive payment for the service.

When the work required to provide a service is substantially greater than ordinarily required, the fact that extra work occurred is identified by adding modifier −22 to the usual procedure code. The ethical question associated with the usage of this modifier is, "How significant or increased does a service have to be before it warrants the addition of this modifier?"

The ethical issues associated with this modifier are double-sided. The modifier may be added inappropriately to services that do not meet the standard of increased services. On the other hand, the modifier may be intentionally disregarded to avoid the "hassle" of attempting to receive payment for additional services. It is unlikely that a provider will have significant success in inappropriately adding the modifier because the documentation has to support the substantial additional work and the reason for the additional work, such as increased intensity, time, technical difficulty, and the severity of the patient's condition. Unless the provider falsifies or exaggerates the documentation associated with the procedure, unethically obtaining reimbursement for modifier −22 is improbable.

The more likely ethical scenario occurs when the provider's staff member chooses not to add the modifier because he or she doesn't want to delay reimbursement—particularly if the person feels that collection performance is being evaluated and his or her job may be at risk if the accounts receivable amount becomes too great. The staff member prefers to take the timely but lesser reimbursement from the unmodified procedure, rather than to struggle for the greater but delayed reimbursement when the modifier is used.

Where is the line that determines whether or not the −22 modifier should be used? There are no defined criteria because two equally qualified evaluators examining the same case can arrive at opposite determinations as to whether additional reimbursement is appropriate. Therefore, you should not use the −22 modifier unless the service provided is *undeniably, significantly greater* than that usually provided.

There are two reasons for this standard—when this modifier is used, payment will be delayed. Therefore, the case should be evaluated to be "increased" by any reasonable reviewer so that reimbursement will not be delayed unnecessarily. Second, because of the time value of money, it may be better to obtain a lesser amount sooner than a slightly greater amount at some significantly later time. A common rule of thumb is that the procedure should be at least 40% greater than the average or usual case before this modifier is used. If this principle is used, the odds of receiving additional reimbursement is greater than if a slightly increased service is submitted and, when additional reimbursement is received, it is sufficient to offset the delay in receiving the payment.

Thinking It Through 6.3

1. Explain how the belief that the primary purpose of modifiers is to increase reimbursement can result in unethical use of modifiers.

2. In your opinion, which modifier associated with surgical procedures is most likely to produce an ethical issue? Why?

3. What are the ethical ramifications of *not* using a modifier when one is appropriate?

6.4 Ethical Choices Regarding Procedure Methods and Unlisted Codes

One of the major recent advances in medical treatment has been the increase in the alternatives that are available when considering treatment options—particularly surgical options. Historically, surgery was an "open" approach by which internal organs were accessed through an incision, which subsequently had to be closed. In the mid-nineteenth century practical clinical endoscopic surgery became possible, with enormous advances made in the latter half of the twentieth century. Laparoscopic surgery was introduced in the 1980s and has exploded in its usage since that time. Robotic surgery was first performed in 1992 and is also increasing in its usage.

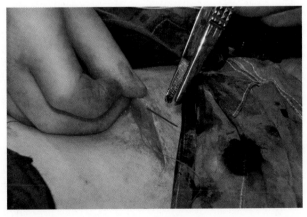

Until the mid-nineteenth century, surgery was usually performed openly through an incision. Some surgeries are still completed this way.

CODING TIP

To properly select a procedure code, the coder must know the method by which the procedure was performed.

Each of these procedures requires different levels of surgical skill for the physician, different types of equipment, and different amounts of time. In recognition of this fact, different CPT codes have been established to enable physicians to accurately report the nature of the services that they provided. This, in turn, allows appropriate RVUs to be assigned to each code.

SELECTING PROCEDURAL CODES BASED ON THE METHOD OR APPROACH

Often a procedure can be performed in different ways. For example, there are three different ways in which a hysterectomy can be performed: abdominally, vaginally, or laparoscopically assisted (Table 6.4).

Similarly, there are four different ways in which an ovarian cyst can be removed and/or drained: with a needle (vaginal), needle (abdominal), open abdominal, or laparoscopy (Table 6.5).

The relative values for each of the hysterectomy codes are substantially different (Table 6.6).

The circumstances are the same for the ovarian cyst codes (Table 6.7).

Correct code selection is critical in being accurately paid for the service provided. For example, if a provider performs a vaginal ovarian cyst drainage but bills for an ovarian cystectomy using 58925, he or she will be paid more than twice the appropriate amount. Whether done intentionally or whether it is done by error produced through ignorance, both are ethically inappropriate.

Table 6.4 Hysterectomy Methods and Associated Codes

Method	CPT Code
Abdominally (open procedure)	58150
Vaginally	58260
Laparoscopically assisted	58553

Table 6.5 Ovarian Cyst Removal Methods and Associated Codes

Method	CPT Code
Needle (vaginal)	58800
Needle (abdominal)	58805
Open abdominal	58925
Laparoscopy	49322

Table 6.6 RVUs for Hysterectomy Methods

CPT Code	Relative Value Units
58150	27.78
58260	23.00
58553	31.71

Table 6.7 RVUs for Ovarian Cyst Removal Methods

CPT Code	Relative Value Units
58800	8.16
58805	11.12
58925	20.56
49322	10.15

The situation becomes a little more complex when there is not a CPT code available that precisely describes the procedure performed. The case study of Megan Overland provides an example.

Example

Megan Overland is a 34-year-old female who is taken to surgery for a diagnostic laparoscopy to identify the causes of her abdominal pain. The surgeon discovers that there are a number of adhesions that require lysis to visualize all portions of the abdomen. While performing the lysis of adhesions, the surgeon inadvertently nicks the patient's bladder.

The surgeon identifies it immediately and is able to perform the repair through the laparoscope. The surgeon sends the operative report to his billing office and the coder selects the following codes:

49320—Diagnostic laparoscopy

51860-51—Cystorrhaphy, suture of bladder wound, injury or rupture; simple

The coding supervisor reviews these code choices and believes that they are incorrect. The primary problem is that the laparoscopic bladder repair was reported using an open repair code. The supervisor believes that the most accurate code for this bladder repair service is 51999—Unlisted laparoscopy procedure, bladder. However, he knows that it will be very difficult to obtain payment for this unlisted code and so he tells the coder to leave the codes as they were because the provider did not attempt to bill for the lysis of adhesions that was done in connection with the billing of the diagnostic laparoscopy (49320).

In this case, it is not sufficient to be "close enough" because even though the supervisor's "compromise" would seem to be fair, there are several problems:

- It is not the most accurate method of reporting the service.
- Many payers would not reimburse the physician for the second procedure because the surgeon caused the injury.
- The proposed billing selection would result in a significant overpayment relative to the amount of work actually performed in conjunction with this procedure, assuming that the surgeon could or should bill for the secondary procedure.

Attempts to be close enough are usually ethically challenged, as indicated in the case of Abby Smith.

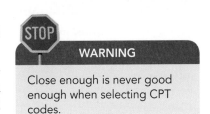

WARNING

Close enough is never good enough when selecting CPT codes.

Example

Abby Smith is a 23-year-old female who has severe pelvic pain caused by fibroids in her uterus. Dr. Parker, an OB/GYN, determines that a myomectomy using a vaginal approach is the best treatment option. While performing the procedure, the fibroid is determined to be larger than originally thought. With skill and extra time, Dr. Parker was able to remove the fibroid vaginally, with a total weight of 262 grams.

Dr. Parker's coder checks the CPT book and finds that no code describes a vaginal myomectomy for a fibroid that exceeds 250 grams. She determines that the most appropriate code is 58999—Unlisted procedure, female genital system (non-obstetrical). Dr. Parker's billing manager objects to the use of this code because unlisted procedures and services with a −22 modifier are underpaid and reimbursement is often significantly delayed. She instructs the coder to bill CPT code 58146 because it is the code that most closely describes the service.

The code that the billing manager is suggesting is 58146—Myomectomy, greater than 250 grams, abdominal approach. The RVUs for that procedure is 31.37. However, if the fibroid was only 12 grams less, the appropriate code would have been 58145, with 14.65 RVUs.

THE PURPOSE AND USE OF UNLISTED CODES

Regarding ethics and procedural code selection, there are two primary ethical concerns—selecting the correct procedural approach and overcoming the avoidance that exists in the use of unlisted CPT codes. In the surgical section of the CPT code book, 89 separate codes are defined as "unlisted" codes. These codes appear in most subsections of the surgical section and give providers and coder the opportunity to report a service for which no specific CPT code exists. Each of these codes is characterized by having "99" as the last two digits and they are immediately adjacent to the specific codes that exist for the relevant organ system. Some examples of the unlisted codes include those listed in Table 6.8.

The overwhelming number of procedures performed by physicians in the United States have CPT codes that accurately describe and facilitate the reporting of the service. However, as time continues and medical advances increase, the number of new procedures for which a CPT code does not exist also increases (Figure 6.13).

The aversion that many providers and coders have in using unlisted codes is that they require the submission of documentation to receive reimbursement. Without the documentation to describe the procedure performed it is impossible for anyone to know what was done, let alone assign a reimbursement value to that service. This process eliminates the advantages associated with electronic claim submission and payment and requires the manual intervention of an individual to review the records, evaluate the service, and assign a reimbursement level.

When unlisted procedures are used, payers have various requirements to obtain payment. One payer's requirements are as follows:

- A clear description of the nature, extent, and need for the procedure or service.

BILLING TIP

Coders must be prepared to submit medical documentation anytime an unlisted code is billed to a third-party payer.

Table 6.8 Examples of Unlisted CPT Codes

Description	CPT Code
Unlisted procedure, breast	19499
Unlisted procedure, leg or ankle	27899
Unlisted procedure, cardiac surgery	33999
Unlisted laparoscopy procedure, stomach	43659
Unlisted procedure, stomach	43999
Unlisted laparoscopy procedure, renal	50549
Unlisted laparoscopy procedure, ureter	50949
Unlisted laparoscopy procedure, bladder	51999
Unlisted procedure, urinary system	53899
Unlisted hysteroscopy procedure, uterus	58579
Unlisted procedure, maternity care and delivery	58999
Unlisted procedure, nervous system	64999
Unlisted procedure, anterior segment of eye	66999
Unlisted procedure, middle ear	69799

- Whether the procedure was performed independent from other services provided, or if it was performed at the same surgical site or through the same surgical opening.
- Any **extenuating** circumstances that may have complicated the service or procedure.
- Time, effort, and equipment necessary to provide the service.
- The number of times the service was provided. (Harvard Pilgram Health Care, 2009)

Extenuating
Explanatory or unusual.

To conduct ethical coding, the use of unlisted codes will almost certainly be required from time to time. Obtaining reimbursement for unlisted codes can be a very frustrating process because it is less efficient than an electronically filed claim with a defined CPT code. Often, substantial disagreement exists between payer and provider as to the equitable reimbursement level for an unlisted procedure. Appeals often must be filed to obtain the reimbursement to which the provider believes it is entitled and, even after appealing, the final reimbursement may be no more than the reimbursement available for a lesser procedure that has

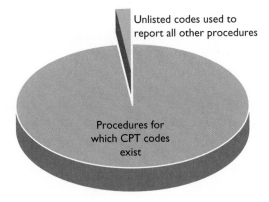

Unlisted codes used to report all other procedures

Procedures for which CPT codes exist

FIGURE 6.13
The majority of commonly performed procedures have a CPT code available for reporting the service.

a CPT code and a defined value. When the delay in reimbursement is considered, the economic deficit for the provider is even greater.

CATEGORY III CODES

To address the issues of emerging technology and the inability of providers to obtain payment for these new, cutting-edge services, the AMA (2009) introduced Category III codes in February 2001. The primary purpose of these codes is to allow data collection regarding emerging technologies, services, and procedures. When providers supply cutting-edge services, they are not limited to the use of unlisted Category I CPT codes, but are required to use the appropriate Category III code. This provides advantages to both the provider and the payer because it helps identify services that are becoming common practice throughout the country and helps define the service delivered—the parties do not have to rely exclusively on the provider's description of the service to identify it.

Prior to the usage of Category III codes, a significant problem existed—a procedure had to be commonly used before a code could be assigned to it, but there was no way to collect data regarding the procedures without a code. The AMA has very strict standards concerning the requirements and criteria that must exist before the creation of a new CPT code. The standards for Category III codes are substantially less (AMA, 2010a). Table 6.9 illustrates the substantial difference between the requirements for a Category I and Category III code.

These codes still do not have RVUs assigned to them and many third-party payers will not reimburse for these particular services because they are deemed to be "experimental," which is often an exclusion associated with health insurance policies. Nonetheless, it is better to have these codes available to move the process forward more quickly in making reimbursable Category I codes for new procedures.

Category III codes are approved for five years. If the Category III code does not meet the criteria for advancement to a Category I code within that time period, the code is removed from the list and it has

> **FYI**
>
> Category III CPT codes are often not payable—but they are helpful in reducing the need for the use of unlisted CPT codes.

Table 6.9 Requirements for Category I Versus Category III CPT Codes

The CPT Advisory Committee and CPT Editorial Panel Require for Category I . . .	The CPT Advisory Committee and CPT Editorial Panel Require for Category III . . .
that the service/procedure has received approval from the Food and Drug Administration (FDA) for the specific use of devices or drugs;	A protocol of the study or procedures being performed;
that the suggested procedure/service is a distinct service performed by many physicians/practitioners across the United States;	Support from the specialties who would use this procedure;
that the clinical efficacy of the service/procedure is well established and documented in U.S. peer review literature;	Availability of United States peer-reviewed literature for examination by the Editorial Panel;
that the suggested service/procedure is neither a fragmentation of an existing procedure/service nor currently reportable by one or more existing codes; and	Descriptions of current United States trials outlining the efficacy of the procedure.
that the suggested service/procedure is not requested as a means to report extraordinary circumstances related to the performance of a procedure/service already having a specific CPT code.	

Table 6.10 Category III CPT Codes That Became Category I CPT Codes

Description	Category III Code	First Introduced	Category I Code	Year of Change
Endometrial cryoablation with ultrasonic guidance, including endometrial curettage, when performed	0009T	2002	58356	2005
Initial pharmacist face-to-face visit, first 15 minutes	0115T	2005	99605	2008
Subsequent pharmacist face-to-face visit, first 15 minutes	0116T	2005	99606	2008
Pharmacist face-to-face visit, each additional 15 minutes	0117T	2005	99607	2008

Sources: Pharmacist Services Technical Advisory Coalition, 2005; Witt, 2005.

reached its "sunset." Several CPT Category I codes have graduated from Category III. Some examples include those listed in Table 6.10.

Some codes that have reached their sunset have been reinstated. For example, CPT code 0059T—Cryopreservation; reproductive tissue, oocyte(s) was introduced in 2004 and was removed from the manual for 2009 because it was determined that oocyte (egg) freezing was not yet common practice to warrant transforming it into a Category I code. However, 0059T was recycled or reinstated for 2011.

Thinking It Through 6.4

1. Explain how advances in medical technology and techniques can create ethical issues in code selection.

2. If a coder in a surgical practice says, "We never use unlisted codes," does it mean he or she is engaging in unethical coding? Why or why not?

3. Discuss the ethical issue associated with a coder *not* attaching a −22 modifier to a surgical procedure.

6.5 Separate Billing of Supplies and Procedures

The Healthcare Common Procedure Coding System (HCPCS), managed by the CMS, is designed to provide codes and descriptors that represent procedures, supplies, products, and services that may be provided to Medicare beneficiaries and individuals enrolled in private insurance programs. Level I HCPCS codes are the CPT codes, and are recognized as a subset of the overall HCPCS coding system (Table 6.11).

Table 6.11 Levels of the HCPCS Coding System

Healthcare Common Procedure Coding System (HCPCS)	
Level I	CPT codes
Level II	HCPCS codes (drugs/supplies)

When HCPCS codes are discussed, the codes most commonly considered are the Level II codes. The Level II codes are focused on items and nonphysician services that are not represented in the Level I codes. For physician practices, the most common usage of Level II codes is to report medical supplies and injectable medications.

The "Surgery Guidelines" section of the CPT code book states, "Supplies and materials provided by the physician (e.g., sterile trays/drugs), over and above those usually included with the procedure(s) rendered are reported separately. List drugs, trays, supplies, and materials provided. Identify as 99070 or specific supply code" (AMA, 2010b). In other words, physicians *can* bill for supplies *if* they are *over and above* those *usually* provided. The primary difficulty in this process is defining "usually provided." In a literal interpretation of the CPT guidelines, two separate physicians may have different protocols in performing the same procedure, meaning that the supplies usually provided may vary from physician to physician. Does this mean that the physician who routinely uses additional supplies, at significantly greater cost, is not able to be reimbursed for the additional expense?

Another common question regarding the billing of supplies is whether or not a service can be billed simply because a supply code exists. Consider the case study of a vascular surgery practice's billing methods.

Example

A vascular surgery practice does a substantial number of abdominal and extremity ultrasounds each day. The practice administrator discovered a HCPCS Level II code for ultrasound gel (A4559—Coupling gel or paste, for use with ultrasound device, per oz.). It was decided that this code would be billed in conjunction with each ultrasound service because the practice, in aggregate, was spending a great deal of money on ultrasound supplies—specifically, ultrasound gel.

When submitting this service to payers, approximately 90% of the claims were rejected because "the supply billed is included as part of the procedure performed." This denial is consistent with the general CPT guidelines. However, about 10% of the payers would issue some payment for this line item, which encouraged the practice administrator to continue the practice. Whenever a claim was denied by the insurer, the practice would write off the charge. However, when it was paid, the practice would keep the money and bill the patient for any coinsurance that might be associated with that service.

1. What is your opinion of this practice?
2. Because a payer will reimburse for a particular service, does it mean that it is ethical to bill for the service? Why or why not?

There are other occasions in which there is no clear-cut answer regarding the use of supplies. Rather, it is often a matter of payer policy concerning code interpretation. For example, CPT code 58300 is defined as "Insertion of intrauterine device (IUD)." Some payers, particularly state Medicaid programs, will include the cost of the device itself (J7300 or J7302) in the reimbursement for this code, meaning that billing for the supply is not separately possible. However, in calculating

RVUs, the Medicare program specifically excludes the supply from the reimbursement of the physician service. This means that most payers will allow the billing as follows:

58300

J7300/J7302

A general rule of thumb for the billing of supplies is that the supply is separately billable if the supply itself is the centerpiece or purpose of the procedure. In the case of an intrauterine contraceptive device (IUD) insertion, it is impossible to perform the procedure without the supply. However, the insertion of the device is the purpose of the procedure and therefore it is legitimate and ethical to bill for the two components: (1) the work involved in inserting the device, and (2) the device itself.

In other cases, there are procedures that are impossible to perform without certain supplies. However, these supplies are a tool to perform the procedure and are not the focus for the procedure itself. An example is a suture repair (CPT code 12002—Simple repair of superficial wounds of scalp; 2.6 cm to 7.5 cm). It is not possible to perform this procedure without the use of suturing materials, but the physician is not able to bill for the suture material itself because it is a component part of the procedure. The closing of the wound is the focus of the procedure, not the sutures themselves. In fact, there are now multiple ways in which to close wounds, including sutures, adhesives, and strip devices.

Provider offices can bill for supplies only when these criteria are met:

1. It is over and above the services usually provided in connection with the procedure, or
2. It is the centerpiece or purpose of the procedure, AND
3. The provider incurs the expense of supplying the device. If the patient or facility supplies the device, it is inappropriate and unethical for a provider to bill for the service.

Example

The patients of Dr. Calender, an orthopedic surgeon, often require crutches when they have a leg injury. For some payers, the reimbursement that Dr. Calender receives is less than the cost of the crutches. When the patients are covered by these payers, Dr. Calender writes a prescription for the crutches and instructs the patient to obtain the device at the next-door pharmacy, which is able to obtain higher reimbursement for the crutches than the physician.

However, the physician's coder is not specifically aware of this arrangement and bills E0114—Crutches, underarm, other than wood, adjustable or fixed, pair, with pads, tips, and handgrips, whenever Dr. Calender bills a procedure where crutches would be necessary for the patient.

This is a perfectly legitimate and ethical way to bill for this service, provided that Dr. Calender purchased the crutches and is billing it to the payer or patient as a "pass-through" expense. Virtually no payers include the cost of the crutches with any other CPT code because of

WARNING

Check with individual payer guidelines prior to submitting claims for supplies.

the wide variety of crutches that are available and variability of cost associated with the devices. However, ignorance within the practice concerning the service being provided can result in unethical overbilling of services.

The only code in the CPT book that facilitates supply billing is 99070—Supplies and materials, provided by the physician over and above those usually included with the office visit or other services rendered (list drugs, trays, supplies, or materials provided). Because this is a single code, it means that it is virtually impossible for the provider to communicate the nature and cost of the device to the third-party payers without submitting a manual claim and, perhaps, submitting an invoice that proves the cost of supplying the device. Therefore, the billing of HCPCS codes is preferable because it communicates to the payers in a far more detailed and specific manner than is possible with the use of 99070. In addition, it is more likely to result in an ethical billing approach because it removes the variability associated with the code reporting.

Thinking It Through 6.5

1. Do you believe that the CPT guidelines for the billing of supplies are sufficiently clear to help coders avoid ethical problems? Why or why not?

2. What are the possible ethical problems associated with different payer rules for the billing of supplies?

3. Why do you believe there is only one code in the CPT book suitable for billing supplies? Is this adequate? Why or why not?

CHAPTER REVIEW

Chapter Summary

Learning Outcomes	Key Concepts/Examples

6.1 Detail the components that are ethically billed in conjunction with global surgical procedure codes. Pages 176–186	• The CPT code book specifies that each of the codes in the surgical section includes eight different components.
	• The services included in these components are broken into three large groupings:
	  1. Preoperative
	  2. Intraoperative
	  3. Postoperative
	• There are substantial differences between the CPT definition of the postoperative period and the Medicare definition of the postoperative period.
	  1. Medicare specifies postoperative period by the number of days; CPT does not.
	  2. Medicare does not allow for billing of complications, unless a return to the operating room is required; CPT allows for billing of complications provided in any setting.

Learning Outcomes	Key Concepts/Examples
6.2 Ethically apply the principles of bundling and unbundling to surgical CPT codes. Pages 186–195	• The principle of bundling is based on the fact that it is not appropriate to bill for every element provided in the course of a procedure. Unbundling is defined as either of the following: 1. Separately billing for the individual components of a single procedure. 2. Billing for multiple procedures when performed during the same encounter, when one or more of the procedures is a component of one of the other procedures. • A separate procedure designation indicates that the procedure is usually performed as part of another, more significant procedure. • A common convention in CPT coding is the concept of parent–child codes. Sometimes codes in this type of relationship can be billed together when performed during the same encounter. However, they often cannot be billed together. • The National Correct Coding Initiative (NCCI) is a tool to identify codes that cannot be billed together when performed during the same encounter.
6.3 List the modifiers used to facilitate ethical billing for services that are normally bundled with another procedure. Pages 195–205	• The purpose of modifiers is to provide a means to report or indicate that a service or procedure that has been performed has been altered by some specific circumstance, but not changed in its definition or code. • Some of the modifiers that are used to facilitate appropriate billing are: 1. −59 2. −24 3. −26 4. −52 5. −53 6. −22
6.4 Explain the ethical risk of improper code selection and the incorrect usage of unlisted procedure codes. Pages 205–211	• Recent advances in medical treatment have increased the number of treatment methodologies available to physicians. Special care must be taken to ensure that the proper code for the method use is selected. • Unlisted codes must be used when there is no specific code that describes the procedure performed. This can often result in unethical behavior by coders because of the difficulties associated with obtaining payment for unlisted procedures. • The introduction of Category III codes has helped reduce the number of unlisted codes that must be used to describe new procedures.
6.5 Evaluate the circumstances in which the separate billing of supplies is and is not ethical. Pages 211–214.	• Supplies that are ordinarily used in the course of a procedure cannot be billed separately by providers. • Supplies that are over and above those ordinarily used in a procedure can be billed separately, usually using HCPCS Level II codes. • Different third-party payers may have specific rules that allow or prohibit the billing of certain supply codes. • The only available CPT code to use for billing of supplies is 99070.

End-of-Chapter Questions

Multiple Choice

Circle the letter that best completes the statement or answers the question.

1. **LO 6.1** In the surgical section of the CPT code book, which section comes next in the following sequence: integumentary, musculoskeletal, respiratory, cardiovascular, _____?

    a. Digestive

    b. Urinary

    c. Hemic and lymphatic

    d. Male genital system

2. **LO 6.1** Which of the following is *not* a concept included in the global surgical procedure?

   a. Preoperative services
   b. Operative services
   c. Postoperative services
   d. Surgical supplies

3. **LO 6.1** When deciding whether a service is included as part of a global procedure code, which of the following is *not* a consideration?

   a. Is the service usually provided in conjunction with the procedure?
   b. Is the service significant and separately identifiable from the primary procedure?
   c. Is the provider qualified to perform the procedure?
   d. Is there documentation of the service in the medical record?

4. **LO 6.1** Which of the following is true regarding procedures with a 10-day postoperative period?

   a. They tend to be minor procedures, such as needle biopsies, endoscopic procedures, and certain laparoscopic codes.
   b. There are two postoperative visits that are built into the reimbursement for these procedures.
   c. The concept of the 10-day postoperative period was created by commercial insurers and does not apply to Medicare patients.
   d. Any service provided within 10 days of the procedure can be billed separately without a modifier.

5. **LO 6.2** Which of the following is *not* true regarding codes with a separate procedure designation?

   a. They usually are procedures that can be done in conjunction with other procedures through the same incision.
   b. They usually represent a procedure carried out as an integral part of a larger procedure.
   c. They can never be billed in conjunction with another procedure.
   d. They occur most commonly with procedures that involve the abdomen or pelvis.

6. **LO 6.2** Which of the following is true regarding parent–child codes?

   a. It is not possible to bill two codes from the same set of parent–child codes.
   b. The primary purpose is to save space in the CPT code book.
   c. The primary purpose is to save space in the ICD-9 code book.
   d. The parent code is not directly associated with the indented child codes.

7. **LO 6.2** It is unethical to bill for multiple procedures during the same operative session when

   a. The lesser procedure was performed, but it was not significant
   b. The lesser procedure is an integral part of the larger procedure
   c. The lesser procedures are not reflected in the operative report
   d. All are unethical

8. **LO 6.3** Which of the following is the primary purpose of modifier usage?

   a. To obtain additional payment for a service
   b. To indicate that a procedure has been altered in some way
   c. To indicate that a claim must be submitted manually (on paper)
   d. To indicate that a specific code does not exist to describe the service provided

9. **LO 6.3** The primary purpose of the −59 modifier is to

   a. Report a discontinued procedure
   b. Report a service separately that is usually bundled with another procedure
   c. Report the technical component of a procedure
   d. Obtain extra payment for a particularly difficult procedure

10. **LO 6.3** The biggest risk of not using a −26 modifier is
    a. Overpayment
    b. Underpayment
    c. Duplicate reimbursement for a single provider
    d. Claim denial

11. **LO 6.3** The −22 modifier should be added to a procedure code when
    a. The service is at least 10% greater than usually provided
    b. The service is at least 25% greater than usually provided
    c. The service is at least 40% greater than usually provided
    d. The provider feels it is appropriate

12. **LO 6.4** The relative values for the same procedure done via different methods are
    a. Widely variable
    b. Approximately the same
    c. Exactly equal
    d. No pattern can be determined

13. **LO 6.4** Category III CPT codes were introduced in
    a. 1992
    b. 1997
    c. 2001
    d. 2005

14. **LO 6.5** The Healthcare Common Procedure Coding System (HCPCS) is managed by
    a. AMA (American Medical Association)
    b. CMS (Centers for Medicare and Medicaid Services)
    c. WHO (World Health Organization)
    d. AHA (American Hospital Association)

15. **LO 6.5** When billing for supplies, the biggest difficulty is defining
    a. Supplies
    b. Medically necessary
    c. Usually provided
    d. The correct HCPCS code

Short Answer

Use your critical thinking skills to answer the following questions.

1. **LO 6.1** Explain why or why not the concept of global procedure billing is an effective means to control inappropriate and unethical billing practices.

2. **LO 6.1** What must occur for a preprocedure service to be separately billable, as opposed to being part of the global service?

3. **LO 6.1** Explain why varying definitions of "typical" postoperative services can result in ethical dilemmas.

4. **LO 6.1** Is Medicare's policy regarding the treatment of postoperative complications fair and effective? Why or why not?

5. **LO 6.2** Discuss the concept of billing all of the services and let the payers determine what they will and won't pay. List and discuss the pros and cons of this philosophy.

6. **LO 6.2** Discuss the issue of code selection and the management of accounts receivable.

7. **LO 6.2** Describe the difference between Column 1/Column 2 edits and mutually exclusive edits in the Correct Coding Initiative.

8. **LO 6.3** Discuss the possible benefits of ICD-10-CM implementation in conjunction with reporting services that require a modifier.

9. **LO 6.3** Discuss the particular ethical risks associated with modifier −52.

10. **LO 6.3** Describe the biggest compliance risk associated with procedural coding and list some possible options for managing that risk.

11. **LO 6.4** Explain why code compromise is or is not a good idea in relation to code selection.

12. **LO 6.4** Explain the risks and benefits in using unlisted codes.

13. **LO 6.4** Describe the factors involved in the performance of a risk versus reward analysis concerning appealing a claim with a −22 modifier attached.

14. **LO 6.5** Describe the three factors that must be met before a supply can appropriately be billed.

Applying Your Knowledge

At the beginning of this chapter, you were introduced to Margaret, who was responsible for billing for services provided by a general surgeon. The issue addressed was the nature and quantity of E/M services billed in connection with surgical services provided by the physician. While on the surface it may appear to be an issue with regard to E/M services, the major issue in this case is the application of billing rules related to procedural billing.

In reviewing this case, it is incorrect to automatically assume that something unethical or even incorrect is taking place. At this point, the only thing known for certain is that billing patterns have changed. It is possible that billing practices prior to the recent changes were incorrect and that the changes are now bringing the practice into compliance with standard billing protocols for surgical services. It is a major error on the part of many coders to assume that errors or unethical behavior is occurring before a full analysis of the circumstances surrounding the billing has been completed.

According to the case study, Margaret is assigning codes for surgical services using the operative reports. However, she is billing for E/M services based on the superbills or charge tickets completed by the physician. Before Margaret can fully decide the appropriateness of the billing practices, she has to see the progress notes for the E/M services that she believes are associated with the surgical procedure.

1. What might Margaret find in the E/M service notes that may confirm or change her opinion regarding Dr. Smitkins's billing for these services that occur after a surgical procedure?

2. Would there be any advantage or disadvantage in looking at the physician's presurgical E/M notes?

3. If the physician is billing inappropriately, what specific issues and supporting documentation should Margaret bring to his attention to convince him to change his billing practices?

4. What are the possible reasons that the physician may choose to bill in an inappropriate fashion?

5. Margaret's job is the sole financial support for her family and she can sense that the physician is becoming agitated regarding the discussion of this subject. What approaches can she take to stop inappropriate billing (if it exists) without losing her job?

Throughout this chapter a number of illustrations of the RBRVS table, as available on the Medicare website at www.cms.gov, are provided. This is the most easily accessible and cost-effective tool available to help facilitate proper and ethical procedure billing. Several elements in Figure 6.14 support ethical billing. Those areas are:

Global Days: This column indicates how many days, postprocedure, are included in the reimbursement for the particular CPT code. Most codes have 0, 10, or 90 global days, although add-on codes such as 58611 (noted as ZZZ) have no global period. Their global period is based on the code to which they are attached. Some codes also have an indication of YYY, which means that the global period is determined by the payer because the unlisted nature of the code makes it quite variable.

Preop, Intraop, Postop: This column reflects what percentage of the total reimbursement for the procedure is allocated to the three components of the service. This is particularly important if a surgeon does not provide the total service. For example, if a surgeon at a major medical center performs an emergency surgery on a patient from a rural area, she may provide the postoperative service for this patient. In that case, the surgeon would bill the service with a −54 modifier (Surgical Care only). The physician would receive only the percentage allocated to intraoperative care.

Multiple Procedure, Bilateral Procedure, Assistant Surgeon, Co-Surgeon: The indicators in these columns reflect if and/or when a procedure can be billed in various circumstances. Table 6.12 supplies the definition of each of these indicators.

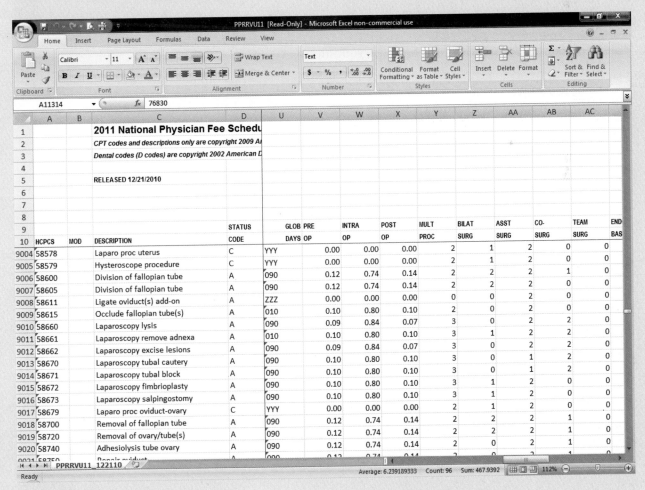

FIGURE 6.14

A small sample of the RBRVS table, which is available on the Medicare website.

Table 6.12 Some RBRVS Table Indicators

Indicator	0	1	2	3
Multiple Procedure	No adjustment for multiple procedures	Rules in effect before 1/1/95 apply	Standard payment rules apply	Special rules for endoscopic procedures apply
Bilateral Procedure	Generally not applicable	150% of primary procedure allowed	Not applicable—procedure is already defined as bilateral	Not applicable—generally applies to radiology procedures
Assistant Surgeon	Allowed only if documentation supports billing	Assistant never allowable	Assistant is allowable	N/A
Co-Surgeon	Co-surgeon not permitted	Co-surgeon can be paid if documentation supports	Co-surgeons permitted	N/A

The accessibility of this information on the Internet is an important tool for providers and coders to submit claims appropriately and ethically.

Look up each of the following CPT codes in the RBRVS table for the current year:

a.   45382

b.   58925

c.   22226

d.   15736

Based on your findings, answer the following questions.

1.   Will there be an adjustment when this procedure is done as part of multiple procedures during the same encounter?

2.   Can this procedure be billed bilaterally?

3.   Can an assistant surgeon's services be billed for this procedure?

4.   Can a co-surgeon's services be billed for this procedure?

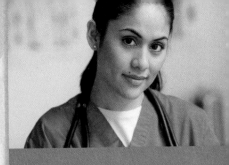

Coding Ethics and Diagnoses

7

LEARNING OUTCOMES

After completing this chapter, you will be able to:

7.1 Summarize the basic principles of diagnosis coding, using ICD-9-CM codes, including the commonly used conventions.

7.2 Interpret the diagnosis coding guidelines that are applicable to various circumstances.

7.3 Evaluate ethical dilemmas associated with the intentional misuse of diagnosis codes, in both the inpatient and outpatient context.

7.4 Analyze circumstances in which ethical dilemmas are created by omitting or failing to report key diagnosis information.

7.5 Differentiate between circumstances that appear to be ethically challenged and circumstances that are ethically appropriate.

Key Terms

Acute condition

Chronic condition

Comorbidity (CC)

Diagnosis-related group (DRG)

Differential diagnoses

Essential modifier

Nonessential modifier

Extrapolation

Late effect

Medical necessity

Neoplasm

Principal diagnosis

Sign

Symptom

CASE STUDY

Evelyn just started her new job as a customer service representative in the Billing Department at a large multispecialty clinic. Her first call was from an extremely irate patient, who believed that his service was going to be covered by his insurance. The claim was denied and he had called the insurer to ask why. The insurance company representative told him that if the provider had used a different diagnosis code, the claim would have been payable. The patient loudly informed Evelyn that the insurance company representative said that "they had used the *wrong* diagnosis!" He insisted that they change the diagnosis and resubmit the claim so that he would not be responsible for this bill.

Evelyn put the patient on hold and asked the person training her about what she should do in this situation. The trainer told her that they were evaluated, in part, on the ratings obtained from the practice's Patient Satisfaction Survey Program. Evelyn was told that it was best to do whatever it took to satisfy the patient. She was not comfortable doing so, but she told the patient that she would forward this request to a person who would find a payable diagnosis for the claim. The patient indicated that he was satisfied and he hung up. Evelyn was uneasy, but soon forgot the matter as she took a series of more patient telephone calls.

1. What are the factors that created this particular situation?
2. Should Evelyn be uneasy about her actions in this case?
3. What is the best way to resolve this type of situation?

Introduction

Assignment of the proper diagnosis code is a critical element of the medical coding process. As indicated in Chapter 1, the purpose of the diagnosis code is to answer the question "Why?" Specifically, "Why is the patient receiving the services that he or she received during the encounter in question?" In the American health care system, the diagnosis code, in large part, supplies the information needed for the payer to determine the medical necessity of a procedure or service. The diagnosis code can indicate either that the patient has a condition that requires the service, or it supplies an explanation as to why the service was provided.

At first glance, this sounds like a reasonable and straightforward process. However, for a number of reasons, there are complications and ethical challenges that exist in the process of selecting diagnosis codes, ranging from the quality and quantity of the documentation provided to the selection of each code itself.

7.1 The Basics of Diagnosis Coding

The diagnosis coding system used in the United States is based on the World Health Organization's (WHO) ninth revision of the International Classification of Diseases (ICD-9). WHO's purpose for ICD-9

> **FYI**
>
> In the United States, the *Clinical Modification* was added to the *International Classification of Diseases, Ninth Revision* (ICD-9) because the standard ICD system is not specific enough for claim reporting.

Table 7.1 ICD-9 Codes Published by WHO Versus the ICD-9 Clinical Modification

ICD-9 Code	Description	ICD-9-CM Code	Description
216	Benign neoplasm of skin	216.0	Skin of lip
		216.1	Eyelid
		216.2	Ear
		216.3	Face
		216.4	Neck
		+ 5 other codes	
451	Phlebitis and thrombophlebitis	451.0	Superficial vessels, lower extremities
		451.11	Femoral vein
		451.2	Lower extremities, unspecified
		451.83	Deep veins of upper extremities
		+ 6 other codes	
640	Hemorrhage in early pregnancy	640.03	Threatened abortion, antepartum
		640.80	Oth specified hemorrhage in early pregnancy, unspec.
		640.90	Unspec. hemorrhage in early pregnancy, unspec.
		+ 6 other codes	
784	Symptoms involving head and neck	784.0	Headache
		784.2	Swelling, mass or lump in head/neck
		784.51	Dysarthria
		784.7	Epistaxis
		+ 17 other codes	
824	Fracture of ankle	824.0	Medial malleolus, closed
		824.4	Bimalleolar, closed
		824.7	Trimalleolar, open
		+ 7 other codes	

is to classify morbidity and mortality information for statistical and other tracking purposes. This system is not sufficient to report services in the clinical setting because of its lack of specificity, which is the reason for the Clinical Modification that has been attached to the basic ICD-9 framework. Table 7.1 offers examples of the additional specificity provided by the CM addition to ICD-9.

THE DESIGN, MAINTENANCE, AND CONVENTIONS OF ICD-9-CM

Modifications to ICD-9-CM are made through the ICD-9-CM Coordination and Maintenance Committee (C&M). This committee is made up of representatives from two governmental agencies within the U.S. Department of Health and Human Services (HHS)—the National Center for Health Statistics (NCHS) and the Centers for Medicare and Medicaid Services (CMS) (Buck, 2010). These governmental agencies receive and welcome input from interested parties, who are instructed to submit requests for modification to the ICD-9-CM codes at least two

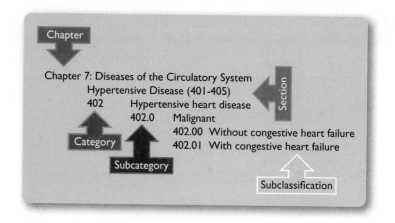

months prior to a scheduled meeting of the C&M Committee, which is open to the public (Centers for Medicare and Medicaid Services [CMS], 2010c). Code change requests need to occur within the context of the primary ICD-9 framework. Therefore, new three-digit code sections can't be created—generally, only greater diagnostic specificity can be achieved by adding a fourth and/or fifth digit to an already existing three-digit ICD-9 code section (Figure 7.1).

In conjunction with the ICD-9-CM codes, the federal government prints the *ICD-9-CM Official Guidelines for Coding and Reporting.* These are specific instructions developed to accompany and support the official conventions and instructions provided within ICD-9-CM itself. The guidelines are formulated in conjunction with four organizations that make up the cooperating parties for ICD-9-CM:

- American Hospital Association (AHA).
- American Health Information Management Association (AHIMA).
- Centers for Medicare and Medicaid Services (CMS).
- National Center for Health Statistics (NCHS).

Changes are made to the diagnosis codes every year, with the changes put into effect on October 1 of that year. Those changes are made in three different ways—additions, deletions, and revisions. Additions include new codes (usually new fourth- and fifth-digit codes within existing categories and subcategories) and additional explanatory information in connection with the codes. Deletions include changing a subcategory code that is valid for use to an invalid code by placing one or more subclassification codes beneath it, or deleting instructional or explanatory notes. For example, in 2010, 999.7 was a valid ICD-9-CM code suitable for usage. It was deleted as a usable diagnosis in 2011 because 10 new codes were added beneath it (999.70, 999.71, 999.72, etc.). Revisions are made when the language of the code itself or the explanatory materials associated with that code are modified in some fashion.

Conventions for the Alphabetic Index. The ICD-9-CM manual is divided into three volumes, as follows:

- Volume 1: Tabular (Numeric) List.
- Volume 2: Alphabetic Index.
- Volume 3: ICD-9-CM Procedure Codes.

Volumes 1 and 2 were designated by the Health Insurance Portability and Accountability Act (HIPAA) for use in all health care settings. Volume 3 procedure codes are used for inpatient procedures reported by hospitals. When the ICD-9-CM code book is obtained, unless specified otherwise, the book is likely a combination of Volumes 1 and 2. In most cases, Volume 2 (the Alphabetic Index) appears first, followed by the Tabular List (Volume 1).

The Alphabetic Index (Volume 2) is substantially larger in size than Volume 1 because it includes a variety of diagnostic terms that could conceivably be used. The Tabular List includes a much narrower set of terminology. The purpose of Volume 2 is to help identify the correct code in Volume 1. It absolutely must not be used as the sole means by which a code is selected, because it can easily result in an incorrect code choice, as in the following example of Diane.

Example

Diane is a 29-year-old female patient who is currently pregnant. The physician wrote on her superbill "cervical abnormality." The physician's coder went to Volume 1 of ICD-9-CM and found the following entry:

Abnormal, abnormality, abnormalities

Cervix

In pregnancy or childbirth 654.6x

Since the patient was still pregnant, the coder assigned diagnosis code 654.63.

If the coder in Diane's case had gone to the Tabular List in Volume 1, he would have found several codes that can describe abnormalities of the cervix. If the coder had reviewed the chart, he would have found that the patient's exact condition was "cervical incompetence." Volume 1 has a code for this specific condition—654.53. While this is not ethically inappropriate, it is a clear indication of improper coding, which resulted from exclusive use of Volume 2.

Several conventions are applicable to the Alphabetical Index that, if followed, will help produce correct and ethical diagnosis code selection. The first convention is "nonessential modifiers." These words are enclosed in parentheses and help explain or clarify the usage of the code. It is not necessary that these modifiers have a complete (or any) relationship to the patient's condition. In short, they supply suggestions as to possible locations or types of a given condition.

Example

Ileus—(adynamic) (bowel) (colon) (inhibitory) (intestine) (neurogenic) (paralytic) 560.1

The condition in the example (an intestinal obstruction) may take a variety of forms and may be found in a variety of locations. The Alphabetic Index provides suggestions as to what some of these variations might be.

WARNING

If a code in the Alphabetic Index has an essential modifier, the patient must have the condition described by the modifier to use that code.

Essential modifier
Describes a condition that must be present to use the parent code.

Nonessential modifier
Describes a condition that may be present, but is not required, for the code to be used.

CODING TIP

When finding codes in the Alphabetic Index, anatomic sites are not primary categories. The key is to look up the condition and then find more specific information under that primary category.

An **essential modifier** is not enclosed in parentheses and does affect the selection of the code. Single codes can have both essential and **nonessential modifiers** within the Alphabetic Index. An example of both essential and nonessential modifiers is the listing for code 787.24.

Example

Incoordination

Esophageal-pharyngeal (newborn) 787.24

To use code 787.24, esophageal-pharyngeal incoordination must exist. Most often it occurs in newborns (hence the nonessential modifier), but it can occur in other patients as well. It is not inappropriate to use this code for an adult, provided he or she has the condition.

The Alphabetic Index is organized by main terms. Those main terms generally fall within one of four categories:

- Diseases—influenza, bronchitis.
- Conditions—fatigue, fracture, or injury.
- Nouns—disturbance or syndrome.
- Adjectives—double, large, small. (Office of Compliance, Privacy & Internal Audit, 2010)

A common mistake made by many users is to look in the Alphabetic Index for anatomic sites. Anatomic sites are usually found as subcategories in the appropriate disease or condition main term. Also, it is important to understand that conditions and the associated ICD-9-CM codes can be found in multiple locations in the Alphabetic Index. For example, ICD-9-CM code 632 (Missed Abortion) can be found under six different major headings in the Alphabetic Index, and more in subheadings.

Example

Abortion (complete) (incomplete) (inevitable) (with retained products of conception)

Missed 632

Dead

Fetus

Early pregnancy (death before 22 weeks gestation) 632

Delivery

Cesarean section

Complicated by

Death of fetus

Early 632

Fetal

Death

Early 632

Intrauterine fetal death

Early 632

Missed

    Abortion 632

Pregnancy (single) (uterine) (without sickness)

    Complicated by

        Intrauterine fetal death

            Early 632

        Missed

            Abortion 632

    Management, affected by

        Fetal

            Death

                Early 632

    Retention, retained

    Dead

        Fetus

            Early fetal death 632

    Products of conception

        Early pregnancy 632

Conventions for the Tabular List. Throughout the Tabular List (Volume 1), conventions appear that provide consistency in instruction and guidance as to the proper usage of the ICD-9-CM codes. The first are designated "notes," which define terms or give coding instruction. An example is found immediately following the first chapter heading in the Tabular List:

Example

1. INFECTIOUS AND PARASITIC DISEASES (001–139)

Note: Categories for "late effects" of infectious and parasitic diseases are to be found at 137–139

Use Additional Code. A second convention in the Tabular List is the instructional term "use additional code." The purpose of this device is to provide a more complete picture of the patient's illness. When the "use additional code" instruction is included and the criteria in the instructions are met, it is not an optional choice—it is required to most correctly and effectively code.

Example

510 Empyema

    Use additional code to identify infectious organism (041.0–041.9)

Empyema is a collection of pus, usually found in the chest. The purpose of the secondary diagnosis is to explain what infectious organism

CODING TIP

Some of the instructions and conventions in the Tabular List are not optional. For example, when phrases such as "use additional code" or "code first" appear in conjunction with a code, more than one diagnosis code is required to properly report the service.

(type of bacteria) is causing the collection of pus. This can be important because, based on the type of bacteria, it can reflect the relative severity of the patient's condition. If a patient has empyema with a fistula (510.0), caused by Methicillin-resistant *Staphylococcus aureus* (MRSA) (041.12), the condition is much more severe than if it were another type of bacteria. In this way, the correct application of diagnosis codes provides the medical necessity support for more intensive treatment. In addition, it provides a more complete and accurate reflection of the patient's condition.

Code First. "Code first" is another nonoptional instructional term. In this case, the code in question is in italics, which indicates that it cannot be a primary code. Instead, it is a secondary code and instructions for finding the possible primary codes are supplied.

Example

366.41 *Diabetic cataract*

Code first diabetes (249.5, 250.5)

If, for example, this code (366.41) is used as a primary diagnosis, the claim would be denied for having an invalid diagnosis. In addition, it provides an incomplete picture concerning the medical necessity for the treatment or services provided.

Code, If Applicable. There is also a coding instruction that is similar to "code first," but is optional or may not be applicable in every situation. This instruction usually appears as "code, if applicable."

Example

428 Heart failure

Code, if applicable, heart failure due to hypertension first (402.0–402.9, with fifth digit 1 or 404.0–404.9 with fifth digit 1 or 3)

If the patient does not have heart failure due to hypertension, then the use of the additional codes is not appropriate or required. The code from this section is appropriate as a primary diagnosis if there is no other coexisting condition.

Excludes. An important term in the tabular section of the book is "excludes." Anytime this language appears beneath a code, it means "do not use this code" if the patient has one of the conditions following "excludes."

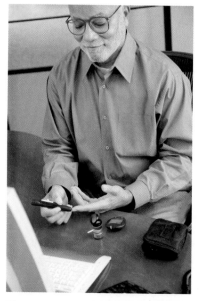

The instructional note to "code first" indicates that a particular condition must be present, documented, and coded before the original term can be reported. In the case of coding for a diabetic cataract, the coder must code first for diabetes, since it is an underlying condition.

Example

150.2 (Malignant neoplasm of) Abdominal Esophagus

Excludes: *adenocarcinoma (151.0)*

Cardio-esophageal junction (151.0)

If the patient has either a neoplasm in the form of adenocarcinoma or it is located at the cardio-esophageal junction, then 150.2 is the incorrect ICD-9-CM code. Specific instruction is given to look at diagnosis code 151.0 if either of these conditions exists.

Includes. Whenever "includes" appears, it is simply a clarification or further definition of the contents of the code. It does not mean that the condition has to exist, but if it does exist, this code should be used to report the condition.

Example

087 Relapsing fever

    Includes: recurrent fever

STOP WARNING

If the word "and" appears in the description of a valid code, then both conditions must be present for that code to be used.

And. In some cases, the word "and" appears in the code description. This can seem somewhat misleading in that if "and" appears as a category header, it can mean that the code can be assigned if the patient has *either* of the two conditions listed or *both* of the conditions listed.

Example

474 Chronic disease of tonsils and adenoids

    474.00 Chronic tonsillitis

    474.01 Chronic adenoiditis

    474.02 Chronic tonsillitis and adenoiditis

However, if the word "and" appears in the code description of a valid code, then *both* conditions must be present for that code to be assigned.

With. If the word "with" appears in the code description, both conditions must exist for a code in that category or subcategory to be used.

Example

366.4 Cataract associated with other disorders

Beneath this subcategory there are additional codes, most of which are in italics, which means that they can be used only as secondary codes to a primary diagnosis. All of those codes have the "code first" instructions beneath them to facilitate correct and accurate coding.

Not Elsewhere Classifiable (NEC). Within the ICD-9-CM coding system, an important term is "not elsewhere classifiable" ("NEC"). This means that the provider has a confirmed diagnosis for a patient, but no code exists that precisely describes the condition. It is impossible for there to be a code that adequately describes every condition that a provider might encounter. However, the framework of the system has sufficient structure to allow for the reporting of diagnoses with reasonable specificity. A common synonym for "not elsewhere classifiable" is "other specified."

An example of an appropriate use of "NEC" is the 43-year-old female who is undergoing infertility treatment. She has been diagnosed with infertility due to her advanced age and her declining ovarian production. There is no specific "infertility" code for this condition. Therefore, the appropriate code is 628.8—Infertility, female, of other specified origin. Otherwise, any codes assigned would be either incomplete or inaccurate.

Not Otherwise Specified (NOS). When a code has "not otherwise specified" ("NOS") or "unspecified" in its description, it means that the patient has a condition that falls within the general category of diagnosis codes, but there is insufficient information known about the patient's condition to assign a specific code. This often occurs in the very early stages of treatment, before a specific diagnosis is assigned. Consider the case of Harold's visit to the emergency department.

Example

Harold, a 73-year-old male, presents to the emergency department with symptoms of heart failure. The ED physician stabilizes the patient and transfers care to the cardiologist on call. The ED physician does not follow the patient any further and, therefore, doesn't know the final diagnosis. Therefore, the ED physician assigns a diagnosis of 428.9—Heart failure, unspecified, for her services.

Another possible usage of the "unspecified" code occurs when the patient undergoes a standard diagnostic workup for a suspected condition, but all diagnostic tests come back normal or have unremarkable information. An example is the patient who is unable to achieve pregnancy, but all diagnostic tests do not provide an obvious cause of the patient's infertility. In that case, the patient's diagnosis (until a definitive diagnosis is identified) is 628.9—Infertility, female, of unspecified origin.

The Effect of ICD-10-CM on Diagnosis Coding. Effective on October 1, 2013, ICD-10-CM must be used, rather than ICD-9-CM. Although ICD-10 has a completely different format for its codes and there are a dramatically larger number of codes than ICD-9, the majority of the basic principles in code usage remain the same. For more specific details, see Chapter 8.

The transition from ICD-9 to ICD-10 produces a significant level of difficulty as coders lose the familiarity with ICD-9 that they developed over a number of years. In addition, ICD-10 requires the development of different communication systems to transmit the higher level of detail concerning the patient's condition from the provider to the coder and biller.

1. Four organizations are involved in managing the ICD-9-CM coding system. Explain the interest of each of these organizations in this code set.

2. Describe the differences between an essential and a nonessential modifier.

3. Explain the purpose of italicized codes. Why can't they be used as primary diagnoses?

7.2 Guidelines for ICD-9-CM Coding and Reporting

To assist both providers and coders in the proper (and ethical) use of ICD-9-CM codes, CMS and NCHS publish the *ICD-9-CM Official Guidelines for Coding and Reporting.* The instructions and conventions described previously are the primary tool by which to make code selections. However, there are occasions in which additional guidance is required and that is the purpose of the published guidelines. If there is ever a conflict between the instructions or conventions and the guidelines, the instructions/conventions take precedence.

The guidelines document is divided into several sections and subsections. Section 1 outlines the conventions, which were previously discussed, the general guidelines, and the chapter-specific guidelines. Section 2 provides guidance regarding the selection of the **principal diagnosis.** Section 3 gives direction concerning the reporting of additional diagnoses, beyond the principal diagnosis, whereas Section 4 focuses on the coding and reporting guidelines for services provided in the outpatient setting.

> **FYI**
>
> The term "principal" diagnosis is used most frequently with inpatient hospital services, while the term "primary" diagnosis is used most frequently with outpatient services. The principal diagnosis is the condition that prompted the hospitalization. The primary diagnosis is the condition that is chiefly responsible for the encounter.

Principal diagnosis
The condition chiefly responsible for causing the admission of the patient to the hospital.

GENERAL CODING GUIDELINES

The coding guidelines begin by reiterating the importance of using both the Alphabetic Index and the Tabular List in code selection. Reliance on only one or the other can easily result in errors in code assignment and, at best, suboptimal levels of specificity in coding (CMS, 2009). Emphasis is also placed on the level of detail required to accurately report services. Diagnosis codes can have three, four, or five digits. If fourth or fifth digits are available, they *must* be reported and it is erroneous to submit a three-digit diagnosis when fourth or fifth digits are available. On the other hand, it is also incorrect to add fourth and fifth digits to codes that are intended to be only three digits in length.

Signs and Symptoms. One of the most important elements of proper diagnosis coding is recognizing that sign and symptom codes are available for use. Most medical education programs instruct medical students to think in terms of **differential diagnoses.** Part of identifying the correct diagnosis is "ruling out" various options. Unfortunately for new providers, there are no diagnosis codes that report the rule-out concept. In cases in which a physician performs or orders a test for the purpose of confirming or ruling out a particular diagnosis, there is no specific code for that particular purpose.

Differential diagnoses
A list of possible diagnoses, based on the symptoms present, that are gradually ruled out until the final diagnosis is determined.

Consider the case of a visit to the emergency room for appendicitis.

Example

A 47-year-old male presented to the ER with severe pain in the lower right abdomen. The physician ordered an ultrasound to determine if the patient had appendicitis. The ordering system requires the physician to put in a diagnosis to justify the purpose of the ultrasound. The physician entered "rule out appendicitis." The coder in the radiology department, using only the information on the order sheet, assigned a diagnosis of 541—Appendicitis, unqualified.

This could be the correct diagnosis and it would likely be a payable diagnosis by most third-party payers. However, it is not the correct diagnosis based on the information available to the coder. In this case, a code for signs or symptoms from the "Sign and Symptom" section of the ICD-9-CM book is the appropriate option.

Signs are physical manifestations that can be felt, heard, measured, or observed by medical professionals. Signs include fever, hypertension, abnormal lab results, and so forth. **Symptoms** are abnormal physical experiences that are subjective in nature. They cannot be seen or confirmed by health care providers, although it does not make them any less real or legitimate. Symptoms include pain, discomfort, vertigo, nausea, and so on.

Sign
Physical manifestation that can be felt, heard, measured, or observed by medical professionals.

Symptom
Abnormal physical experience, subjective in nature, that cannot be seen or confirmed by health care providers.

Ethical Responsibility in Diagnosis Code Usage

The Health Insurance Portability and Accountability Act (HIPAA) of 1996 requires that ICD-9-CM be used as the definitive diagnostic code set for the submission of claims in the United States. However, HIPAA does not require the parties who use these codes to interpret them in a consistent fashion or to use them in any sort of standard format. It is also not possible to know, without individual review of each record, whether the most specific possible diagnosis has been used.

One element of ethical behavior is being aware of your responsibilities and conducting yourself in a professional manner. Being unfamiliar with coding rules and guidelines and being unfamiliar with codes, by design or by accident, has unethical overtones. If it is done by design, it is clearly unethical. If it is done by accident and ignorance, it is also unethical because insufficient attention to professional responsibility will often result in outcomes that benefit the party, but harm those to whom a duty is owed.

The payer has a responsibility to both the patient and the provider to properly process claims with proper diagnoses. If a payer improperly denies a claim based on the diagnosis submitted, the payer benefits but the provider (and possibly the patient) loses. Providers are also harmed if the payer does not properly consider the diagnosis and pays a claim that should not be covered under the terms of the patient's policy. If the provider submits a claim with an improper diagnosis, the provider "wins" but the payer loses.

Providers often submit inaccurate or incomplete diagnoses simply because the correct diagnosis does not appear on the provider's superbill. Some practices take the shortcut of using only the diagnoses that are on the superbill and, if the patient has a different diagnosis that is not on the superbill, the "closest" diagnosis is used. This is not ethical because it mischaracterizes the nature of the encounter and may cause harm to the patient in the future because the billing and the medical record are not consistent.

The three parties in the transaction (patient, provider, and payer) all have ethical responsibilities related to diagnosis code usage. While little can be done, beyond education, to influence the patient's ethical outlook, the payer and provider, as professionals, do have a significant responsibility to the others (Figure 7.2).

Responsibility in Diagnosis Code Assignment

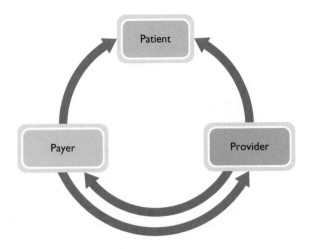

These sign and symptom codes are found in Chapter 16 of the ICD-9-CM book, which spans ICD-9-CM codes 780–799. These codes cover anything from a loss of consciousness, to fever, to swelling, to pain, to abnormal lab results, and many other possible issues. In the example of the patient with abdominal pain, the correct diagnosis, based on the information available, is 789.03—Abdominal pain, right lower quadrant. The diagnosis is sufficient to obtain payment for services rendered, but it does not overstate, misstate, or mischaracterize the patient's condition. If a diagnosis of 541 was assigned and the patient did not actually have appendicitis, an incorrect diagnosis would have been submitted.

This can be a much more significant problem if certain diagnoses are assigned to a patient in the absence of that condition. For example, if a patient went to her OB/GYN to have a Pap smear to screen for cervical cancer and the coder assigned a diagnosis of 180.0—Malignant neoplasm of the cervix, endocervix, instead of V76.2—Special screening for malignant neoplasms, cervix, the patient could experience significant difficulty in obtaining insurance (either health or life) at some point in the future. In this case, the incorrect assignment of a diagnosis could negatively impact the patient because it mischaracterizes her condition, interfering in some future activity or preventing her from receiving a needed service in the future. It also could cause claim denials or, at best, delay payment. Consider the case of Allan's visit to his physician.

WARNING

Selecting an incorrect diagnosis code can not only result in claim denials, it also can cause serious problems for the patient in attempting to obtain health or life insurance in the future.

Example

Allan, a 67-year-old man, went to his family practice physician to follow up on a previous incidence of liver enlargement. The diagnosis marked on the superbill was 789.1—Hepatomegaly. However, when the charge was entered, it was posted as 798.1—Instantaneous death. The claim was denied by the insurer because it felt it unlikely that the physician would bill a Level 3 E/M code in connection with a patient who died in the office. The insurer also submitted an inquiry to the provider because it wanted to know how the patient who died in the office received more E/M services three days later.

Signs and symptoms are not exclusively limited to Chapter 16 of the ICD-9-CM book. They can be found throughout the book, in context in the various chapters, based on the disease and/or organ system. Some examples include:

286.6x—Elevated white blood cell count

338—Pain, not elsewhere classified

369.6x—Profound impairment, one eye

611.72—Lump or mass in breast

626.4—Irregular menstrual bleeding

In each case, the diagnosis reports a sign or a symptom but it does not explain the underlying condition, nor does it require that the underlying condition or its cause is even known.

Conditions and Their Relationship to the Disease Process. The ICD-9-CM coding guidelines indicate that it is not appropriate to report sign or symptom diagnoses that are a standard part of a given disease process, unless the instructions within the code book specifically instruct the coder to do so. On the other hand, if the patient has a condition that is not routinely associated with a disease process, it should be reported.

Example

A 17-year-old male is in an automobile accident, in which he experiences a severe fracture of the right arm. The diagnosis assigned is 813.18. The coder also assigned a diagnosis of 338.11—Acute pain due to trauma.

The 338.11 code is unnecessary because acute pain is a standard part of the original injury. The only reason to report acute pain due to trauma is if it is the primary reason for the encounter or it is beyond that which is normally a part of the condition.

Multiple Diagnosis Coding for a Single Condition. A common misconception among providers and coders is that more diagnoses are preferable to fewer diagnoses. This idea is, in part, derived from the payment system on which most inpatient hospital services are reimbursed—**diagnosis-related groups (DRGs).** To prevent the delivery of unnecessary procedural services provided solely to collect additional revenue, most inpatient hospital services are delivered on the basis of the patient's diagnosis. The concept is that the hospital is reimbursed based on the severity of the patient's condition, not how many procedures and services it can perform and deliver. Unfortunately, this establishes a whole new set of ethical dilemmas as it pertains to diagnosis code selection.

In the outpatient office setting, the number of diagnoses is not the focal point of generating reimbursement. In fact, in the outpatient world, diagnoses have nothing to do with the quantity or level of reimbursement. Instead, diagnoses are a gateway to reimbursement. Appropriate diagnoses must be supplied to justify the payment of the respective services provided to the patient. Therefore, adding multiple diagnoses to obtain higher reimbursement is a fruitless and wasteful task.

CODING TIP

Every service requires at least one diagnosis code, but it is inappropriate to report more diagnoses than are necessary to accurately describe the patient's condition at the time of service.

Diagnosis-related group (DRG)
A payment system for inpatient hospital services in which payments are issued based on the patient's diagnosis, not on the quantity of service provided to the patient.

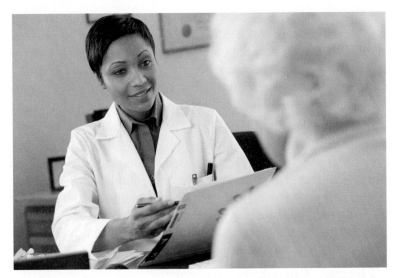

Diagnosis codes are the gateway to payment for services delivered in the outpatient setting. A provider will not receive greater payment for using one diagnosis than for another. However, if sufficient diagnoses are not provided to put the provider through the payment gateway, it is possible that no payment will be received, until and/or unless an adequate diagnosis is supplied to support the service.

The question is often asked, "How many diagnoses do I need to accurately report a service?" The answer to that question is widely variable, based on the circumstances. A simple answer to the question is, "As many as it takes to accurately characterize and report the reason for the service." Depending on the circumstance, a highly complex medical condition can be reported with a single diagnosis code while, in other cases, a relatively minor condition may require three or four diagnoses to accurately supply the medical necessity for the procedure or service.

There are certain occasions in which multiple diagnoses are required to pass the gateway. That occurs when instructions are provided to "use additional code," or "code first," or "code, if applicable" any causal condition first. Multiple codes may also be needed to report late effects, complication codes, obstetric codes, and any other condition that is not adequately described by a single code.

Acute and Chronic Conditions. An **acute condition** is one in which the symptoms are sharp, severe, or intense in effect. Examples of conditions that could be acute are appendicitis, the onset of a stroke, the onset of a myocardial infarction (heart attack), or a grand mal seizure. **Chronic conditions** are those that are constant or habitual, but may or may not be particularly intense at any given time. Examples of chronic conditions include diabetes, hypertension, depression, and urinary tract infections.

The primary difference between an acute and a chronic condition is the level of intensity or severity at the time of the encounter. An acute condition may require a higher intensity of service than a chronic condition. However, the diagnosis should correctly characterize the patient's condition. In the inpatient setting, higher reimbursement is provided for acute conditions because of the higher degree of service intensity that is required.

Acute condition
Condition in which the symptoms are sharp, severe, or intense in effect.

Chronic condition
Condition that is constant or habitual, but may or may not be particularly intense at any given time.

The situation becomes slightly more complex when a patient's chronic condition becomes acute. For example, a patient with chronic laryngitis (476.0) may completely lose his or her voice (464.0). To properly code this service, the acute condition is coded first, followed by the chronic or subacute condition. This reports the intensity of the current situation (complete loss of voice) while providing context to the situation—the patient's ongoing struggle with laryngitis.

Combination Codes. A combination code is a single code that describes two diagnoses *or* a diagnosis with a secondary process or manifestation *or* a diagnosis with an associated complication. An example of a combination code is 474.02—Chronic tonsillitis and adenoiditis. To properly use this code, the patient must have both or all of the conditions described by the particular code. If there is no combination code that supplies sufficient specificity, additional codes should be added as needed.

Late Effects. **Late effects** are remaining conditions that exist after the acute phase of an injury or illness is over. There is no time limit on late effects, and it is theoretically possible that a patient could experience late effects of an illness for the remainder of his or her life. However, it is rare for late effect codes to be used in the absence of a present symptom or illness. In that case, the current illness or symptom should be reported first, with the late effect diagnosis reported second. Basically, the secondary late effect diagnosis explains why the primary diagnosis exists or, at the very least, provides context to the current illness.

Late effect
Condition that remains after the acute phase of an injury or illness is over.

Example

Mary, a 32-year-old female, is experiencing partial fecal incontinence and smearing (787.62). She has struggled with this condition since the birth of her last child five years ago. At that time, she had a fourth-degree perineal laceration (664.31). The appropriate way to report this service is to describe her current condition (787.62), with a secondary diagnosis of 677—Late effect of complication of pregnancy, childbirth, and the puerperium. She does not have a current laceration, but she is experiencing the effect of that laceration five years after the fact.

There is no firm definition as to when a provider should begin to use a late effect code, as opposed to a current condition code. In general, the late effect code should be used when the active treatment phase is complete. The provider is responsible for making that determination.

Impending or Threatened Conditions. One challenge faced by coders occurs when confirmation of a particular condition does not exist, yet the symptoms are pointing in the direction and, if the patient doesn't yet have the condition, he or she may have it in the near future. The guidelines for selecting codes are:

- If the condition did occur, use the code as a confirmed diagnosis.
- If the condition does not actually occur, determine if there is a code for an "impending" or "threatened" condition. If so, use that code.
- If the condition does not occur and there is not a code for "impending" or "threatened," the underlying condition, signs, or symptoms should be reported. The actual condition code should never be used if the condition never occurs.

WARNING

Do not assign a diagnosis code to a patient unless there is clinical certainty that the patient actually has that condition.

Example

Consider the case of a 24-year-old woman who is 10 weeks pregnant and is experiencing significant vaginal bleeding. Given the possible outcomes, the appropriate coding pattern is as follows:

- If the patient has a miscarriage, it is coded as 634.90—Spontaneous abortion, without complication.

- If the patient does not have a miscarriage, it is coded as 640.03—Threatened abortion.

- If the threatened abortion code did not exist, the symptom code of 640.93 would be used—Unspecified hemorrhage in early pregnancy.

It is important not to assign a diagnosis code that describes a condition that the patient does not have. In the previous example, it could cause the patient significant trouble in the future if a miscarriage is reported when it never occurred. Similarly, malignant **neoplasms** should never be assigned to patients until a definitive diagnosis has been determined. Until that time, a diagnosis with an "unspecified" or "uncertain behavior" should be used. If it is determined that the patient does not have a malignant neoplasm, the patient's record does not improperly reflect a serious diagnosis that may inhibit his or her ability to obtain insurance in the future.

Neoplasm
Abnormally fast-growing tissue. Malignant neoplasms are considered cancerous in nature.

CHAPTER-SPECIFIC CODING GUIDELINES

In addition to the general coding guidelines previously discussed, there are also chapter specific coding guidelines. These guidelines apply only to codes in the section being referenced. For example, one of the first chapter-specific guidelines is related to HIV. It states that "only confirmed cases" should be assigned the HIV diagnosis code. The instructions clarify that confirmation does not mean that a positive laboratory test is required—the provider's diagnostic statement is sufficient.

The chapter-specific guidelines may give guidance as to unusual diagnosis ordering, specific coding rules for individual disease processes, or defining acute versus chronic in specific circumstances that may vary from the general guidelines. Providers and coders should be thoroughly familiar with the published ICD-9-CM coding guidelines to ensure that they are coding properly. Special attention should be paid to codes frequently used within their practice.

Thinking It Through 7.2

1. How does medical school training factor into diagnosis determination and the use of ICD-9-CM codes? How might this present a challenge for coders?

2. Explain why it is important to differentiate between acute and chronic conditions.

3. What is the risk associated with assigning a diagnosis code to a patient when he or she does not have the condition?

7.3 Ethical Issues: Intentional Misuse of Diagnosis Codes

The ethical struggle associated with the use of diagnosis codes tends to be more problematic than that of procedure codes. There are several reasons for these ethical problems:

1. **The selection of diagnosis codes is more variable in nature, compared to the selection of procedure codes.** Procedure codes are very clearly defined. Either a procedure was performed or it was not. The ethical problems with procedures are generally associated with circumventing the boundaries of what is and is not acceptable billing practice or misstating the level of service provided in the case of an E/M code. On the other hand, diagnoses are more open to interpretation, such as acute versus chronic, screening versus diagnostic, or symptoms versus definitive diagnosis.

2. **Assigning diagnosis codes seems less ethically important than selecting a procedure code.** Diagnoses are either a gateway to payment or are the determining factor in establishing payment levels when claims are submitted to a third-party payer. Physicians and coders who may be uncomfortable with falsifying the fact that they performed a procedure may have a lower discomfort level with selecting a diagnosis that is not completely false, but doesn't tell the entire story.

3. **Assigning a less than accurate diagnosis code seems to be a "victimless crime."** In fact, the selection of a particular diagnosis code over another may actually benefit the patient because it reduces or eliminates his or her personal financial responsibility in paying for the service. Justification for diagnosis modification can be based on several premises:

   a. The insurance companies are making too much profit.

   b. The patient's coverage should reimburse for this service—changing the diagnosis is only obtaining the benefit to which the patient is entitled.

   c. Provider reimbursement is too low—"appropriate" diagnosis code selection is only "righting" the wrong of inadequate reimbursement.

THE OBJECTIVE OF DIAGNOSIS CODE ASSIGNMENT

As indicated in Chapter 1, the purpose of the diagnosis code is to answer the question "Why?": Why was the provided service delivered? To put it in clinical terms, "What was the medical necessity that justified the service?"

An important issue, as it pertains to diagnosis code assignment, is the definition of **medical necessity.** The definitions can vary widely. For example:

- *Recommended AMA Managed Care Contract Definition*: "Health care services or products that a prudent physician would provide to a patient for the purpose of preventing, diagnosing, or treating an illness, injury, disease or its symptoms in a manner that is: (a) in accordance with generally accepted standards of medical practice;

FYI

Ethical dilemmas can often arise more easily related to diagnosis codes than procedure codes.

Medical necessity
The provision of services that are appropriate to treat the patient's condition.

(b) clinically appropriate in terms of type, frequency, extent, site and duration; and (c) not primarily for the convenience of the patient, physician, or other health care provider" (American Medical Association [AMA], 1999).

- *Medicare Definition in Layman's Terminology:* "Services or supplies that are needed for the diagnosis or treatment of your medical condition, meet the standards of good medical practice in the local area, and aren't mainly for the convenience of you or your doctor" (CMS, 2010b).
- *Formal Medicare Definition:* "No Medicare payment shall be made for items or services that are not reasonable and necessary for the diagnosis or treatment of illness or injury or to improve the functioning of a malformed body member" (Cinquino, 2010).

Some payers, including the Medicaid program, do not have a specific definition of medical necessity. Each state has the responsibility for defining what is and is not "medically necessary" (Sindelar, 2002). Similarly, each payer may have a different definition of "medically necessary," some that are more stringent than others. Therefore, that which is medically necessary in the eyes of one payer may be determined to be medically unnecessary in the eyes of another.

The purpose of assigning an ICD-9-CM code is to characterize, in the most accurate manner possible, the reason for the encounter. This can become an ethical issue when the reason for the encounter is not medically necessary, according to the payer's definition. Consider the case of Helena's routine visit to her physician.

Example

Helena, a 38-year-old woman, was scheduled for a "routine physical" with her primary care physician—an internal medicine physician. The physician billed the service as 99395—Preventive medicine exam, with a diagnosis of V70.0—Routine general medical examination. The claim was denied because, earlier in the year, the patient went to her OB/GYN to have a pelvic exam (the internal medicine physician does not perform pelvic exams). That physician billed the service as 99395—Preventive medicine exam, with a diagnosis of V72.31—Routine gynecological exam.

The insurer denied the claim because it was not medically necessary. According to its policy and definition of medical necessity, only one routine medical exam per year is necessary. For that reason, Helena was notified that no benefits would be payable for the service received at the internal medicine physician office.

This was the first time Helena ever had this experience because her previous OB/GYN did not code the claims for her pelvic exam as a routine service. Therefore, when the internal medicine physician billed the routine service, it was paid by the insurer.

Helena called the internal medicine physician billing office and demanded that the claim be resubmitted in whatever fashion necessary to have the claim paid. Helena told the billing representative that she is on a maintenance dosage of hypertension medication and that hypertension (401.9) should be the primary diagnosis.

Compliance and Diagnosis Coding

Diagnosis code assignment is a critical component of any provider compliance program. The focus of compliance and procedure code assignment is ensuring that the services provided are accurately reported and documented. The focus of compliance and diagnosis coding is ensuring that:

- The most specific possible diagnoses are used.
- The diagnoses that most accurately characterize the patients' conditions are assigned.
- All relevant diagnoses are included.
- All nonrelevant diagnoses are excluded (Figure 7.3).

In the American health insurance system, the payer determines whether a service is medically necessary, as it defines the term in its contract with the patient and/or the patient's employer. The provider also has a contract with the payer and, in most cases, the contract requires the provider to adhere to the payer's definition. The fact that the payer covers one routine (well-visit) exam per year indicates that it believes that there is sufficient medical necessity to warrant that service. Also, nearly everyone in the field of women's health agrees that periodic pelvic exams, including the collection of a Pap smear, are medically necessary. Therefore, almost everyone would agree that both of these services could be medically necessary. This claim denial is primarily a function of claim processing systems that track the quantity of services delivered within a given timeframe.

A greater challenge generally exists in working with diagnosis codes versus procedure codes. The primary reason is there is greater interpretation involved in determining the relevance and accuracy of a diagnosis compared to determining whether or not a procedure was performed. To establish an effective diagnosis compliance program, it is essential that protocols for reporting specific disease states, to which adherence is closely monitored, be established. It is not possible to be

FIGURE 7.3

Four elements of compliance must be considered when examining diagnosis codes: specificity, accuracy, completeness, and relevance. If any of the four elements is lacking, it is probable that the diagnosis coding is inappropriate.

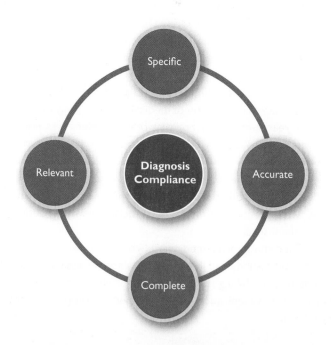

compliant in a circumstance when all parties within the office or facility are not aware of the baseline requirements.

PATIENT-DRIVEN ETHICAL CHALLENGES

Referring back to the example of Helena, while most would agree that both of these services, independently, are medically necessary, the payer's definition and policy establishes that the second service is not medically necessary. The patient feels that this problem can be resolved by changing the diagnosis (and procedure code in this particular case). The patient believes that this is not an ethical problem because she is asking them to assist her in obtaining the benefit to which she is entitled.

This sounds reasonable and almost noble. However, it has a significant ethical component to it because assigning diagnoses that don't precisely represent the purpose of the visit or the nature of the patient's condition is simply a shortcut to solving a different problem—a payer claim processing system issue. Instead of working with the patient and the insurance company to discuss the situation and arrive at a solution that, if not acceptable, is understood by all parties, the patient and the provider are tempted to circumvent the problem by changing the diagnosis.

WARNING

Patients often make requests concerning the changing of diagnosis codes that are clearly unethical. Unfortunately, the patients either don't see it that way or they don't care.

This is problematic because it results in a claim filing that is inconsistent with the medical record. If the chart is audited by the payer or governmental agency, the provider may be subject to claim recoupment and other contractual or legal penalties. The provider is taking a substantial risk, although many providers appear willing to take this risk or don't fully understand the nature of the risk they are assuming.

This is a difficult situation because the provider has the responsibility of reporting accurate claims to the payer while trying to maintain a satisfied customer. It is often a difficult balancing act because the patient will often threaten to leave the practice because "Dr. X's office down the street said that it would submit the claim to get paid." Unfortunately, this claim may be true. Providers that choose to conduct themselves in an ethically appropriate manner are often working in an environment where unethical diagnosis reporting occurs. Patients may use knowledge of that situation to their advantage.

PROVIDER-DRIVEN ETHICAL CHALLENGES

Not all ethical challenges stem from the coder's selection of diagnosis codes. Some may be motivated by physicians. Consider the following case of Dr. Walter Janke.

Example

Dr. Walter Janke and his wife operated two companies—Medical Resources, LLC, and America's Health Choice Medical Plans. America's Health Choice was a Medicare Advantage program, which delivered services to Medicare patients on behalf of Medicare. Medical Resources was the primary care arm of that health plan.

On November 26, 2010, Dr. Janke and the district attorney for the Southern District of Florida agreed to settle fraud allegations for $22.6 million. The government accused Dr. Janke of submitting false diagnosis codes to obtain higher reimbursement than would otherwise be payable. Dr. Janke adamantly denied the allegations, but stated that he settled the claims to avoid the cost of additional litigation.

"Patients seeking health care should be able to rely on the diagnoses they are given," said Tony West, assistant attorney general for the Justice Department's Civil Division. "We will aggressively pursue those who falsify medical diagnoses in order to receive taxpayer funds to which they are not entitled" (Mattise, 2010).

There are occasions in which providers will be tempted to make unethical choices regarding diagnoses, not by patients, but by their own need or desire to obtain additional revenue. In most cases, this occurs when the patient will choose not to receive the service unless someone else (usually an insurer) pays for it. If a provider's patient base is heavily weighted toward patients who are covered by government programs (e.g., Medicare or Medicaid), the provider does not have a practical option to tell the patient that he or she is financially responsible for the charge because of a nonpayable diagnosis. In many cases, the patient is unwilling to make payment for medical services and, in some cases, he or she is completely unable to make payment.

INPATIENT FACILITY DIAGNOSIS CODE ASSIGNMENT

For years, inpatient hospital services have been based on DRGs (diagnosis-related groups). DRGs were adopted by the Medicare program in 1983 as the means by which payment levels for inpatient hospital services were determined. All patients were classified into 1 of approximately 500 groups (Medical-Billing-Coding.org, 2006). The payment levels for each patient in a particular group are the same because the concept is based on the assumption that each patient in that group has a similar condition (Figure 7.4). The theory is that the cost of delivering services to these patients is approximately the same in that the patients will use approximately the same number of resources, be in the hospital approximately the same number of days, and so on. In this manner, the Medicare program attempted to control costs by discouraging hospitals from providing more intensive services than required to generate additional revenue. In fact, hospitals were encouraged to discharge patients more quickly because they received the same amount of payment for the patient whether the patient was hospitalized for the average amount of time, less than average time, or more than average time.

Many claimed that this process was not fair because patient conditions could be widely variable, even if they have the same general diagnosis. Therefore, on October 1, 2007, the Medicare Severity Diagnosis Related Groups (MS-DRG) were introduced. This increased the total number of DRGs from 538 to 745 (CMS, 2008).

Under the new system, the primary difference between the DRGs was whether or not the patient had complications and **comorbidities (CCs)** or major complications and comorbidities (MCCs). For example, a patient

Comorbidity (CC)

A coexisting but unrelated disease process.

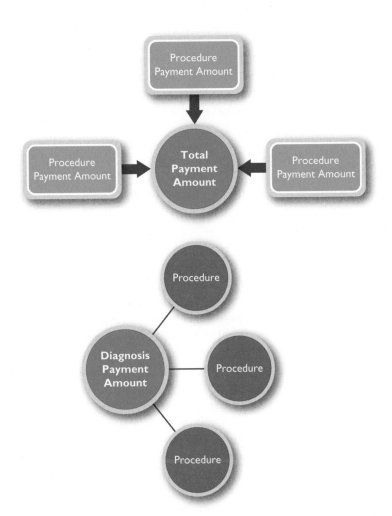

FIGURE 7.4
In the physician payment model, each procedure or service is assigned a reimbursement value. Generally, the more procedures performed, the greater the revenue received by the physician. In the hospital payment model, the number of procedures is less important than the diagnosis assigned to the patient, since the payment level is attached to the diagnosis, not the procedure.

with bleeding in the upper gastrointestinal tract would be assigned to one of the three DRGs for that condition, as shown in Table 7.2.

Unfortunately, the ethical problems associated with medical reimbursement did not go away through the introduction of DRGs. Although the problem of delivery of unnecessary services to obtain additional payment was addressed, a new problem was created—"creative" diagnosis assignment. Hospitals recognized that they would receive a higher amount of reimbursement if the patients had more significant or severe illnesses. The government also recognized that some diagnosis groups may be more susceptible to upcoding than other groups. As a result, data and trend analysis were included as part of the Office of Inspector General's Work Plan for Fiscal Year 2008, in an effort to identify incorrect, unethical, or fraudulent classification of a patient's diagnosis (CMS, 2008).

Table 7.2 Subset of the DRG Code Listing for Patients with Upper Gastrointestinal System Bleeding

DRG	Condition
377	UGI Hemorrhage with MCC
378	UGI Hemorrhage with CC
379	UGI Hemorrhage without CC

In Table 7.2, a hospital would receive higher reimbursement for a patient who had major complications and comorbidities than a patient who had an uncomplicated case. In some instances, coders were instructed to search the patients' record for anything that could be classified as a complication, to upgrade the DRG and thereby upgrade the reimbursement for the patient's care.

The largest settlement in history under the False Claims Act was paid by Tenet Health Care in 2006 in relation to charges of manipulating outlier payments to Medicare, paying kickbacks, upcoding DRG codes, and engaging in bill padding (Fraud Prevention, 2010). A total of $900 million in penalties were paid to the federal government in conjunction with this case.

The ethical issues related to DRGs are generally more significant than those related to procedural and service coding because the line between appropriate and inappropriate coding is not so clear. In the case of a procedure, either it was provided or it was not. Billing for a procedure that did not occur is clearly wrong. However, in the case of a DRG assignment, whether a patient has a complication or comorbidity can be open to interpretation. Highly qualified reviewers can have significant, legitimate disagreement concerning the diagnosis assignment for a patient with a lengthy hospital stay and numerous variables.

Another major issue regarding appropriate DRG assignment is that the only way to ensure accuracy is to review the medical records on case-by-case basis. This is a time-consuming and inefficient process. In a best-case scenario, a tiny minority of all medical records are reviewed and, therefore, hundreds of millions of dollars are paid inappropriately on an annual basis because of inappropriate DRG upcoding.

The most efficient way for payers to review inappropriate inpatient hospital diagnosis assignment is to perform data analysis. The usage of DRGs by individual providers is compared to the average of providers that have similar characteristics, such as geographic location, patient mix, socioeconomic conditions, and other factors. Whenever a provider has a significantly higher percentage of patients with a particular DRG than would be expected based on the available benchmarks, this is a signal of a potential problem. This causes the payer to investigate the provider's records to determine if overpayments were issued to the provider.

Extrapolated
Making an assumption about an entire group based on a relatively small sample of that group.

In most cases, it is impossible to check every record of every patient who is assigned a particular DRG by a facility, especially if it is a large facility. Most payers resolve this issue by reviewing a sample of the charts for coding accuracy and appropriateness. When inappropriate coding is found, the erroneous coding percentage is **extrapolated** to the entire patient population. The payer then asks for a refund, based on this calculated figure, because it assumes that if cases were overcoded in 10% of the sample, then they must be overcoded in 10% of all payments (Figure 7.5).

Many providers strongly object to this methodology in calculating overpayments because they claim that it is unfair to assume that errors are made at a given rate throughout an entire facility based on a relatively small sampling. Payers agree that the error rate may not be the same throughout the facility—they indicate that it could be higher. However, they are willing to accept the results of the extrapolation because it is the most accurate way to estimate error rates.

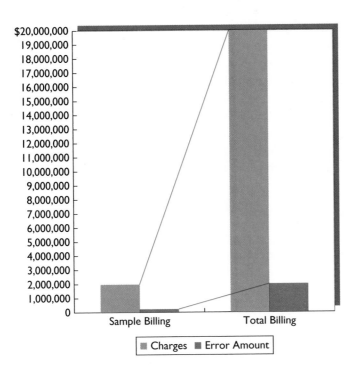

FIGURE 7.5

In this case, a particular provider received $20,000,000 in payment for a given DRG. A sample of this billing was reviewed and the total payment received for the sample cases was $2,000,000. There were $200,000 in overpayments in the sample, representing a total of 10%. It is assumed that all of the provider's billings produced overpayments in a similar amount, which would result in a request for overpayment of $2,000,000.

The element often missed in the debate over the calculation of overpayments is the amount of time and expense dedicated to the review of claims—particularly for providers that consistently make a good-faith effort to code appropriately. A provider, whose audit returns a 0% overpayment rate, still does not win because it incurs the costs associated with cooperating with the payer audit and none of these funds do anything to improve patient care. This is another case where inaccurate or unethical coding submitted by providers, which admittedly occurs, adversely affects providers who always engage in ethical coding. The bad behavior of others forces ethical providers to absorb the expense of audits and defending legitimate coding disagreements.

FYI

Many providers object to third-party payer methods of calculating improper billing. Some payers use small samples and apply the percentage of erroneous billing found in the sample to all of the provider's billings. Providers believe that this is not an accurate method of calculating liability.

Thinking It Through 7.3

1. Of the three causes of ethical problems related to diagnosis coding listed at the beginning of this section, what is the most significant in your opinion?

2. Explain the importance of all four elements when considering diagnosis codes and compliance programs.

3. Explain the different role that diagnosis codes play in outpatient versus inpatient coding.

7.4 Ethical Dilemmas: Omitting or Misleading Information

Ethical dilemmas related to diagnosis coding are often a function of actively choosing one code over another. For example, diagnosis A most accurately reflects the patient's condition, but it is not payable.

Diagnosis B is a payable diagnosis. The question for the coder is, "Do I select diagnosis A or diagnosis B?"

However, another type of ethical dilemma related to diagnosis code assignment also exists. This dilemma does not involve choosing one code or another. Instead, the dilemma involves the intentional omission of diagnoses that are highly relevant to the patient's condition or the intentional use of a diagnosis that mischaracterizes the nature of the services provided. In each case, the purpose of the code selection (or omission) is to mislead or misreport the patient's true diagnosis.

FAILING TO REPORT RELEVANT INFORMATION

When selecting diagnosis codes, a coder may sometimes fail to report relevant information, often to obtain higher reimbursement. Consider the case of Mary's fertility treatment.

Example

Mary, a 38-year-old, has two children ages 12 and 10. At the time of the birth of her second child, she elected to have a tubal ligation because she and her husband did not want any additional children.

Mary and her husband divorced three years later. She is now in a new relationship and desires to have a child with her new husband. Her insurance policy specifically excludes coverage for any infertility treatment that occurs following a previous voluntary sterilization procedure.

The provider submits claims for infertility treatment services to the patient's insurer, which is a different insurer than she had at the time of her sterilization 10 years ago. The provider uses a diagnosis of 628.2—Infertility, of tubal origin. This diagnosis is accurate, in that the patient is infertile because of her "tied" tubes. The insurer pays the claims for the infertility treatment.

In this case, the diagnosis code selection could be either provider-driven or patient-driven. The provider may choose to use this diagnosis because it knows that the patient will not continue with treatment because she is unable to afford the care using her personal funds. The provider is willing to accept the insurance company's payment for the services, rather than completely lose the opportunity to provide treatment to the patient. The patient may insist that the provider submit the claim with a "payable" diagnosis because she doesn't want to pay for the service on an out-of-pocket basis and feels that she pays a significant amount in premiums to the insurer—she should be getting her money's worth now that she needs the service. The patient states that if a "payable" diagnosis is not used for the claims, she will go elsewhere to another clinic that is willing to code in that fashion.

The diagnosis used in this case (628.2) does not tell the whole story. A diagnosis code exists to report that a patient had a previous tubal ligation: V26.51—Tubal ligation status. By failing to report this code, the service becomes potentially payable because the payer may not be aware of the cause of the patient's condition which, in this case, was a voluntary decision made years ago.

The failure to report the tubal ligation status of the patient results in an unethical and inappropriate claim, not because a false diagnosis was submitted, but because the failure to report the tubal ligation diagnosis creates, in effect, a false impression and a false diagnosis.

In the theology of most major religions, there are two overarching types of acts—acts of commission and acts of omission. Acts of commission are wrongdoing done through the purposeful performance of an act. Acts of omission are wrongdoing that occurs through the *failure* to perform an act that the individual should have done. Unending debates have occurred regarding which is worse, although most would agree that both are wrong. However, the general consensus is that acts of commission are worse because they are more obvious and require clear specific intent.

MISSTATING THE SEVERITY OF A CONDITION

Ethical dilemmas in coding can arise if a coder misstates the severity of a condition, often to justify a procedure's medical necessity. Consider the case of Brittany's plastic surgery.

Example

Brittany, a 22-year-old aspiring model, was told by her agent that she needs a "nose job" to obtain the most lucrative modeling jobs. The agent referred her to a local plastic surgeon, who told Brittany that she had a congenital deviation of her septum (diagnosis code 754.0). Because of this physical problem with her nose, the doctor advised Brittany that the claim could be submitted to her parents' insurance company and she would not have to pay out-of-pocket for the cosmetic procedure. Brittany was not previously aware that she had a deviated septum and had no previous complaints with her breathing.

WARNING

Improper use of diagnosis codes can make a noncovered cosmetic procedure look like a covered, medically necessary procedure.

In Brittany's case, the legitimate argument could be made that Brittany had a deviated septum and, therefore, the diagnosis code assigned was correct. However, the assignment of diagnosis code 754.0 misstates the severity of the condition and mischaracterizes the medical necessity of the procedure (30420—Rhinoplasty, primary; including major septal repair). Because Brittany had no symptoms, such as wheezing (786.07) or respiratory insufficiency (786.09), few payers would acknowledge this procedure as medically necessary or payable. In short, the fact that a patient has a particular condition does not mean that it requires medical intervention, unless it is symptomatic or has the risk of creating harm to the patient in the future, if untreated.

In addition, the failure to use diagnosis code V50.1—Other plastic surgery for unacceptable cosmetic appearance, also facilitates the mischaracterization of the treatment necessity. If V50.1 were used, the payer would know with certainty that the claim was not medically necessary. By disregarding the use of this code, the physician has created an unethical and inappropriate claim that could result in incorrect payment for the service.

GIVING CORRECT, BUT INCOMPLETE, INFORMATION

Omitting information when selecting diagnosis codes also leads to ethical problems and denied claims. Consider the case of Marian's in-vitro fertilization (IVF) treatment.

Example

Marian and her husband desire to have children and have completed six unsuccessful intrauterine insemination treatment cycles. They require the more aggressive IVF treatment, but their insurance policy does not cover the service. They state that they are unable to afford the IVF treatment.

The financial representative at the fertility clinic indicates that she understands their situation and that she can help. Many of the procedure codes that report services that are part of the treatment process are also the same procedure codes used to report services that are part of insemination treatment or diagnostic services. Less than half of the total cost of the process is attributable to services that are unique to IVF—the remainder of the costs are for services that appear identical to other services that are covered by insurance.

The representative agreed to submit the claims for the IVF monitoring services, using the diagnosis that was used for the insemination cycles: 628.8—Infertility, other specified cause. The IVF-specific services would not be submitted to the insurer. The patient and her husband agreed to this plan.

In Marian's case, the diagnosis codes that were proposed for submission were not incorrect—in fact, they had been submitted appropriately for previous artificial insemination claims. The patient continues to have the same fertility problems and the same diagnosis that she had previously. The only difference is that the form of treatment has been changed to a more aggressive therapy—one that is not covered by the patient's insurance.

The problem is that the diagnosis code is not the best code that describes the reason for the encounter the patient is having prior to the actual egg retrieval procedure, which is the key to the IVF process. The best diagnosis is V26.81—Encounter for assisted reproductive fertility procedure cycle. This diagnosis better describes the reason the patient is visiting the office on each of the days the patient is preparing for the egg retrieval than does the infertility code.

The primary purpose for *not* using V26.81 is to obtain benefits on behalf of the patient to which she is not entitled. This is unethical because the purpose is to mislead the insurer into paying a claim that it would not pay if the diagnosis code was used appropriately. One element in proper, ethical code selection is to answer the question, "Why am I using/not using this particular code?" If the answer has anything to do with misleading the insurer or hiding information, then it is not ethical.

USING NONSPECIFIC DIAGNOSES WHEN MORE DETAIL IS AVAILABLE

Coders must code to the greatest level of detail to describe a particular encounter, based on the available documentation. This can

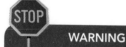

WARNING

The use of an accurate, but misleading, diagnosis code can result in an unethical action.

lead to ethical dilemmas, especially when the level of detail would limit reimbursement for a procedure. Consider the case of Margaret's depression.

Example

Margaret is a 63-year-old female who was widowed about three months ago. She is coming to the office today with complaints of malaise and fatigue. After talking with the patient for a few minutes, the physician determines that the patient is having an adjustment reaction to the recent loss of her husband and is experiencing related depression. He prescribed an antidepressant and referred the patient to a local grief support group. The best diagnosis for this encounter is 309.0—Adjustment disorder with depressed mood.

However, Margaret's insurer has subcontracted all mental health services to another company, which has specific requirements and forms that must be submitted for payment to be issued. Claims with a diagnosis from Chapter 5 of the ICD-9-CM manual (290–319) must be forwarded to the subcontractor for approval. The physician, who was aware of this insurer's policy, avoids using any of these diagnosis codes. In this situation, he used 780.79—Other malaise and fatigue.

The physician chose the diagnosis code based on what he perceived would be the fastest route to payment. The most accurate and specific diagnosis code was not used because it would result in delayed payment and an increased "hassle factor." The diagnosis reported to the insurer is not consistent with the diagnosis reflected in the patient's chart—unless the physician also ensured that the mention of depression or adjustment disorder was not part of the progress note. Either way, it was not an appropriate code selection, done for the wrong reason.

Thinking It Through 7.4

1. In your opinion, which is worse in the field of diagnosis coding—a sin of commission or a sin of omission?

2. Do you believe that these types of dilemmas related to diagnoses are more patient-driven or provider-driven? Why?

3. Is it possible that the improper use of nonspecific diagnoses is the result of inadequate training or poor coding tools? If so, does this influence whether the code selection is unethical? Explain your position.

7.5 Analyzing Ethically Challenging Situations

An ethically challenging situation is a circumstance that appears to be ethically wrong or inappropriate, but is not wrong. These situations can occur because coding—particularly diagnosis coding—is an art as opposed to being a science. Unusual circumstances may have the appearance of impropriety, but are not incorrect.

NOT INCLUDING ALL POSSIBLE AND RELEVANT DIAGNOSES

Significant controversy exists among coders regarding the submission of claims that correctly describe the patient's primary condition, but do not report every possible relevant diagnosis. Some argue that the primary diagnosis is sufficient and it is frequently difficult to determine the diagnoses that are or are not relevant. Others believe that it is essential to include *every* relevant diagnosis and failing to do so results in an improperly submitted claim.

Example

Janice is a 24-year-old in her first pregnancy, who is receiving global OB care from Dr. Jones. Janice calls the office during her 13th week, reporting symptoms of a urinary tract infection. Dr. Jones's nurse asks her to come in later that same day for evaluation of her symptoms and any necessary treatment. During that visit, Dr. Jones confirms a urinary tract infection.

Because this visit was not part of the global OB package (UTI is not part of a "routine" pregnancy), the service is separately billable. Dr. Jones's coder bills 9921x, with a primary diagnosis of 599.0 and a secondary diagnosis of V22.2 (Pregnancy, incidental). The claim is filed to the payer and it is denied as part of the global package. Dr. Jones's coder contacts the payer and she is advised that the claim was denied because it had a diagnosis of "pregnancy" attached to it. The payer representative says that if V22.2 was not attached to the claim, it would have been paid. The coder is not comfortable with this advice because she feels it is not ethical.

> **FYI**
>
> Coding guidelines, in themselves, do not hold the force of law. Therefore, not following coding guidelines precisely is not necessarily unethical—particularly if it results in the patient receiving benefits to which he or she is entitled.

The coder's supervisor disagreed with the coder and said that V22.2 should not be included on the claim. His justification was that coding guidelines do not have the force of law and that failing to follow coding guidelines does not automatically make it unethical or inappropriate. In fact, the supervisor pointed out to literature published by the provider's specialty organization, which supported the elimination of V22.2 from the claim (American Congress of Obstetricians and Gynecology, 2010). In this case, the "solution" recommended does not include falsifying a claim—it means being less than complete in reporting.

To determine whether a circumstance appears ethically challenged or if it is ethically inappropriate, two key questions need to be asked and answered:

1. Does the patient have a benefit for this service?
2. Is the provider entitled to payment for this service?

If the answer to both questions is yes, then it is not ethically inappropriate to submit a claim and receive payment for that service, even if it appears inappropriate. Another way to look at the situation is to ask the question, "What is the physician's objective in leaving off V22.2?" In this case, the objective is to receive payment to which the provider is entitled and for which the patient has benefits. The obstacle to that payment is the settings in the payer's claim payment system, which causes a denial of a payable claim.

ALLOWING AN UNUSUAL CIRCUMSTANCE THAT IS NOT PAYABLE—ORDINARILY

It is frequently said that there is an exception for every rule. Is this the case in coding? Using the previous example involving the case of Mary, consider whether an exception in this case is appropriate. The circumstances of the case are the same, except Mary's husband has a medical condition that contributes to the situation.

Example

Mary is now in a new relationship and desires to have a child with her new husband. Her insurance policy specifically excludes coverage for any infertility treatment that occurs following a previous voluntary sterilization procedure. However, her new husband has oligospermia, which means that he has very few usable sperm. Their physician advises them that it is impossible for them to achieve pregnancy without in vitro fertilization, due to the husband's poor sperm count.

As indicated on the discussion on page 246, the appropriate diagnosis in this case is V26.51, which indicates that the female partner had an elective sterilization. This condition makes the desired treatment a noncovered service, according to the terms of the patient's benefits.

Some payers will completely refuse to offer benefits for the IVF service because of the elective sterilization. However, others will sometimes allow benefits for services when the patient has a comorbidity that makes the service necessary, regardless of the patient's sterilization status. In this case, the husband's poor sperm count would make IVF necessary, with regard to her previous tubal ligation. Therefore, leaving off diagnosis code V26.51 would be appropriate to allow for payment—in addition to a discussion with the payer and obtaining a specific prior authorization or preapproval. The correct/payable diagnosis in this case would be 628.8—Female infertility, other specified cause (the husband's poor sperm count).

It is important to remember that diagnosis code selection is not a legally binding activity—failure to adhere to all coding guidelines is not necessarily illegal or even unethical. You begin to approach the line of ethical versus unethical when there is an intention to deceive or mislead someone that is involved in the process.

As indicated in Figure 7.6, the objectives of coding are (1) to accurately report the services provided and the reason for those services and (2) to facilitate the payment of services to which the patient and provider are rightfully entitled.

In the case studies in this section, the use of all correct or appropriate diagnoses meets objective 1 but fails objective 2. While it would be desirable to meet both objectives at all times, it is not realistic. In some

COMPLIANCE TIP

When the intent of diagnosis code selection is to deceive or mislead, then the action becomes unethical and potentially illegal.

The objectives of diagnosis coding are to:

- Accurately report the services provided and the reason for those services

AND

- Facilitate the payment of services to which the patient and provider are rightfully entitled

FIGURE 7.6

A statement of the objectives of diagnosis coding.

cases, insurer rules make adherence to precise coding rules impractical. The theoretical objective of precise coding guideline adherence is admirable, but if the patients are not receiving the benefits to which they are entitled and the provider is not receiving payment to which it is entitled, the guideline adherence will become irrelevant in that the practice will have difficulty maintaining its existence as an ongoing business.

Providers and coders should always ask, before assigning a diagnosis, "What is my purpose in this choice?" If the answer is honorable and consistent with the objectives of accuracy and obtaining proper benefits, then an ethical choice will result. If the answer is merely to obtain payment without regard to accuracy and honesty, then an unethical choice will likely result.

Thinking It Through 7.5

1. Do you agree with the coder's conduct in the case of Janice and the urinary tract infection during pregnancy? Why or why not?

2. Why is the two-part consideration of objectives in coding important?

CHAPTER REVIEW

Chapter Summary

Learning Outcome	Key Concepts/Examples

7.1 Summarize the basic principles of diagnosis coding, using ICD-9-CM codes, including the commonly used conventions. Pages 222–231	• The ICD-9-CM coding system is based on the World Health Organization's (WHO) system. However, the WHO system is not specific enough for reporting services for payment to third-party payers.
	• Diagnosis codes are divided into chapters, sections, categories, subcategories, and subclassifications.
	• The ICD-9-CM manual is divided into three sections:
	  1. Volume 1—Tabular (Numeric) List
	  2. Volume 2—Alphabetic Index
	  3. Volume 3—ICD-9 Procedure Codes
	• There are conventions that appear in the Alphabetic Index. They are:
	  1. Essential/nonessential modifiers
	  2. Organization by main terms
	    • Diseases
	    • Conditions
	    • Nouns
	    • Adjectives
	• The conventions in the Tabular List are:
	  1. "Use additional code"
	  2. "Code first"
	  3. "Code, if applicable"
	  4. "Excludes"
	  5. "Includes"
	  6. "And"
	  7. "With"
	  8. "Not elsewhere classified" ("NEC")
	  9. "Not otherwise specified" ("NOS")

Learning Outcome	Key Concepts/Examples
7.2 Interpret the diagnosis coding guidelines that are applicable to various circumstances. Pages 231–237	• Diagnosis coding guidelines require that both the Alphabetic Index and Tabular List be used in code selection. • Codes should not be assigned to a patient until confirmation of a condition has been received. Without confirmation, sign and symptoms codes should be assigned. • Symptoms that are a standard part of a disease process should not be reported. • There is no rule as to the number of diagnosis codes that are required. Using multiple diagnoses is not better if it results in a mischaracterization of the patient's condition. • Diagnosis codes are a gateway to payment. Physicians do not receive greater payment by using one diagnosis versus another, but without an appropriate diagnosis, they may not receive any payment. • Differentiating between acute and chronic conditions is important in accurately reporting the nature and severity of a patient's condition. • Chapter-specific coding guidelines provide information regarding unusual diagnosis coding protocols.

7.3 Evaluate ethical dilemmas associated with the intentional misuse of diagnosis codes, in both the inpatient and outpatient context. Pages 238–245	• There are several reasons that ethical issues can arise in conjunction with diagnosis coding:
	  1. Selecting diagnosis codes is more variable in nature, compared to selecting procedure codes.
	  2. Assigning diagnosis codes seems less ethically important than selecting procedure codes.
	  3. Assigning a less-than-accurate diagnosis code seems to be a victimless "crime."
	• Four components to the evaluation of diagnosis coding in any compliance program are:
	  1. Specificity
	  2. Accuracy
	  3. Completeness
	  4. Relevance
	• Ethical dilemmas in diagnosis coding can be either patient-driven or provider-driven.
	• Inpatient facility coding provides an increased opportunity for unethical diagnosis coding, because diagnoses are the basis of the payment system.

7.4 Analyze circumstances in which ethical dilemmas are created by omitting or failing to report key diagnosis information. Pages 245–249	• Unethical diagnosis coding can occur even without actively reporting incorrect codes by:
	  1. Failing to report relevant information.
	  2. Misstating the severity of a condition.
	  3. Providing correct, but incomplete information.
	  4. Using nonspecific information when more specific information is available.

7.5 Differentiate between circumstances that appear to be ethically challenged and circumstances that are ethically appropriate. Pages 249–252	• Some unusual circumstances regarding diagnosis coding have the appearance of impropriety but are not unethical:
	  1. Not including all possible and relevant diagnoses.
	  2. Allowing unusual circumstances that are not payable—ordinarily.
	• There are two objectives in coding—both of which are equally important:
	  1. Accurately reporting the services provided and the reason for those services.
	  2. Facilitating the payment of services to which the patient and provider are rightfully entitled.

End-of-Chapter Questions

Multiple Choice

Circle the letter that best completes the statement or answers the question.

I. **LO 7.1** The diagnosis code supports the _____ concerning the procedure.

  a. Prior authorization

  b. Medical necessity

  c. Retrospective review

  d. Payer's policy

2. **LO 7.1** Which of the following items are tracked through WHO's International Classification of Diseases?

   a. Morbidity, mortality
   b. Severity, morbidity
   c. Complexity, severity
   d. Mortality, complexity

3. **LO 7.1** What is the order of ICD-9-CM organization, from *least to most* specific?

   a. Category, subcategory, subclassification, chapter, section
   b. Section, chapter, category, subcategory, subclassification
   c. Chapter, section, category, subcategory, subclassification
   d. Category, subcategory, chapter, section, subclassification

4. **LO 7.1** Which is recommended to be used for assignment of diagnosis codes?

   a. Alphabetic Index
   b. Tabular List
   c. Alphabetic Index, followed by Tabular List
   d. Tabular List, followed by confirmation in Alphabetic Index

5. **LO 7.1** Which of the following is *not* a category in which codes are organized in the Alphabetic Index of the ICD-9-CM code set?

   a. Diseases
   b. Organs
   c. Conditions
   d. Adjectives

6. **LO 7.1** When a code has the instruction "code first" attached to it, the code is designated by

   a. Italics
   b. Bold text
   c. Underlining
   d. Parenthesis

7. **LO 7.2** Which of the following is *not* a sign or symptom code?

   a. Abdominal pain
   b. Appendicitis
   c. Fatigue
   d. Nausea

8. **LO 7.2** In the outpatient setting, diagnosis codes are

   a. The determining factor in the amount of reimbursement
   b. A gateway to reimbursement
   c. Not a factor in the reimbursement process
   d. Used in the same way as they are in the inpatient setting

9. **LO 7.3** The selection of diagnosis codes are _____ in nature.

   a. Precise
   b. Variable
   c. Arbitrary
   d. Limited

10. **LO 7.3** In the American health care system, the _____ determines medical necessity.

    a. Physician
    b. Payer

c. Coder

d. Patient

11. **LO 7.3** The Medicare Severity Diagnosis Related Groups (MS-DRGs) were introduced in 2007 because

    a. The number of DRGs needed to be decreased.

    b. The previous DRG system did not recognize the additional days that some people remained in the hospital.

    c. The previous DRG system did not sufficiently differentiate between more complex and less complex conditions.

    d. The number of DRGs needed to be increased.

12. **LO 7.4** Unethical diagnosis coding through omission can occur through

    a. Pressure from the patient

    b. Decisions made by the provider

    c. Both a and b

    d. Neither a nor b

13. **LO 7.4** The omission of diagnosis codes can result in all of the following *except*

    a. Failing to report relevant information

    b. Misstating the severity of a condition

    c. Overpaying hospitals

    d. Giving correct, but incomplete information

14. **LO 7.5** Which of the following is *not* a question that should be asked when considering a diagnosis code?

    a. Does the patient have benefits for the service?

    b. Is the provider entitled to receive payment for the service?

    c. Will the payer not be able to identify an improper diagnosis code?

    d. What is the objective of using this code?

Short Answer

Use your critical thinking skills to answer the following questions.

1. **LO 7.1** Why is the American system of diagnosis code reporting based on WHO's ICD system? What are the advantages and disadvantages of this system?

2. **LO 7.1** Discuss the content and purpose of each volume of the ICD-9-CM code set. Make note of the order in which each volume is usually published.

3. **LO 7.1** Describe the difference between essential and nonessential modifiers in the Alphabetic Index of the ICD-9-CM code set. How can proper interpretation of their usage be important in ethical coding?

4. **LO 7.1** Why can codes in italics *not* be used as primary diagnoses?

5. **LO 7.1** Discuss the differences between "not elsewhere classified" and "not otherwise classified."

6. **LO 7.2** How is it possible that a lack of familiarity with diagnosis code usage could be considered an ethical problem?

7. **LO 7.2** What are the differences between acute and chronic conditions? Why is this distinction important in assigning a diagnosis code?

8. **LO 7.2** What are the risks associated with assigning a diagnosis code to a patient's condition when the patient does not actually have the condition?

9. **LO 7.3** List and discuss the various factors that make people think that unethical diagnosis assignment is a "victimless" crime.

10. **LO 7.3** What are the ramifications of complying with a patient's request to improperly change a diagnosis code?

11. **LO 7.3** Why is diagnosis code assignment so much different for the inpatient setting than for the outpatient setting?

12. **LO 7.3** Distinguish between a complication and a comorbidity. Why are they important in DRG selection?

13. **LO 7.3** How are providers who assign diagnosis codes appropriately penalized because of providers that are unethical in their coding?

14. **LO 7.4** Why might a provider user a nonspecific diagnosis when a more specific diagnosis is available?

15. **LO 7.5** What are the objectives of diagnosis coding? Discuss the importance of these objectives and how they relate to each other.

Applying Your Knowledge

In August 2007, a 45-year-old physician in Jersey City, New Jersey, died of a heart attack. This tragedy was not seen as unusual, until the Hudson County public safety complex began receiving numerous phone calls from various police officers in different law enforcement agencies and jurisdictions. The officers were calling to confirm the details of the physician's death, asking "Is it true? Is he dead?" The physician had no known ties—formal or informal—to any law enforcement or governmental agency.

An investigative report by the *Newark Star-Ledger* revealed that the physician, who was operating an unremarkable medical practice, was actually serving as a supplier of illegal prescriptions for steroids and human growth hormones. A total of 248 law enforcement officers from 53 different agencies were found to be patients of this physician.

Further investigation revealed that these illegally provided steroids and hormones were paid for by the patients' health insurance. The physician submitted claims for his services and wrote the prescriptions using a diagnosis of low testosterone (257.2) or low human growth hormone (253.3). The use of these diagnosis codes facilitated significant payments to the physician and various pharmacies, with little or no cost to the officers. Since all public servants in New Jersey are covered by self-insured plans, ultimately the taxpayers were supplying medications for illegal use (Brittain & Mueller, 2010).

Clearly, serious illegal activity was taking place. However, the whole scheme was funded by fraudulent insurance claims, built on improper diagnosis code submission. Consider the following questions concerning this situation.

1. Based on the material in this chapter, what *type* of improper diagnosis code submission occurred?

2. Do an Internet search on the frequency of low human growth hormone and low testosterone levels in otherwise healthy males. Could the claim payers have identified a problem? What should they have done?

3. If you were the coder in this physician office, how would you respond if you saw this activity taking place? List specifically the actions, in order, that you would consider.

4. Are there any other parties in the process that should have been aware of this situation? If so, who are they and what should they have done?

The Internet has made accessibility to ICD-9-CM codes a simple process (Figure 7.7). Numerous vendors provide virtual ICD-9-CM and CPT code books online. The use of these formalized tools usually requires the purchase of a subscription or paid access of some form. For those who do not want to pay for ICD-9-CM code information, ICD-9 code information can even be found in commonly accessed places such as Google or Wikipedia.

When using free services, great care must be taken to ensure and confirm that the information is correct. While the Internet is a remarkable tool, there is no guarantee that the information provided is correct. The use of search tools and general information sites should be limited to initial investigations and locating of specific codes, which then are confirmed through more reliable sources.

The Medicare website does provide valuable information regarding diagnosis codes. Specifically it provides links to the Centers for Disease Control and Prevention (CDC) website, which supplies both the official ICD-9-CM guidelines and a conversion table that shows the changes that occurred each year over the past 24 years and illustrates the codes that were previously used to report a diagnosis prior to the creation of the new code.

Although it is not particularly user-friendly, a complete listing of all current ICD-9-CM codes is provided on the Medicare website in a Microsoft Excel spreadsheet format (Figure 7.8). The first column provides a list of all valid diagnosis codes and the second column provides the full (long) description of the

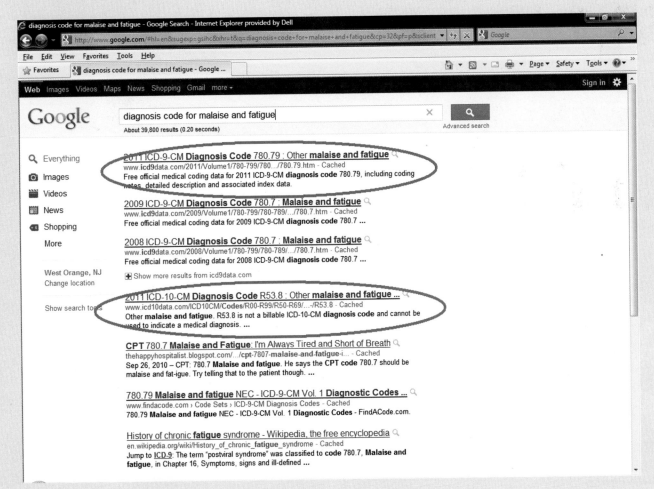

FIGURE 7.7

Diagnosis codes can be found by using basic Internet search tools such as Google. As illustrated here, searching for "diagnosis code for malaise and fatigue" produced more than 90,000 results and provides information about both ICD-9 and ICD-10 codes for these conditions.

Chapter 7 | Coding Ethics and Diagnoses

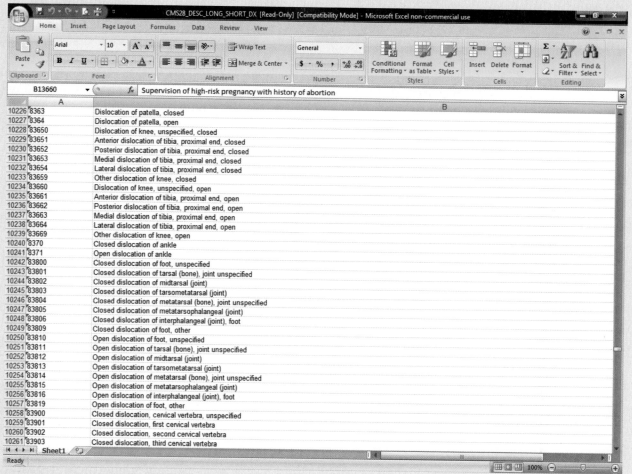

FIGURE 7.8

The full listing of 14,432 ICD-9-CM codes, effective on October 1, 2010 (CMS, 2010a).

diagnosis. Successful use of this tool requires advanced knowledge of the Excel program because there is no punctuation (specifically, periods) in the code set. Punctuation can be added using tools within the Excel program.

1. Select three different ICD-9-CM codes from the diagnosis Tabular List. Enter the code numbers in Google and select the first result that you obtain. Does the description you find match the code description from the ICD-9 code book? Summarize your findings for all three codes.

2. Discuss your opinion concerning the quality of the website(s) from which you obtained the information in question 1. On what do you base your opinion?

3. What are the greatest risks associated with using a website that is free and not subscription-based? Does the use of a subscription-based website guarantee accuracy in diagnosis information? Why or why not?

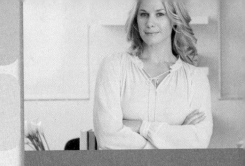

ICD-10 and Coding Ethics

8

LEARNING OUTCOMES

After completing this chapter, you will be able to:

8.1   Describe the ICD-10-CM code set and the transition
      process from the ICD-9-CM code set.

8.2   Explain the similarities and differences between ICD-9
      and ICD-10 and the available tools for facilitating the
      transition.

8.3   Evaluate the practical ethical challenges that health care
      providers and organizations will face in the transition to
      ICD-10-CM.

8.4   Design protocols to address and avoid the ethical
      challenges created by the use of ICD-10-CM.

CASE STUDY

The billing office staff at North Mountain Ophthalmology Associates gathered for their regular staff meeting in January 2012. Their supervisor, Olga Simonetti, had just returned from a conference on the topic of the transition from the ICD-9-CM code set to the ICD-10-CM code set. The physicians at the practice had heard about the upcoming transition and they wanted their billing supervisor to obtain more information. One of the items on the agenda for the billing office staff meeting was Olga's summary about what she learned at the meeting. Specifically, she was going to speak about the effect of ICD-10 on the billing office function.

As the meeting started, Olga mentioned what a wonderful time she had at the resort where the meeting was held. She hinted that she may have spent more than a little time on the beach and some of the staff members got the impression that Olga hadn't attended all of the meetings at the conference. One staff member whispered to another, "They should have sent me—I can skip meetings just as well as she can!"

Olga explained the following major points that she heard at the meeting:

- The use of ICD-10 codes is required effective October 1, 2013. The presenters at the meeting strongly recommended that providers do not wait until that date to prepare—a timeline should be created and followed, particularly regarding training throughout the organization.

- ICD-10 has a significantly higher level of specificity than does ICD-9. There are many more codes in the ICD-10 code set.

- The presenters at the conference recommended a couple of software programs that help providers make the transition from ICD-9 to ICD-10. They demonstrated how it was possible to enter an ICD-9 code and the corresponding ICD-10 code would be provided.

- The presenters at the meeting indicated that this was going to be a highly significant event in the U.S. health care system—much more significant than the possible Y2K issues faced in 2000.

Following the presentation of the highlights, Olga began to explain how she thought this information should be applied in the context of the North Mountain Ophthalmology practice. She stated her opinion that:

1. This was not going to be a "big deal." The Y2K issue was a great deal about nothing and this will probably be the same.

2. Ophthalmology practices use a relatively small subset of diagnosis codes. Therefore, the transition from small ICD-9 subset to the larger ICD-10 subset will not be significant, since there will probably be equivalent codes for nearly all of the codes they use frequently.

3. There is no need to spread this information widely across the practice—especially with the doctors. Since the old codes will be exchanged with new codes, it will appear about the same for the noncoders. In fact, a special effort can be made to ensure the charge ticket looks identical, except for the code numbers.

4. There is no need to address this issue in the near future—preparing too far in advance will be counterproductive because new codes will be forgotten if they are not used regularly. The current focus should be on the installation of the new EHR (electronic health record) later this year. Since she now has the necessary information, Olga said that significant attention will be paid to ICD-10 around July 1, 2013.

A few of the certified coders in attendance at the meeting spoke up, indicating that they had received training at a local coding chapter meeting about ICD-10. The information they received was consistent with what Olga had heard at her meeting, but they strongly disagreed with her interpretation and the application for their practice. Olga said, "You are just believing the 'Chicken Littles' who think everything will be a disaster. You don't need to worry about this—that's why I'm the supervisor and it's my job to take care of this."

1. What have you heard to date about the ICD-10-CM code set? From what sources have you received that information?

2. Based on this case study, what is your opinion of Olga's leadership style? What do you think of her interpretation of the information she received at the conference?

3. Provide a brief analysis of the strengths and weaknesses of Olga's communication with her staff. What do you think may be accurate and what might not be accurate?

Introduction

The transition from the ICD-9-CM code set to the ICD-10-CM code set on October 1, 2013, represents the most significant change in the practice of health care coding since the January 1, 1992, introduction of evaluation and management (E/M) codes to the Current Procedural Terminology (CPT) code set. However, the replacement of one code set with another has a greater impact on every health care entity in the country than any other single event related to coding. It is more significant on this occasion because the last time a change of code sets occurred, coding was largely a voluntary process, used by a relatively limited number of providers and health care entities. Therefore, the impact on the health care industry at that time was comparatively minor.

With any change comes a significant amount of discomfort, primarily because of a lack of knowledge and a fear of the unknown. An entire generation of coders has functioned with the CPT-4 and ICD-9-CM code sets during their careers. This change takes half of their knowledge base and turns it upside down. Coders who had large sections of the diagnosis code book memorized now must learn new codes from scratch.

This type of change has significant impact on the operational capability of all health care organizations. This is an instance in which an externally imposed reduction in operational capacity (the implementation of ICD-10) presents a significant opportunity for ethical

FYI

The conversion from ICD-9 to ICD-10 is the most significant change ever in medical coding in the United States. The most recent comparable change was the introduction of E/M codes in 1992.

challenges in the health care industry. While those in health care fight to maintain profitability as efficiency inevitably declines, one of the perceived solutions to their problem is to take ethical shortcuts to offset the productivity and revenue reductions.

8.1 The ICD-10-CM Code Set and the Transition from ICD-9-CM

When major transformation occurs, fear and misinformation are common byproducts, regardless of the industry or setting in which the change occurs. The magnitude of the transition to the ICD-10-CM code set has the potential to produce significant amounts of fear and misinformation, which can either lead to paralysis and inaction or to **overzealousness** in the discussion of the issue, resulting in the inefficient execution of the change. To ensure that accurate and realistic information is the basis for the discussion of this transition, pertinent information is required concerning the history of the change, the necessity of the change, and the benefits of the change.

HISTORY OF THE TRANSITION

The World Health Organization (WHO) originally published the *International Classification of Diseases*, Tenth Revision (ICD-10), in 1993. This coincided with the recognition by the National Committee on Vital and Health Statistics (NCVHS) in 1993 that ICD-9 was no longer sufficient for its purpose (Grider, 2010). Since that time it has been used around the world for tracking morbidity and mortality data. Over the years, ICD-10 has been gradually adapted for use in clinical service reporting (e.g., to third-party payers) by several major countries. This was possible in large part because most of these countries have single payer models for their citizens' health coverage.

Although ICD-10 has been used in the United States since 1999 for reporting mortality data, ICD-9 continues to be the code set used to report morbidity data and used by hospitals and other health care providers to report diagnostic information to third-party payers for claim payment. The primary reason for the delay in implementation is the relative complexity of the U.S. health care system—particularly the third-party payer component. There was great resistance by most parties involved because of the fear of the transition process.

Significant and repeated delays occurred in the transition from ICD-9 to ICD-10. The first formal implementation date was announced in 2008 as October 1, 2011. Because of concerns expressed by medical societies and health care organizations of all sizes regarding the aggressiveness of the schedule, the implementation date was postponed. The *Federal Register* published the final rule on January 16, 2009, announcing that ICD-10 would go into effect on October 1, 2013. However, the need to convert from ICD-9 to ICD-10 had been a major topic of discussion in the health care community for more than a decade.

Two primary reasons exist for the delay in implementation of ICD-10:

- Direct costs to be experienced in all sectors of the health care industry.

Overzealousness
Excessive interest in or commitment to a cause.

CODING TIP

Services provided on September 30, 2013, must be coded using ICD-9, while services provided on October 1, 2013, must be coded using ICD-10. The only exception is for patients who are in an inpatient status at midnight on October 1, 2013. Their services are to be coded with ICD-9 until their discharge.

Table 8.1 Cost Estimates for ICD-10-CM Implementation

Study	Implementation Costs	Lost Productivity Costs	Notes
Robert E. Nolan Consulting Firm (2003)	$5.5 to $13.5 billion	$752 million to $1.4 billion	Lost productivity costs include only hospitals and physician practices, not long-term care, labs, payers, and others
RAND Corporation (2004)	$475 million to $1.53 billion	$5 to $40 million	Most commonly cited study
Dept. of Health and Human Services (HHS)–led Research	$849 million to $3.05 billion	$572 million	Participating organizations were HHS, CMS, CDC, ONCHIT,* Veterans' Affairs, and Department of Defense

*ONCHIT = Office of the National Coordinator for Health Information Technology.

Source: Conn, 2008.

- Dramatically reduced productivity during the education and orientation process.

It is agreed that the direct costs will be substantial, but there is significant disagreement about exactly how much it will cost. A variety of studies put the range of costs from $475 million to $13.5 billion (Table 8.1). Most of the variation occurs because of differences in the ways that the costs are calculated.

Every entity that touches a diagnosis code will incur expense associated with this transition. Providers will incur expense in revising their practice flow and systems to accommodate the new codes and expense in training staff and physicians. However, for providers, the biggest possible expense is the reduction in productivity and possible loss of revenue due to payment slowdowns. Claim error rates are conservatively estimated to rise to 6 to 10% following ICD-10 implementation, when the standard claim error rate is 3% following the annual updates to the ICD-9 code set (Conn, 2008). Based on the experience of other countries that have transitioned to ICD-10, the Department of Health and Human Services (HHS) expects the productivity and accuracy levels to return to a more normal state within six months.

Payers will incur substantial expense because they will need to modify their claim processing systems to accept the new ICD-10 codes. Moreover, it will take substantial time to review every payment policy that requires the use of a particular diagnosis code for a claim to be paid. In addition, all payer staff members who work in claims, medical review, or prior authorization will need training in ICD-10.

Billing software vendors, electronic health record (EHR) vendors, and claims clearinghouses will incur significant expense in rewriting their software to facilitate the use of ICD-10 codes. The ICD-9 code set, which uses codes of three to five digits in length (largely numeric), will be replaced by ICD-10, which uses alphanumeric codes of three to seven digits in length. The length of the diagnosis code field will need to be increased and the capability of the field to handle alpha characters throughout the field will be the largest challenge. Whether the vendors can recoup the cost of these modifications will largely depend on the terms of the contract between the vendor and the provider. Many vendor contracts provide assurance that their

COMPLIANCE TIP

All entities in the health care system are affected by the change to ICD-10 and, therefore, they all have compliance issues to address.

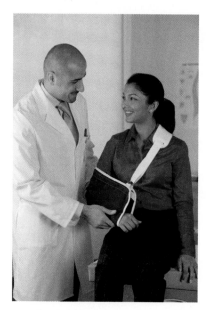

Pay-for-performance programs require detailed data on physicians' performance. One way to track performance is to analyze diagnosis codes. ICD-10 can provide more detailed data than ICD-9, enabling more exact tracking of physicians' performance and, in many cases, improved patient care.

Pay-for-performance
Program in which providers are compensated by payers based on the quality of care that they deliver, not simply the number of procedures.

system will facilitate claim submission to third-party payers and that the change to ICD-10 is simply keeping the program compliant with the contract. Vendors will need to identify alternative methods of financing this expense if they are unable to charge it to their existing clients.

REASONS FOR THE CHANGE TO ICD-10

In light of the tremendous expense incurred by all parties during and after the transition, many have questioned the necessity of the change. As mentioned previously, the need for change was recognized as early as 1993, by the National Committee on Vital and Health Statistics (NCVHS). The specific reasons given for the change at that time were:

- Lack of space for expansion (no room for new codes related to conditions for which codes already exist, within the context of the existing framework).
- Overlapping and duplicative codes (similar codes appearing in separate sections).
- Inconsistent and noncurrent use of terminology.
- Lack of codes for preventive services (a lack of specificity regarding the new types of preventive services that are now provided).
- Insufficient specificity and detail (many services must be reported as "unspecified" or "not otherwise specified").
- Insufficient structure to capture or recognize new technology (National Committee on Vital and Health Statistics, 2003).

Since the time these reasons were expressed in 1993, **pay-for-performance** has become a key reimbursement issue. The ICD-9 code set does not provide sufficient detail or specificity to easily evaluate a physician's performance based on the claim data submitted for payment. ICD-10 provides sufficient information to make qualitative decisions related to the care provided, supplying another reason for the transition from ICD-9 to ICD-10.

BENEFITS OF THE CHANGE TO ICD-10

The risks and expenses associated with the transition to ICD-10 are substantial, but there are also significant benefits in changing to the new code set. From a public health perspective, ICD-10 will improve the quality of the nation's health care data. The increased specificity afforded by the new code set will allow public health officials to better track disease trends and will help identify the spread of communicable disease in the United States and around the world (Grider, 2010). Since the United States is one of the few countries in the world not using ICD-10 for tracking morbidity data, it has not been able to participate in worldwide data sharing. This is critical, given that increased traveling and immigration have made the world a much smaller place, so that the spread of disease can be more easily identified.

From the perspective of a health care provider in the United States, there are three specific benefits in using ICD-10 as the diagnosis code set: (1) more precise documentation of clinical care, (2) more accurate coding, and (3) a contribution to health care quality improvement initiatives.

More Precise Documentation of Clinical Care. Frequently, ICD-9 requires the use of multiple codes to fully report a disease or condition. Unless the coder is highly skilled and understands the principles of multiple code usage, the additional codes may not be used. In addition, some payers recognize only one diagnosis code per procedure, even when multiple diagnoses are supplied. With ICD-10's code specificity, there are many occasions in which a single diagnosis code can fully and accurately describe a patient's condition.

For example, under ICD-9, a patient with acute cor pulmonale and a septic pulmonary embolism would have the condition reported as:

Example

415.0   Acute cor pulmonale AND

415.12   Septic pulmonary embolism

Under ICD-10, this condition would be reported with a single code:

Example

126.01   Septic pulmonary embolism with acute cor pulmonale

In addition to potentially reducing the number of codes used, the nature of the treatment is communicated more clearly. For example, if a patient has acute tonsillitis caused by the streptococcal virus, the provider is required to report the ICD-9 diagnosis as 463—Acute Tonsillitis and 041.10—Staphylococcus, unspecified. If the patient returns four months later with another incidence of acute tonsillitis, the same ICD-9 diagnosis codes would be used. If the ICD-10 code set was used, the visits would be coded as follows:

Example

Visit 1   J03.00   Acute streptococcal tonsillitis, unspecified

Visit 2   J03.01   Acute recurrent streptococcal tonsillitis

This coding scenario provides a much clearer picture to anyone reviewing this person's claim because the reviewer would know that the infection is recurrent just by looking at the diagnosis for the second visit. The only way this would be possible previously with ICD-9 is if the reviewer studied multiple claims for the same patient.

More Accurate Coding. Throughout the ICD-9 code book there are many codes with fourth and fifth digits of "8" or "9."

CODING TIP

ICD-10 codes provide the opportunity to supply substantially more detailed information about the patient's condition than do ICD-9 codes.

Example

277.8 **Other specified** disorders of metabolism

277.9 **Unspecified** disorders of metabolism

The same pattern is found throughout the ICD-9 code set. Codes with an "8" as the fourth digit represent situations in which the provider knows what the patient's disorder is but there is no code that accurately describes the condition. Codes with a "9" as the fourth digit indicate that the provider has not yet definitively diagnosed the patient's condition.

This situation will occur less frequently in the ICD-10 code set. Because there are more codes available, there will be fewer "other specified" diagnoses. There will still be occasions in which the provider doesn't have a definitive diagnosis and the use of "unspecified diagnoses" will be required. However, the increased specificity in the system prompts providers to be more accurate in their coding, as opposed to defaulting to an unspecified code, which often happens with the use of ICD-9.

The greater degree of accuracy is illustrated in the following case. In ICD-9, the first visit for a patient with a torus fracture of the right arm radius would be coded as:

Example

813.45   Torus fracture of radius (alone)

Unfortunately, the same diagnosis would be used for each and every encounter associated with this condition. In addition, there is no way to know which arm was affected by the fracture. In ICD-10, the service is coded as S52.521A. Each of the digits represents a different element of the condition, as follows:

Example

S52 Fracture of forearm

   S52.**5** Fracture of **lower end of radius**

      S52.52 **Torus** fracture of lower end of radius

         S52.52**1** Torus fracture of lower end of **right** radius

            S52.521**A** Torus fracture of lower end of right radius, **initial encounter for closed fracture**

Contribution to Health Care Quality Improvement Initiatives.   The ability to be highly specific in diagnosis coding through ICD-10 allows reviewers and payers to understand the frequency and circumstances in which patients are treated for a given condition and helps providers justify the services that they provide. For example, using the case of the patient with recurrent tonsillitis, if a physician submits a claim with an ICD-10 diagnosis of J03.01 four times in a six-month period, conclusions may be able to be drawn regarding the quality of the physician's care—why was a tonsillectomy not performed by now? This information can be collected from claims data, without an expensive and labor-intensive chart review. Of course, there may be a valid reason for delaying surgery, but the potential outlier is identified much sooner than it would otherwise be noticed.

Similarly, the use of J03.01 could justify the performance of a tonsillectomy after just one office encounter. The patient sought a second opinion from this physician, who recommends an immediate tonsillectomy. Using ICD-9, the only option this physician would have for a diagnosis is 474.00—Chronic tonsillitis. However, that does not fully paint the picture that the physician is encountering, given that there is an acute episode of tonsillitis presently occurring. The ICD-9 code set does not support the quality of the physician's decision as well as does ICD-10.

COMPLIANCE TIP

ICD-10 will facilitate the more aggressive use of pay-for-performance payment methodologies, which will increase the attention that needs to be paid to related compliance issues.

Thinking It Through 8.1

1. What surprised you the most about the transition from ICD-9 to ICD-10 that you did not previously know?

2. What is your opinion of the cost estimates regarding the transition to ICD-10? Which one do you feel is most reliable? Why?

3. Of the reasons for change provided by the NCVHS in 1993, which do you believe is the most compelling? Why?

8.2 Similarities and Differences Between ICD-9 and ICD-10 and Tools for Transition

Much of the fear associated with the transition to ICD-10 is that it is a "new" system with a substantially larger number of codes within the code set. Seasoned coders have significant sections of the code books memorized and, in the ordinary course of events, they are able to supply a procedure or diagnosis code on demand. The comfort that comes from that level of knowledge will be lost on the implementation of ICD-10 because it will take months, if not years, to achieve that level of familiarity again. Also, many question if it will be possible to become as familiar with the sheer quantity of ICD-10 code set as they were with the ICD-9 codes.

COMPARING THE CODE SETS

A substantial difference exists between the two code sets, as illustrated in Table 8.2.

Table 8.2 Comparison of ICD-9-CM and ICD-10-CM

	ICD-9	ICD-10
Number of characters	3–5 characters in length.	3–7 characters in length.
Number of codes	Approximately 13,000 codes.	Approximately 68,000 available codes.
Types of characters	First digit can be alpha (E or V) or numeric; digits 2–5 are numeric. Most codes are all numeric.	Digit 1 is alpha; digits 2 and 3 are numeric; digits 4–7 are alpha or numeric.
Code capacity	Limited space for adding new codes.	Flexible for adding new codes.
Specificity	Lacks detail.	Very specific.
Laterality designations (right vs. left)	Lacks laterality.	Has laterality.

Source: American Medical Association [AMA], 2010.

Laterality
The side of the body on which a disease is located or a procedure is performed.

Sequelae
Negative effects of a previous disease.

CODING TIP

Once the patterns of the ICD-10 coding structure are learned, identifying proper codes may be easier than in ICD-9, even though there are a substantially larger number of codes from which to choose.

The most daunting of the differences is the sheer number of diagnosis codes in ICD-10—more than five times as many as in ICD-9. However, the differences are not as overwhelming as they might seem. The biggest reason for the large number of additional codes is the specificity offered by the codes, including **laterality** and other differentiating factors such as trimester when reporting pregnancy services or reporting the type of encounter (initial, subsequent, or **sequelae**). The number of fundamental base codes is not dramatically different. Once coders learn the repeating code patterns, coding may actually become easier.

ICD-10-CM codes may consist of up to seven digits, with the seventh-digit extensions representing visit encounter or sequelae for injuries and external causes. Figure 8.1 demonstrates the function of each of these digits.

Moreover, many of the conventions of ICD-9 coding continue to be used in the same fashion in ICD-10. For example, the following conventions are exactly the same in ICD-10 as they are in ICD-9:

- Includes.
- Not otherwise specified.
- Excludes.
- Code first underlying disease.
- Use additional code.
- Colon.
- Brackets.
- Parentheses.

FIGURE 8.1
Code Structure of ICD-10-CM Versus ICD-9-CM

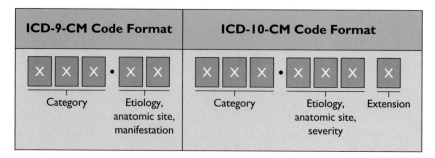

Source: Barta, McNeill, Meli, Wall, and Zeisset, 2008.

The "notes" convention is similar, except ICD-10 has an additional feature that allows the differentiation between "with" and "without," which allows more specificity in coding. The only new conventions are the "excludes1" and "excludes2" features, which define codes that are mutually exclusive and conditions that require two diagnoses, respectively. Table 8.3 compares the differences between instructional notes as they are used in ICD-9-CM and ICD-10-CM.

Table 8.3 Convention Comparison Between ICD-9-CM and ICD-10-CM

Convention	ICD-9-CM	ICD-10-CM
Notes	Further define terms, clarify information, or list choices for additional digits.	Further define terms, clarify information, or list choices for additional digits. *With/without* notes are the options for the final character of a set of codes; the default is *without*. For five-character codes, 0 as the fifth-position character represents *without*, and 1 represents *with*. For six-character codes, the sixth-position character 1 represents *with*, and 9 represents *without*.
Includes	Notes that further define or provide examples and can apply to a chapter, section, or category.	Same as ICD-9-CM.
Not otherwise specified	Used when the information at hand does not permit a more specific code assignment.	Same as ICD-9-CM.
Excludes	Notes that indicate terms that are to be coded elsewhere. They can be used for three reasons: 1. The condition may have to be coded elsewhere. 2. The code cannot be assigned if the associated condition is present. 3. Additional codes may be required to fully explain the condition.	Same as ICD-9-CM.
Code first underlying disease	Used in categories not intended as the primary diagnosis.	Same as ICD-9-CM.
Use additional code	Appears in categories in which further information must be added by using an additional code, to provide a more complete picture.	Same as ICD-9-CM.
Colon	Used after an incomplete term that needs one or more of the modifiers that follows to make it assignable to a category.	Same as ICD-9-CM.
Brackets	Enclose synonyms, alternate wording, or explanatory phrases.	Same as ICD-9-CM.
Parentheses	Enclose supplementary words that may be present or absent, without affecting the code number to which it is assigned.	Same as ICD-9-CM.
Braces	Enclose a series of terms, each of which is modified by the statement appearing at the right.	Not used in ICD-10-CM.
Excludes1	Not used in ICD-9-CM.	Indicates that the code excluded can *never* be used at the same time as the code to which the excludes list applies. For example, a congenital condition and acquired condition cannot coexist.
Excludes2	Not used in ICD-9-CM.	Indicates that the condition is not included as part of the code. If the patient has both conditions, a separate code must be used to report it.

Source: Grider, 2010.

Table 8.3 clearly illustrates that most of the coding principles used in ICD-9 are the same as those in ICD-10. If a person understands ICD-9 conventions, learning the ICD-10 conventions will not be a difficult task. The greatest challenge will be learning the organization of the ICD-10 code set, which is more intuitive and logical than the organization of ICD-9.

USING GEMS—A TOOL FOR IDENTIFYING THE NEW CODES

Given that there are five times more ICD-10 diagnosis codes than ICD-9 diagnosis codes, it is logical that coders will need assistance in identifying comparable codes in the new code set. To that end, the National Center for Health Statistics created the General Equivalence Mapping (GEMs) files. The purpose of GEMs is to map ICD-9 codes to the comparable ICD-10 codes *and* to map the ICD-10 files to the comparable ICD-9 codes.

This is somewhat challenging, in that it is not always possible to directly map codes on a one-to-one basis. Several possible variables can occur that may complicate mapping:

- A single unspecified ICD-9 code could map to one of dozens more specific ICD-10 codes.
- A single ICD-10 code could map backward to two or more ICD-9 codes.
- An ICD-9 code may not have an equivalent code in ICD-10.
- An ICD-10 code may not have an equivalent code in ICD-9.

The key element to understand with regard to mapping is that it is not always acceptable to create a crosswalk for use that simply exchanges the ICD-10 code for an ICD-9 code. While this may seem to be the easiest solution to the problem, it will result in improper coding that may have a significant negative impact in the future.

For example, if a patient has sciatica (pain caused by nerve irritation), the diagnosis code in ICD-9 is 724.3. Using the GEMs resource, the ICD-10 code that corresponds with 724.3 is M54.30—Sciatica, unspecified side. However, the ICD-10 code book lists the codes for this condition as follows:

Example

M54.3 Sciatica

    Excludes1: lesion of sciatic nerve (G57.0)

        sciatica due to intervertebral disc disorder (M51.1-)

        sciatica with lumbago (M54.4-)

    M54.30 Sciatica, unspecified side

    M54.31 Sciatica, right side

    M54.32 Sciatica, left side

Proper coding, in this circumstance, would dictate that the most specific information possible be reported. The physician would know on which side of the body the patient was experiencing the pain. Therefore, adequate coding under ICD-9 (724.3) would be insufficient in ICD-10.

Another example demonstrates issues related to both laterality and encounter status. For example, a patient who had a subsequent visit for an abrasion of the left elbow would have the diagnosis assigned in ICD-9 as 913.0—abrasion or friction burn of elbow, forearm, and wrist, without mention of infection. The GEMs crosswalk links that code to the three following ICD-10 codes:

Example

S50.319A Abrasion of unspecified elbow, initial encounter

S50.819A Abrasion of unspecified forearm, initial encounter

S60.819A Abrasion of unspecified wrist, initial encounter

However, none of these would be correct for this circumstance— the correct code is S50.312D—Abrasion of left elbow, subsequent encounter.

GEMs and other crosswalks are vital tools in learning the relationship between ICD-9 and ICD-10 codes. However, they cannot be relied on as the sole means of new code selection. Insufficient specificity will be a guaranteed result if the coder attempts to assign codes without further investigation and research in the codes.

Thinking It Through 8.2

1. Summarize the reasons why the substantial increase in the number of codes is not as overwhelming as it might seem.

2. Most of the conventions in ICD-10 are the same as those in ICD-9. Which ones are different and which is the most significant change? Why is it most significant, in your opinion?

8.3 The Ethical Challenges of ICD-10-CM

There is nothing about ICD-10 or any other code set that automatically makes its use ethically challenging. In the case of ICD-10, most of the possible ethical challenges come about as the result of the lack of familiarity with the system and the complexity that comes with every party in the U.S. health care industry having to adapt to a new system on an abrupt basis on October 1, 2013. To analyze these challenges, the types of challenges and the parties in the process both must be reviewed.

FYI

It is more likely that ethical lapses related to ICD-10 coding will be the result of unintentional actions, as opposed to actively choosing to be unethical. However, this does not change the responsibility of the individuals involved in the process to ensure that their coding is ethical.

Affirmative unethical act
An active choice to engage in an unethical act.

Affirmative Unethical Acts.
An **affirmative unethical act** occurs when a person or organization says, "I/We choose to conduct ourselves in a manner that is intentionally unethical." This type of decision will be reasonably rare as it pertains to ICD-10. However, as the parties involved in the health care process are reviewed, it will become clear that this type of decision is conceivable.

Unintentional Unethical Acts.
The "unintentional" unethical act is the opposite of the affirmative unethical act. Unintentional unethical acts occur when

1. The parties do not recognize or realize that their actions are creating ethical challenges for themselves or others.
2. The parties do not take reasonable steps or precautions to prevent adverse outcomes for themselves or others.

These acts are significantly more likely to occur in relation to the implementation and use of the ICD-10 code system than are affirmative unethical acts.

THE PARTIES IN THE PROCESS

Ethical dilemmas develop, in large part, out of relationships between parties. The code sets used in medical coding also are a key component of relationships between parties—they are the means of communication of the medical necessity of services provided from one party to another. The intersection of the issues of ethical dilemmas and ICD-10 codes occurs in this environment of relationship.

Providers.
When discussions occur regarding ICD-10 implementation, most of the attention is focused on the provider, whether a small physician practice, a large hospital or health system, or any other entity in the health care delivery process. This focus on providers exists because they, generally, are least equipped to effectively implement a change of this magnitude while simultaneously maintaining ongoing operations. Another factor that focuses attention on providers is the sheer number of individuals who are part of provider organizations, relative to health plans, software vendors, and other interested parties. The larger the number of people involved in the process, the more complex it becomes. However, the larger the organization, the more resources the organization has to accomplish the change.

Ultimately, as it relates to coding, the provider is responsible for the codes that are assigned to the claim. However, the other parties have responsibility to the provider (Figure 8.2). Administration is responsible for setting up appropriate systems to facilitate proper billing. Administration is also responsible for providing resources to the billing/coding staff to give them the ability to properly serve the provider. The billing/coding staff is employed to serve the provider, but the provider must be cooperative in communicating with the billing/coding staff to make the coding accurate and effective—particularly in relationship to ICD-10 coding.

Since the provider's name is listed on the claim form submitted to third-party payers as the party that delivered the service, it is

BILLING TIP

The provider is the centerpiece of the responsibility for the ICD-10 transition within the provider office because its name is on the claim.

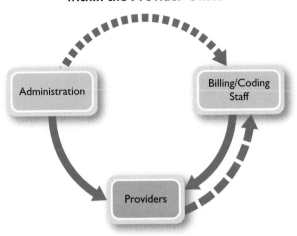

ICD-10 Relationship Responsibilities within the Provider Office

Administration

Billing/Coding Staff

Providers

FIGURE 8.2

The relationship between the various parties within the provider's office.

responsible for the codes that appear on the claim. It is not possible for a physician, nurse practitioner, physician assistant, or any other provider of service to fulfill their responsibility to submit accurate claims on behalf of the patient without knowledge of the ICD-10 coding system. In whatever fashion is necessary and suitable for the setting, the provider must become familiar with the proper usage of the ICD-10 code set.

In most circumstances, the administration of the provider practice bears the responsibility of educating all parties within the organization, including the physicians. Whether that training occurs through internal sources or external sources, the training must occur because of the changes in codes and, more significantly, the change in code specificity. Although certified coders who work in the billing/coding department are going to have significant access to ICD-10 training by virtue of their relationship with their certification organization, many practices do not have certified coders and the practice's administration must obtain appropriate training for the coding/billing personnel.

Perhaps the most difficult element of the transition from ICD-9 to ICD-10, beyond the educational process, is the necessity of system modification and change in communication processes. The marking of superbills as a means of providers communicating procedures and diagnoses to the billing staff is generally no longer reasonably viable because of the sheer number of codes that would be required to accurately report even the most basic of common diagnoses. The American Academy of Family Practice states that it is theoretically possible to have a paper superbill, but it illustrates its unlikelihood by demonstrating the difference in code selection for the common condition of right lower quadrant abdominal pain (Table 8.4).

If a single ICD-9 code must be reported using one of a significant variety of ICD-10 codes, there will not be any feasible way to prepare a superbill/charge ticket that satisfactorily encompasses all of the codes needed. Therefore, provider offices will be forced to either (1) find an alternative method of selecting and communicating diagnosis codes, or (2) maintain the superbill system, but include only generic ICD-10 codes, resulting in an unacceptable lack of specificity.

FYI

The biggest challenge in ICD-10, after the educational process, is adjusting systems and methods of communication to ensure that proper coding occurs.

Table 8.4 ICD-9 and ICD-10 Coding Options for Abdominal Pain

ICD-9-CM	ICD-10-CM Possible Options
Abdominal pain, right lower quadrant—789.03	Abdominal pain, unspecified—R10.9
	Lower abdominal pain, unspecified—R10.30
	Right lower quadrant pain—R10.31
	Tenderness, right lower quadrant abdomen—R10.813
	Rebound tenderness right lower quadrant abdomen—R10.823

Source: American Academy of Family Practice, 2011.

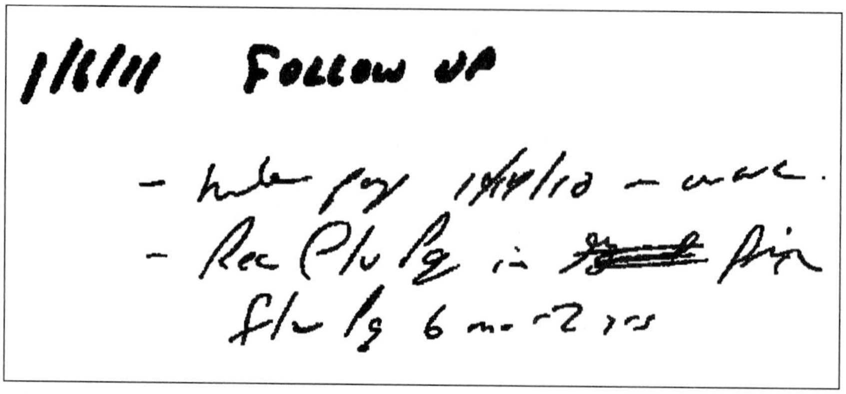

FIGURE 8.3

This progress note indicates that the patient is having a follow-up Pap smear, but there is no explanation as to why. In ICD-9, the best possible diagnosis code, based on this record, is 795.09—Other abnormal Pap smear of cervix. While this is suboptimal in ICD-9, the situation becomes worse in its lack of specificity in ICD-10.

Abstractor
A billing/coding professional who is responsible for identifying diagnosis codes by reviewing the medical record.

Moreover, the instances of inadequate documentation, which frequently occur now, will simply be unacceptable in the future. If the practice determines that it will not educate physicians on ICD-10, but codes will be selected by **abstractors** or coders who review the medical record, then the record has to be sufficiently detailed to allow the best possible code selection. This will require additional training so that providers know what is required in the record to supply the coders with the necessary information (Figure 8.3).

The ethical issues associated with ICD-10 for providers will usually not be the result of an intentional unethical action. Instead, they will most likely occur because of unintentional actions that result in incorrect codes that mischaracterize or are grossly inadequate in their specificity. Table 8.5 lists possible reasons for unethical behavior.

Health Plans/Third-Party Payers. Because third-party payers are the recipients of the claim forms that include ICD-10 codes after October 1, 2013, they must be as prepared, if not more prepared, for the

Table 8.5 Reasons for Unethical Behavior

Provider	Administration	Biller/Coder
Unethical toward patient in delaying or preventing benefits for patient due to improper coding	Unethical toward provider (employer) in development of adequate systems, which results in inadequate coding and decreased/delayed reimbursements	Unethical toward patient in delaying or preventing benefits for patient due to improper coding
Unethical toward billing/coding staff because of resistance to assist them in performing their job	Unethical toward billing/coding staff because of provision of inadequate resources	Unethical toward provider (employer) in development of adequate systems, which results in inadequate coding and decreased/delayed reimbursements

transition than providers. If a provider is unprepared for the ICD-10 transition, only the provider and its patients are harmed. However, if a third-party payer is not ready, the scope of the damage can be extensive as it could affect every provider that submits claims to the payer.

Third-party payers are ethically obligated to be ready to receive these claims and process them properly, according to the terms of the patient's benefits agreement. Devastating harm can result for providers if they see a dramatic decrease in cash flow because the payer is not ready to receive and properly pay claims ICD-10 diagnoses and procedures. In addition, significant financial harm is possible for patients if they lose benefits to which they are entitled because claims are not properly processed or payment is delayed.

Moreover, payers and health plans should not use this transition as an opportunity to improve their cash flow by reducing their claim payouts. To be sure, providers are obligated to submit correct claims. However, it is to be expected that providers will face challenges in adjusting to the new system. If payers construct payment policies that are excessively strict regarding the diagnoses that are required to document the medical necessity for a given procedure, they may receive a windfall profit because of the nonspecific claims that providers may submit during the transition. The denial of these claims will inevitably lead to the nonpayment of otherwise payable claims because of the large number of claims denials that providers could experience. If providers are overwhelmed with denials, some of these claims may exceed claim submission or follow-up deadlines, making them ineligible for payment and allowing the payer to keep the claim payment amount.

The goal of the implementation of ICD-10 is to increase the specificity of diagnosis codes and it is quite reasonable to expect payers to tighten their payment policies, in accordance with the principles of ICD-10. However, it is not ethical for payers to intentionally establish initial guidelines that ensure an excessive number of claim denials, resulting in direct economic benefit to the payer. Payers should partner with providers in the transition process by learning the new system together and communicating openly about the gradual tightening of payment rules, which is completely appropriate (Figure 8.4). Consider the case of Adam Jackson's efforts to prepare his organization for ICD-10.

ICD-10 Relationship Responsibilities

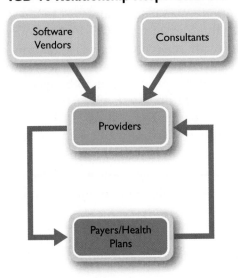

FIGURE 8.4

The relationship and responsibilities between various parties in the health care reimbursement process.

Example

Adam Jackson is Vice President for Claims Processing for American Intercontinental Health Insurance Company. He was meeting with the senior leadership of the organization. Among several major items on the agenda was the need to increase the quarterly dividend that is paid to the shareholders; another was a discussion about the need to prepare for ICD-10. The CEO, Susan Avillar, was very upset as Adam explained the costs associated with the transition. "How do you expect us to spend that much money on claim processing and still make our shareholders happy?" she asked loudly.

Adam admitted that there were initial costs associated with the transition, but he emphasized that, in the long run, there would be a reduction in claim-processing costs. Because ICD-10 specificity would reduce the amount of manual intervention needed, eventually fewer claim reviewers would be necessary. This did not satisfy Susan because the savings would not come soon enough. Adam realized that this conversation was not going well and his colleagues were beginning to avert their eyes away from him. To save face he said, "It's our expectation that the number of denied claims will increase after ICD-10 is implemented because providers won't provide sufficient specificity when they submit the claim. We are planning to gradually implement the more stringent claim payment guidelines."

"Nonsense," interrupted Susan. "Implement those guidelines immediately in October 2013—we'll report that plan at the next shareholders' meeting—that should help our stock valuation."

Adam tried to explain his plan, but it was quickly clear that the meeting had moved on to the next topic.

Software Vendors. Software vendors also have a significant challenge associated with the transition to ICD-10, because it will require substantial changes to their software. They have an extreme ethical obligation to their clients because their products are critical to the effective functioning of provider operations. They must ensure that their software will work properly on and after the transition date. Moreover, the software must be able to operate using both code sets because claims with service dates prior to October 1, 2013, will need to be entered using ICD-9 codes, even after that date. A system that fails to accommodate this change would result in catastrophic harm to the provider.

The unethical vendor may also attempt to charge its clients an additional fee for the transition to ICD-10. This may be permissible under some contracts between vendors and providers, but most contracts have a provision of an **implied warranty of merchantability,** meaning that the product has to be usable for its intended purpose. If the software does not allow the use of ICD-10 codes, then it is no longer usable. In most cases, the changes must occur to maintain the implied warranty, unless the contract is specifically written otherwise.

Consultants. Consultants and other agencies offering advice to providers have an ethical obligation to provide information that is

- Accurate.
- Timely.
- Scalable to the size of the organization.

Implied warranty of merchantability
The principle that a product or service must do what it is advertised to do.

Some consultants and publishers have issued information and publications that were excessive or unnecessary at the time they were sold to customers. Some providers have been convinced that they need to expend substantial sums of money on services that were not needed for a group of its size—the services delivered were not timely and were excessive. Providers have a duty to ensure that they are obtaining education and resources from reliable sources.

Thinking It Through 8.3

1. Figure 8.2 shows that providers are the centerpiece of responsibility in relation to ICD-10 implementation and use. Why is this the case? Do you agree with this assertion?

2. What do you feel is the most difficult element of the transition from ICD-9 to ICD-10? Why?

3. Which is worse—unethical behavior resulting from affirmative actions or unethical behavior resulting from unintentional actions? On what do you base your opinion?

8.4 Addressing and Avoiding Ethical Challenges Associated with ICD-10

The best way to address and avoid ethical challenges in any situation is to accurately predict the circumstances that can create ethical problems and effectively prepare for them. The transition to ICD-10-CM is a prime example in which ethical challenges are foreseeable. Given that the federal government provided over four years' notice of the change (January 16, 2009–October 1, 2013), there is no reason that the ethical problems can't be avoided.

The actions necessary to prepare for the transition to ICD-10 fall within three broad categories:

- Preparation/planning
- Financial investment
- Training/awareness

All of these elements work together to promote the effective transition from ICD-9 to ICD-10. To be effective, the approach must be systematic and must go beyond only learning the codes. Figure 8.5 shows the various key steps that are required, grouped by category.

The amount of time, money, and effort involved in the process will vary substantially, based on the size and nature of the organization. A small physician practice will be able to do this with a small team and a relatively small budget. A large health care system will require a large multidisciplinary team and, perhaps, an investment of millions of dollars.

Regardless of the size or type of organization, all potential ethical issues can be resolved by disciplined preparation, detailed analysis, and persistent training, implementation, and follow-up.

FYI

The best way to address and avoid ethical challenges in any situation is to accurately predict the circumstances that can create ethical problems and effectively prepare for them.

FIGURE 8.5

The steps involved in the transition from ICD-9 to ICD-10, grouped by category. Failure to execute each of the steps will open the door to severe operational difficulties and potential ethical problems.

Preparation/Planning
- Organize a project team
- Conduct a preliminary impact analysis
- Create an implementation timeline
- Analyze documentation needs
- Conduct business process analysis

Financial Investment
- Develop an ICD-10 implementation budget

Training/Awareness
- Develop a communication plan
- Develop a training plan
- Complete information systems design and development
- Conduct needs assessment

Source: Grider, 2010.

Thinking It Through 8.4

1. In your opinion, is the federal government's notice of the transition from ICD-9 to ICD-10 sufficient? Why or why not?

2. Which key element among the recommended steps for preparing for ICD-10 has the greatest potential for ethical issues if it is not performed properly? Why?

3. Which do you believe would be easier—participating as part of the ICD-10 implementation team in a large organization or being in charge of the ICD-10 team in a small practice? On what do you base your opinion?

CHAPTER REVIEW

Chapter Summary

Learning Outcomes	Key Concepts/Examples
8.1 Describe the ICD-10-CM code set and the transition process from the ICD-9-CM code set. Pages 262–267	• The transition from ICD-9 to ICD-10 will be the most significant change in the practice of health care coding. • ICD-10 was first introduced in 1993, at the same time that ICD-9 was found to be insufficient for future use. • The first date for implementation of ICD-10 was October 1, 2011, but it was moved ahead to October 1, 2013. • The reasons for the delays in implementation of ICD-10 are: 1. The direct costs experienced in all sectors of the health care industry. 2. The indirect costs associated with the loss of productivity during the transition. • The change to ICD-10 must occur because of: 1. Lack of room for expansion. 2. Inconsistent use of terminology. 3. Overlapping or duplicate codes. 4. Insufficient specificity and detail. • The benefits of change are: 1. More precise documentation of clinical care. 2. More accurate coding. 3. The contribution to health care quality improvement initiatives.

Learning Outcomes	Key Concepts/Examples
8.2 Explain the similarities and differences between ICD-9 and ICD-10 and the available tools for facilitating the transition. Pages 267–271	• Many are concerned about the transition to ICD-10 because seasoned coders have large sections of ICD-9 memorized. It will take a significant amount of time before that level of knowledge is regained. • Significant differences exist between the code sets, the biggest difference being the larger number of codes in ICD-10. The code format is also different, along with the level of detail in code assignment. • The conventions of ICD-9 and ICD-10 are generally quite similar. • The General Equivalence Mapping files (GEMs) are a valuable tool for helping coders learn the use of the ICD-10 system, but it is not a replacement for learning the code set.
8.3 Evaluate the practical ethical challenges health care providers and organizations will face in the transition to ICD-10-CM. Pages 271–277	• The types of ethical challenges are: 1. Affirmative unethical acts. 2. Unintentional unethical acts. • The parties in the ICD-9 to ICD-10 coding process are: 1. Providers. 2. Health plans/third-party payers. 3. Software vendors. 4. Consultants.
8.4 Design protocols to address and avoid the ethical challenges created by the use of ICD-10-CM. Pages 277–278	• The best way to address and avoid ethical challenges is to accurately predict the circumstances that will create them. • The actions necessary to prepare for the transition to ICD-10 are: 1. Preparation/planning. 2. Financial investment. 3. Training/awareness. • The amount of time and effort involved to make the transition will vary based on organization size and nature.

End-of-Chapter Questions

Multiple Choice

Circle the letter that best completes the statement or answers the question.

1. **LO 8.1** The effective date of the transition to ICD-10 is (was)
   a. January 1, 2013
   b. October 1, 2011
   c. October 1, 2013
   d. Not definitively established

2. **LO 8.1** Which of the following is *not* part of the transition to ICD-10 in the short term?
   a. Fear
   b. Misinformation
   c. Overzealousness
   d. Increased efficiency

3. **LO 8.1** What is the reason for the wide variance in cost calculations for the transition to ICD-10?
   a. Different methods of calculating costs
   b. Inflation
   c. Economic uncertainty
   d. Organizations of different size

4. **LO 8.1** Which of the following is *not* a reason for the transition to ICD-10?

    a. Lack of space for expansion

    b. Code sets needing to be updated regularly—ICD is overdue

    c. Overlapping and duplicative codes

    d. Insufficient specificity and detail

5. **LO 8.2** ICD-10 has approximately _____ more codes than ICD-9.

    a. 120,000

    b. 90,000

    c. 55,000

    d. 30,000

6. **LO 8.2** The most daunting of the differences between ICD-9 and ICD-10 is

    a. The sheer number of codes

    b. The significant difference in the use of coding conventions

    c. The lower capacity for adding new codes in ICD-9

    d. The code format

7. **LO 8.2** Mapping of codes between ICD-9 and ICD-10 is complicated by all of the following *except*

    a. A single ICD-10 code could map backward to two or more ICD-9 codes.

    b. A single ICD-9 code could map to one of dozens of specific ICD-10 codes.

    c. An ICD-10 code may not have an equivalent code in ICD-9.

    d. Sometimes a single ICD-9 code maps to a single ICD-10 code.

8. **LO 8.3** Who is the most important party in ensuring proper ICD-10 coding within the provider office?

    a. Administration

    b. Billing/coding personnel

    c. Front office staff

    d. Providers

9. **LO 8.3** Unethical actions related to ICD-10 coding will likely occur because of

    a. Inadvertent or unintentional actions

    b. Affirmative decisions to be unethical

    c. Excessive specificity in code selection

    d. Excessive preparation for the transition

10. **LO 8.4** The best way to address and avoid ethical challenges is to

    a. Have effective disciplinary programs in place

    b. Have effective educational programs in place

    c. Accurately predict the circumstances that can create ethical problems and effectively prepare for them

    d. Limit the number of people involved in the process

Short Answer

Use your critical thinking skills to answer the following questions.

1. **LO 8.1** Do you agree that the implementation of ICD-10 is the most significant change in the history of medical coding? Why or why not?

2. **LO 8.1** Explain the difference between morbidity and mortality data. Why is it important that countries around the world use ICD-10 for both data elements?

3. **LO 8.1** What is the most significant cause of the delay in implementation of ICD-10? Do you believe that the reasons for the delay are reasonable?

4. **LO 8.1** Explain why every entity involved in the health care finance process is influenced by the change to ICD-10.

5. **LO 8.1** Who has the most significant challenge in the change to ICD-10—providers, payers, or software vendors?

6. **LO 8.2** Of the convention differences between ICD-9 and ICD-10, which do you believe will be the most difficult to learn? Why?

7. **LO 8.2** Explain why you can't just use the GEMs files to select an ICD-10 code.

8. **LO 8.3** Describe the obligation that providers have to the billing/coding personnel to ensure ethical selection of ICD-10 codes.

9. **LO 8.3** Describe the most difficult element of the transition from ICD-9 to ICD-10, after the educational process. How does the consideration of ethics affect this issue?

10. **LO 8.4** Examine Figure 8.5 on page 278. Which do you believe is the most critical step? Why?

Applying Your Knowledge

The two coders who had participated in the billing department meeting with Olga, the supervisor, were still unhappy following the discussion about the transition to ICD-10. They were talking about the issue while they were walking to their break. They were surprised when they heard a voice behind them. "What are you guys talking about?" asked clinic administrator James Hu. The two coders looked at each other in panic, both thinking, "What should we say?"

Finally, one of them said, "We were just talking about what we need to do to get ready for ICD-10."

"We just sent Olga to a conference about that, didn't we?" asked James. "So what do you think—are we going to be ready?"

"We talked about it at our staff meeting," said one of the coders. The other one quickly interjected, "I just read some great material on preparing for ICD-10. Can I share it with you?"

"Sure," said James, as he got on the elevator.

The two coders exchanged glances as the door closed. "Wow, that was close. Do you think we responded appropriately, or did we go too far? What happens if Olga finds out?"

1. What is your opinion of the coders' response to the administrator's question? Was it disrespectful of their supervisor or dishonest to the administrator? Explain your answer.

2. After studying this chapter, are you more or less concerned about North Mountain Ophthalmology's preparation for the change to ICD-10 than when you originally read the case study?

3. Early in the case study, Olga, the billing manager, suggested that ICD-10 is not that significant an issue for ophthalmology practices. Do you think this assessment is accurate, after reading the material in the chapter?

Internet Research

Information on ICD-10 is available from a wide variety of sources, including books, websites, and other publications. One of the best sources for information is the Medicare website, which is available to the public at no cost (Figure 8.6). This information is particularly valuable and reliable because of the role that CMS and other related governmental agencies play in the development and maintenance of ICD-10-CM.

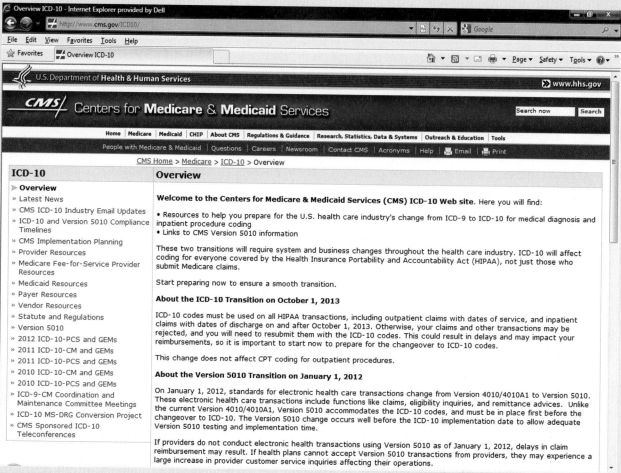

FIGURE 8.6

The Medicare website provides significant information about the transition to ICD-10, including historical information, various resources, and the GEMs files.

A wide variety of resources are available at the CMS website, including implementation information, guidelines for payers and providers, as well supplementary information for vendors and other interested parties. The original regulations are also available from this site, so that the parties can see how the regulations can be applied practically.

Review the materials on the Medicare website at **www.cms.gov/ICD10/** and answer the following questions:

1. What is Version 5010 and what is its relevance to the ICD-10 conversion?

2. Are the GEMs files helpful as they are presented, or could they be presented in a more effective manner? If so, how?

3. What is the most valuable information that you found at this website? Why?

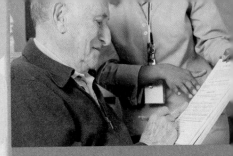

Ethics and the Revenue Cycle

Key Terms

LEARNING OUTCOMES

After completing this chapter, you will be able to:

9.1   Identify the five stages of the revenue cycle, their purpose, and their influence on the subsequent stages.

9.2   Recognize the possible ethical issues that exist when scheduling patients for appointments, registering them, and assigning financial responsibility.

9.3   Discuss the activities related to billing and coding that occur while the patient is receiving treatment.

9.4   Describe the potential ethical issues that can arise in the assignment of codes during the billing process.

9.5   Evaluate ethical situations that occur in relationships with third-party payers.

9.6   Determine the ethical impact of provider behavior and patient response in the patient billing and statementing process.

CASE STUDY

Jason graduated from his medical billing and coding program, obtained his coding certification, and almost immediately found a job as a coder with a local neurosurgery practice. He worked there for approximately three years and enjoyed his experience. However, he was not satisfied with his pay increases (or lack thereof) and he didn't feel that he had any opportunity for advancement or promotion at that practice. He began looking for another position.

He saw an opportunity on a job search website for a position as billing manager for the largest internal medicine practice in the next county. He applied for the position and the practice contacted him about a week later to schedule a telephone interview. Jason was very excited at the possibility. He was familiar with the practice by reputation, but he didn't know a great deal about the physicians or the operation of the clinic itself.

To do some research, he went online and reviewed the practice's website, which included information about the staff and some of its financial policies. Recognizing that he might not be getting a balanced picture, he used a search engine to see what sort of comments had been posted about the practice, like those illustrated in Figure 9.1. He was disturbed by some of the things that he found.

Many of the comments made by patients were related to their experience in waiting in the reception area because the doctors were always running behind, complaints about the behavior of the office staff, and complaints about the billing practices. Generally, the reviews about the physicians personally were good, but there were a disturbing number of complaints about their business practices.

Jason was still looking forward to his interview, but there were some questions in the back of his mind. Were the patient claims true? If the clinic's business practices were so offensive to some patients, was the clinic aware of it or did it not care? Jason decided that he had to find out before he would accept a position with this practice.

1. Using an Internet search engine, locate some information about a practice in your local area. Does the information you find seem consistent with your personal experience and/or the reputation of the practice? What seems to be the focus of the comments?

2. If you were the manager of a practice and discovered complaints about your business practices, how would you respond to what you found?

3. Discuss how these types of complaints could possibly be interpreted as an ethical problem with some of the business practices at the clinic.

Introduction

Revenue cycle
The period of time that occurs between the initiation of service and the time that payment for service is received.

All businesses have a revenue cycle. The **revenue cycle** is the period of time that occurs between the initiation of service and the time that payment for service is received. The length of the revenue cycle can vary

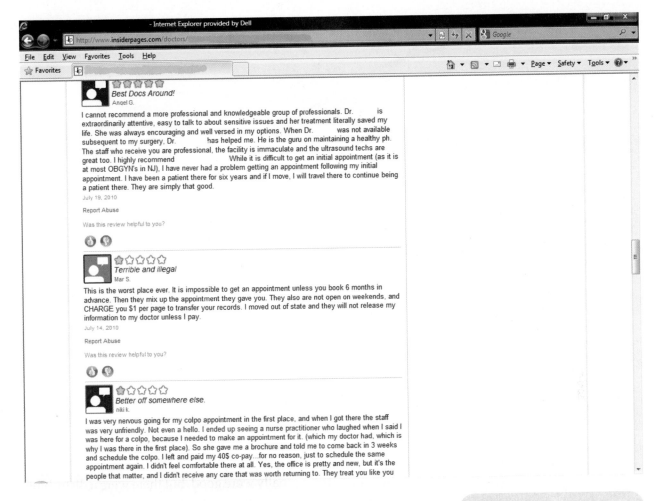

★★★★★
Best Docs Around!
Angel G.

I cannot recommend a more professional and knowledgeable group of professionals. Dr.   is extraordinarily attentive, easy to talk to about sensitive issues and her treatment literally saved my life. She was always encouraging and well versed in my options. When Dr.   was not available subsequent to my surgery, Dr.   has helped me. He is the guru on maintaining a healthy ph. The staff who receive you are professional, the facility is immaculate and the ultrasound techs are great too. I highly recommend   While it is difficult to get an initial appointment (as it is at most OBGYN's in NJ), I have never had a problem getting an appointment following my initial appointment. I have been a patient there for six years and if I move, I will travel there to continue being a patient there. They are simply that good.

July 19, 2010

Report Abuse

Was this review helpful to you?

👍 👎

★☆☆☆☆
Terrible and illegal
Mar S.

This is the worst place ever. It is impossible to get an appointment unless you book 6 months in advance. Then they mix up the appointment they gave you. They also are not open on weekends, and CHARGE you $1 per page to transfer your records. I moved out of state and they will not release my information to my doctor unless I pay.

July 14, 2010

Report Abuse

Was this review helpful to you?

👍 👎

★☆☆☆☆
Better off somewhere else.
niki k.

I was very nervous going for my colpo appointment in the first place, and when I got there the staff was very unfriendly. Not even a hello. I ended up seeing a nurse practitioner who laughed when I said I was here for a colpo, because I needed to make an appointment for it. (which my doctor had, which is why I was there in the first place). So she gave me a brochure and told me to come back in 3 weeks and schedule the colpo. I left and paid my 40$ co-pay...for no reason, just to schedule the same appointment again. I didn't feel comfortable there at all. Yes, the office is pretty and new, but it's the people that matter, and I didn't receive any care that was worth returning to. They treat you like you

widely between types of businesses, ranging from no "cycle" to cycles that range to 30, 60, or 90 days or more. In addition, the complexity of the cycle can vary widely, from simple to highly complex and detailed.

An example of the simplest revenue cycle would be that which occurs when a person purchases gasoline from a local station. When the person drives into the station, he is not allowed to leave the station before making payment for the gasoline he put into their car.[1] In fact, in some circumstances, the customer is required to pay for the gasoline *before* he has access to the pump. In this case, the revenue cycle is zero because there is no passage of time between the provision of service and the payment for service (Figure 9.2).

Other businesses do not require the customer to pay at the time of service. In some cases, it is not practical to do so, such as utility providers. There is no practical way for a utility company to collect payment for its services at the time of service because the services are delivered on a continuous basis. For the revenue cycle to be zero, customers would have to make continuous payments on a minute-by-minute basis. As a result, the customer is billed on a regular (usually monthly)

FIGURE 9.1
The Internet provides the ability for patients to report their opinions about their physician and their experiences at the physician office. This can be valuable information for prospective patients, but it can also be concerning to physician practices, who have little opportunity to defend themselves against unreasonable or false claims.

---

[1]Many people use credit cards to pay for their gasoline and other purchases and so there is no transfer of money from the customer to the business at that moment. However, the customer's financial obligation to the business is met through a separate arrangement with the credit card company—which, by design, has a completely different type of revenue cycle.

FIGURE 9.2

The revenue cycle of a business in which payment is received at the time of service.

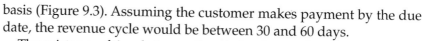

FIGURE 9.3

The revenue cycle of a business in which the customer does not pay at the time of service, but is billed, with the expectation of payment within a specified period of time.

Billing cycle
The amount of time that passes between each billing statement.

BILLING TIP

Each medical practice should ensure that the length of its billing cycle is appropriate. Billing cycles that are too long or too short can be equally ineffective and potentially wasteful.

basis (Figure 9.3). Assuming the customer makes payment by the due date, the revenue cycle would be between 30 and 60 days.

The existence of time between the service date and payment date usually requires the business to bill the customer, which creates the necessity of a **billing cycle,** which is a component part of the revenue cycle. The billing cycle is the amount of time that passes between each billing statement. In most cases it is approximately a 30-day cycle, although it can vary by circumstance and industry.

9.1 Stages of the Medical Revenue Cycle

Some industries have very long revenue cycles, by design. In most cases, long revenue cycles occur when there is the sale of physical products—most often when the product has a high price tag. For example, wholesalers may not require retailers to pay for their product for 90 days or more to give the retailer the opportunity to sell the product and collect the money necessary to pay the wholesaler for their original purchase price.

However, health care revenue cycles are perhaps the longest of any service industry. These are the five stages and 10 individual steps in the medical revenue cycle (Figure 9.4):

Stage 1: Scheduling, registration, and determination of financial responsibility.

Step 1: Preregister patients.

Step 2: Establish financial responsibility.

Medical Revenue Cycle

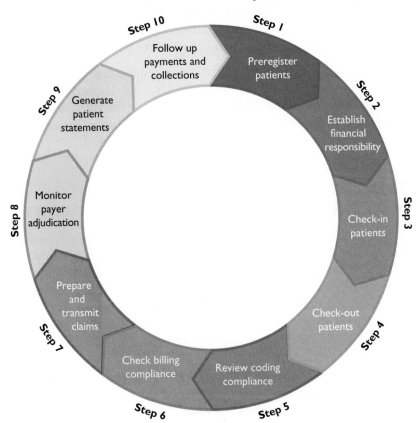

FIGURE 9.4
The 10 steps in the medical revenue cycle. Step 1 begins when information is gathered from the patient prior to his or her encounter with the provider. The cycle is completed following step 10, when payment in full is received.

Stage 2: Patient encounter at the facility or clinic.
> Step 3: Check-in patients.
> Step 4: Check-out patients.

Stage 3: Coding and billing.
> Step 5: Review coding compliance.
> Step 6: Check billing compliance.

Stage 4: Filing of claims with the third-party payer.
> Step 7: Prepare and transmit claims.
> Step 8: Monitor payer adjudication.

Stage 5: Billing of the patient for balances due.
> Step 9: Generate patient statements.
> Step 10: Follow up payments and collections.

Two primary reasons exist for the long revenue cycle:

1. *The intervention of a third party in the payment process.* In a traditional retail outlet, such as a grocery store, no one would expect to be able to walk out of the store with his or her purchases and state, "I'm not paying you now—XYZ Company will pay you for these items at some point in the future." However, this is exactly the scenario faced by health care providers that participate with insurers and other third-party payers.

2. *The complexity of the process, introduced by the third-party involvement.* Because the third party is not physically present for the transaction (e.g., in the room during a patient visit), the details of that visit

have to be communicated to the third-party payer through CPT and ICD-9 coding. Beyond selecting the right codes, the service provider must also learn and adhere to the payer's billing rules, which can vary significantly from payer to payer.

The length and complexity of the revenue cycle creates a significant assortment of opportunities for ethical dilemmas. These dilemmas can occur as the result of the actions of the patient, the provider, and the payer. Before discussing the ethical dilemmas, it is necessary to describe and review the process, from beginning to end.

STAGE 1: SCHEDULING, REGISTRATION, AND DETERMINATION OF FINANCIAL RESPONSIBILITY

The initiation of the relationship between patient and health care provider is different than that of most any other consumer–vendor relationship. Traditionally, customers identify the possible sources of whatever product or service they desire and then evaluate the various factors that can influence their decision-making process. Factors can include items such as total cost, selection, convenience, and quality of service. These factors are weighted and considered and a vendor is chosen based on those results.

Health care, on the other hand, is more complex because of the existence of third-party payers. The element of cost is in large part removed from the equation and "coverage" is put in its place. Because of insurance coverage, customers are less concerned with the actual cost charged by the provider and are very concerned about whether or not the provider participates with their insurer. Based on the type of plan held by patients, the financial responsibility can range from little or nothing if they see a "participating" provider to as much as 100% financial responsibility if they see a "nonparticipating" provider. In a best-case scenario, the patient who sees a provider that is not in his or her insurer's "network" will have significantly higher costs, in copayment and deductibles, than if he or she sees an "in-network" provider.

Because insurers often offer a wide variety of plans, it is sometimes difficult to know whether a particular provider is able to see the patient as a participating provider. Patients often do not understand their insurance and provide inaccurate or erroneous information to the staff of the provider regarding the nature of their coverage, or even the identity of their insurer. The provider staff must capture a significant amount of identifying information concerning the patient to prepare for the patient's first visit to the clinic. This is significantly different than the relatively simple, anonymous transaction that occurs when a customer walks into a grocery store, selects an item, purchases the items, and then leaves. The first step of the revenue cycle is, in effect, determining whether the patient can even "come in."

Table 9.1 illustrates a situation in which a provider's participating status with an insurer can have a more substantial impact on a patient than a difference in retail price. Provider A participates with the patient's insurance company and provider B does not. Because of the terms of the insurance plan, the patient is responsible for payment that is 1,500% higher if he or she sees provider B instead of provider A. In the case of the electronics store, the customer pays 10% more at

Table 9.1 Comparison of Out-of-Pocket Expenses: Retail Store Versus Health Care Provider

	Electronics Store Retail Charge		Health Care Provider Retail Charge	Patient Financial Responsibility
Item cost—location A	$500	Service cost—Participating provider A	$1,000	$ 50
Item cost—location B	$550	Service cost—Non-participating provider B	$ 750	$750

location B than if he or she purchased the item at location A. While there are factors that might explain why a customer would willingly pay 10% more for a product (e.g., better repair service, more knowledgeable salespeople, more convenient location), it would be rare for someone to knowingly incur dramatically higher expense to this degree, regardless of other possible factors.

At a minimum, the provider must attempt to make the patient aware of his or her possible financial responsibility for a service, prior to the initial visit. The degree to which the provider goes to obtain this information and inform the patient will depend on a number of factors, such as familiarity with insurance company policies, degree of certainty about the information received from the patient, and the possible expense associated with the proposed service.

STAGE 2: PATIENT ENCOUNTER AT THE FACILITY OR CLINIC

Once the patient arrives at the provider's facility or clinic, the revenue cycle continues with the confirmation of the patient's insurance information—usually by collecting copies of insurance documentation, such as the patient's insurance card. In addition, if called for by the patient's insurance policy, the provider will often collect the copayment for the service. Then the service must be provided to the patient.

A copayment is a fixed dollar amount that is owed by the patient for each encounter. Copayment amounts can generally range from $5 to $50, although they have trended higher in recent years. The purpose of the increasing copayment is twofold: (1) to increase the financial responsibility for the patient and reduce the responsibility for third-party payers, and (2) to provide a disincentive for people to seek out medical care, unless it is truly necessary. Payers have increased copayments to even higher levels for more expensive services, such as $100 per encounter for an emergency room visit or $500 per day/stay for an inpatient hospital service.

Because the amount due from the patient is fixed and known, most practices collect the money before the patient is seen. This is done for two reasons:

1. To ensure that payment is received. This avoids the scenario of the patients denying that they don't have the money, left their wallet at home, and so on, after they have already received the service.

2. To expedite the check-out process and move patients out of the clinic more quickly.

As an alternative to the copayment, many payers require that patients pay a **coinsurance** amount. Coinsurance is usually a percentage

Coinsurance
An amount, usually a percentage of the total or allowed charge, that is due from the patient for medical care.

Chapter 9 | Ethics and the Revenue Cycle   **289**

Allowed amount
The maximum payable amount, as determined by the payer.

WARNING

It's important to understand the basis on which a payer calculates the patient's coinsurance. If it is based on the billed charge, it is easy for the provider to determine at the time of service. If it's based on the "allowed" amount, the provider has to know the exact contractual reimbursement amount by that payer for each CPT code billed.

FYI

Because patients are responsible for greater amounts of their health care expense, providers are developing new and creative ways of collecting money at the time of service.

CODING TIP

Evaluation and management (E/M) services cannot be automatically billed each time that a procedure is performed.

amount of either (1) the total retail charge of the provider, or (2) the **"allowed amount,"** as determined by the payer. For many office-based services, the coinsurance amount is larger than a copayment amount. However, coinsurance amounts can't be collected until the service is provided because the coinsurance is based on the actual services provided, which can't be determined until the services are completed.

As health care costs continue to increase, more and more payers are offering plans that have significant deductibles. A deductible is an amount of expense that must be incurred by the patient before the insurer will make any payment toward the patient's claims. To make premiums more affordable, many are offering "high-deductible" plans that require patients to make a significant contribution to their health care expense before the insurer pays any amount. This is a substantial shift in the paradigm that was developed over the past 30 years, in which patients had little or no out-of-pocket expense for their medical care. The principle is that consumers will be more responsible with their health care spending if they have a meaningful out-of-pocket cost.

For providers, this creates a dilemma because, like coinsurance, it can't be collected until after the completion of service. This becomes more difficult because most payers consider only the "allowed amount" toward the deductible expense, thereby limiting what the provider can collect. Unless the provider carefully tracks what each different insurance company allows for each CPT code for each different plan it offers, the provider doesn't know how much to collect at the time of service. In most cases, providers elect to wait until the payer processes the claim and advises them of the amount that is due. This delays the reimbursement process for providers because they can't collect any amount until the payer completes adjudication of the claim. Another complicating factor that prevents providers from collecting at the time of service is that they don't know if the patients have met their deductible for the plan's fiscal year (Table 9.2).

STAGE 3: CODING AND BILLING

To accurately code and bill for services provided, a detailed decision tree must be followed to determine the correctness or accuracy of the billing. To determine what type of services were provided, it must be defined whether:

- An evaluation and management (E/M) service was provided.
- A procedural service was provided.
- Both types of services were provided.

Table 9.2 Amounts and Timing of Collection in Different Scenarios

	Retail Charge	Patient Responsibility	Insurer Allowed	Insurer Responsibility	Time Collected		
					Time of Service	Insurer Bill	Patient Bill
Copayment	$200	$25	$125	$100	20%	80%	0%
Coinsurance	$200	20%	$125	$100	0%	80%	20%
Deductible	$200	100%	$125	$ 0	0%	0%	100%

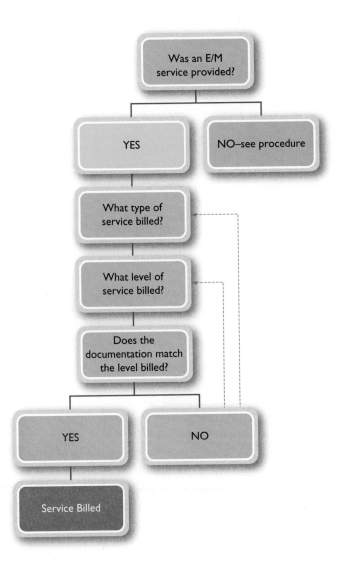

FIGURE 9.5
Steps that must be followed when determining what type of service should be billed *and* ensuring the proper level of E/M service is selected, when appropriate.

If only an E/M service was provided, the decision tree illustrated in Figure 9.5 must be followed. The first element is the type of service provided. Does it meet the criteria for a consultation or is it an office or outpatient service? Is the patient a new patient or an established patient? The answers to these questions will in large part define what section of the code book is used to report the service.

Once the type of service is identified, the level of service must be selected. The process of correctly identifying a level of service is discussed in significant detail in Chapter 5. The key to ensuring the billing of the proper level of service is compatibility with the medical record. In other words, does the documentation match and support the level of service billed?

If the documentation does not support the level of service billed, the billing should be adjusted to reflect the same level of service supported by the documentation.

If an E/M service was not provided and the only service delivered was a procedure, then the second decision tree in Figure 9.6 must be followed. The key element in this tree is also whether or not the documentation supports the procedure being billed. If it does not, then the documentation must be obtained *or* the service should not be billed. If both an E/M service and procedure are provided, then both decision

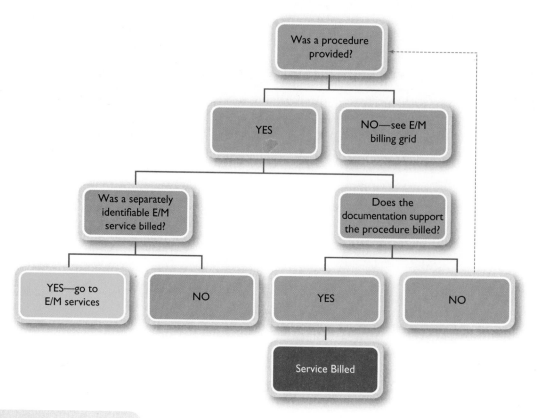

FIGURE 9.6

An illustration of the protocol to be followed to ensure correct coding when a procedure is provided.

trees must be followed and compatability between the billings and medical records must be ensured.

Before the billing process is completed, the provider office must ensure that the billings are in compliance with standard billing rules. This was referenced in Chapter 6, and refers primarily to service unbundling, preoperative and postoperative billing, and other payer-specific billing requirements.

STAGE 4: FILING OF CLAIMS WITH THE THIRD-PARTY PAYER

Once services are properly coded and the charges are entered into the provider's practice management system, claims are generated and electronically transmitted to claims clearinghouses (Figure 9.7). From there, claims are then distributed to the various payers for consideration. After the claims have been processed, the payers issue payment and a corresponding remittance advice (RA) back to the providers. This can occur in a number of different ways:

- Traditional check and paper RA sent via U.S. Mail.
- Check deposited directly into the provider's bank account and the accompanying paper RA sent via U.S. Mail.
- Check deposited directly into the provider's bank account and the accompanying RA retrieved electronically from the Internet by the provider.
- Check deposited directly into the provider's bank account and the accompanying claim adjudication information electronically transferred directly into the practice's billing system.

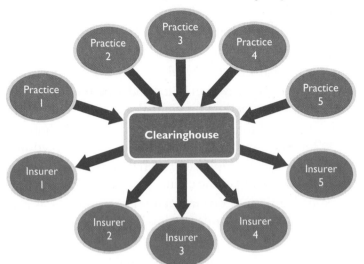

Claim Submissions to Third-Party Payers

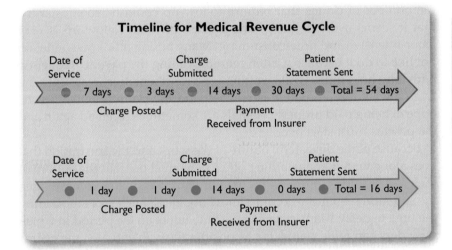

Timeline for Medical Revenue Cycle

Date of Service		Charge Submitted		Patient Statement Sent	
7 days	3 days	14 days	30 days	Total = 54 days	
Charge Posted		Payment Received from Insurer			

Date of Service		Charge Submitted		Patient Statement Sent	
1 day	1 day	14 days	0 days	Total = 16 days	
Charge Posted		Payment Received from Insurer			

After the initial setup is complete, the transmission of claims can be one of the fastest elements of the entire revenue cycle (Figure 9.8). Most payers confirm receipt of claims within two or three business days, which is a dramatic improvement over the past in which claims were sent via U.S. Mail and there was no method by which to confirm that the payer had received the claim. The use of technology has shortened the revenue cycle by weeks compared to as little as 10 to 20 years ago.

Historically, one of the complaints providers had regarding payers was the unreasonable length of time that it took payers to process claims and the practice of some payers to pend or otherwise delay payment of claims. To address this issue, many states have implemented "Prompt Payment" laws, which require payers to process and pay claims within a specified amount of time—usually 30 to 45 days for a **"clean claim."** If claims are not paid within this timeframe, payers incur some sort of penalty—most commonly, they are required to pay interest to the provider. In most cases, these laws have been highly effective in shortening the payment cycle.

BILLING TIP

Providers must carefully monitor the payments that are received from third-party payers.

Clean claim
A claim that has no errors that originated in the provider office.

However, one area of contention that remains between providers and payers is the accuracy of claim payments. Providers claim that payers do not pay claims appropriately in some of the following ways:

- Reimbursing for particular CPT codes at a rate lower than that called for by the contract between the payer and provider.
- Denying payment for certain billed codes by bundling them with other services provided on the same date.
- Denying payment for services as noncovered, even though authorization for the service was obtained prior to the procedure.
- Denying claims as a "duplicate," even though there is no record of an initial adjudication of the claim.
- Requesting additional documentation to support the claim, although thousands of similar claims have been processed previously, without documentation.

The most significant area in which the revenue cycle for practices is extended is the failure of the practice to appropriately follow up on inappropriate or incorrect claim denials. Depending on the practice, the number of claims that require follow-up could be so substantial that it seems overwhelming. The process of claim follow-up is very labor-intensive and time-consuming. Many billing office personnel do not like to do it because it often requires calling the payers, frequently with long hold times while waiting for a representative to assist them. Even after a representative is reached and the claim is refiled in the hope of being paid properly, denials are sometimes received again and the process must start over.

Because of the distasteful nature of the work and the frustration that goes along with it, many billing office personnel put it at the bottom of their list of things to do. As the pile of denied claims becomes larger, the situation seemingly becomes more hopeless, further compounding the urge to delay. Many payers have time limits on the period in which providers can refile claims for reconsideration. Eventually, the claims are too old to refile and the insurer is no longer obligated to pay the claim. This is unfortunate for the provider because most contracts with payers prohibit the provider from billing the patient for any services that were not paid as a result of a failure to file or refile the claim in a timely fashion.

STAGE 5: BILLING OF THE PATIENT FOR BALANCES DUE

The final step in the revenue cycle is the forwarding of a final billing statement to the patient, if a balance remains following the insurer's processing of the claim(s). Ideally, the provider will have collected all of the payment required of the patient at the time of service. However, for a variety of reasons this is not always practical.

In deciding on the patient billing or statement process, the provider must ask several questions:

- If the patient does not pay following the first statement, how many more statements or notices will the provider send out?
- If the patient continues not to pay for the service, will the practice attempt to conduct collection activities (e.g., letters, phone calls, etc.) using the employees of the practice's billing office?

- Whether or not the practice does "in-house" collections, will the practice use an outside agency to collect bills from patients if the bills remain unpaid?
- What type of agency does the practice want to engage and what types of actions does the practice authorize the agency to perform (aggressive telephone calls, series of letters, reporting to credit bureaus, etc.)?

These are all philosophical questions that the practice must ask and answer before it has a substantial amount of past-due patient balances. Unless the entire revenue cycle philosophy is consistent and coherent, it will be less likely to be successful.

Thinking It Through 9.1

1. Coding is a critical part of the entire revenue cycle, but it is not the only part. Rank the five stages of the revenue cycle in order, from most important to least important. Explain the basis for your opinion.

2. Based on your personal experience with the medical industry, where have you seen the most significant problems in the revenue cycle of the practices from which you have received services? What caused you to form this opinion?

3. Failure to have an effective revenue cycle can have an obvious financial impact. What other possible effects could an ineffective revenue cycle have on nonfinancial elements of the practice?

4. Before we examine the ethics of the revenue cycle, what do you think is the most significant opportunity for ethical issues within the cycle? Why?

9.2 Ethical Issues in Registering Patients and Assigning Financial Responsibility

The first stage in the medical revenue cycle would seem, on the surface, to be free of potential ethical problems or dilemmas. However, as deeper examination occurs, the opportunity for ethical issues becomes clearer. Part of the ethical dilemmas are attributable to the number of parties who are involved in the transaction and their varying responsibilities (Table 9.3), whereas the remaining dilemmas are attributable to the complexity of the process (Figure 9.9).

Table 9.3 Responsibilities of the Parties in the Registration–Financial Process

Patient	Provider	Payer
Honesty	Full disclosure/education	Accurate information
Cooperation	Due diligence	Member education
	Follow through on "red flags"	

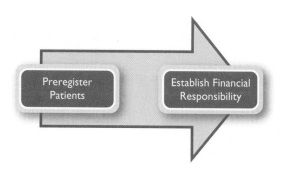

There are four elements to the initial process that require clarification before the next stage in the revenue cycle can occur.

- The patient's identity.
- The patient's insurance coverage, if any.
- The provider's participation status with the patient's insurers, if any.
- Communication of expectations concerning payment responsibility by the patient.

PATIENT IDENTITY

In a cash transaction at a convenience store, the customers' identity is not of concern to the business, unless the product being purchased requires that the purchaser be of a certain age. In those cases, businesses don't necessarily care about the specific identity of their customers—they simply wish to confirm that the customers are of the required age. If the customers produce suitable proof of their age, the transaction continues. The degree to which the businesses confirm the validity of the proof varies significantly, as indicated by teenagers who are successfully able to obtain certain products through the use of false identification.

In a credit transaction, the customers' specific identity is of greater concern to businesses because they wish to have a degree of certainty that the person presenting the credit card, for example, is the owner and/or authorized user of the card. Some businesses require identification to confirm the identity of a customer, but most do not. They presume that the card is being used appropriately because, if the card had been reported stolen, the credit card company would not approve the transaction.

The Patient. In the past, a discussion of the identity of the patient would have been unnecessary in relationship to health care providers. However, changes in society and changes in the economics of health care have made this a serious concern. Providers can no longer be certain that the person who is contacting their office is the same person who has coverage under the insurance plan that is presented.

Identity Theft. Identity theft has increased substantially in the past few years. In addition to the traditional identity theft that has always existed (stealing of a purse or wallet), electronic means of stealing identities has broadened the abilities of those inclined to commit the unethical and illegal act of misrepresenting who they are. Sometimes

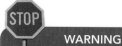

WARNING

The greater incidence of identity theft requires health care providers to be more diligent in ensuring the patient's identity.

the identity theft occurs to access health care services that would be unaffordable without health insurance. By presenting health insurance information, the door to health care services seemingly opens.

Cooperation in Identity Deception. In some cases, a legitimate holder of health care coverage participates in deceiving providers and payers by supplying his or her insurance information (and even the insurance card) to a friend or family member who does not have coverage. The result is the same as when involuntary identity theft occurs—individuals receive access to health care benefits to which they are not contractually entitled. The difference is that the insured person allows and participates in the fraud that occurs. Most often this cooperative deception is justified in the minds of those engaging in it; they believe that the person without insurance truly needs care and would not otherwise receive it without this action.

The Provider. The question must be asked, "How much responsibility does the provider have in confirming the identity of a person presenting insurance information?" There is a continuum of possible approaches, ranging on one end from a total disregard and zero interest to conducting Secret Service–level security checks on the other end. The ideal approach is something in the middle, where the provider takes action as it becomes aware of suspicious activity or unexplained circumstances (Figure 9.10). This represents an appropriate level of **due diligence.**

Due diligence
An appropriate level of job performance.

THE PATIENT'S INSURANCE COVERAGE

A critical component of the initial stage of the revenue cycle is identifying the patient's insurer and the details of the coverage that the insurer provides. Questions must be answered, such as:

- Is the insurance coverage in effect for the proposed date of service?
- Is the patient eligible for benefits under that coverage? If so, what are the limitations (if any) of those benefits?
- Does the patient have other insurance coverage?

Each party to this transaction has responsibilities in facilitating the collection of this vital information.

The Patient. Most people would agree that it is highly unethical for a patient to present an insurance card, representing that the coverage is in effect, when the person knows that the coverage has been terminated. However, the ethical question becomes a little less clear when the patient doesn't have detailed knowledge about his or her health

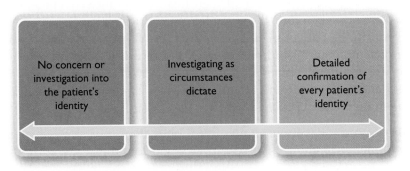

FIGURE 9.10
An illustration of the range of potential depth into which health care providers may research the identity of the patients to whom they are providing care.

It's Not What You Think

A female patient phoned a fertility clinic to schedule an appointment for her and her boyfriend to receive treatment. She provided insurance information to the clinic, indicating that they both had individual, single coverage for their own charges.

In accordance with standard procedure, the clinic called the insurance company to confirm benefits. The insurance company reported that the patient had coverage and that she was the holder of the insurance policy. The provider representative asked, "Is that a single policy?" The insurance representative said, "No, it's a family policy—she has a dependent on the plan." After some further questioning, it was learned that the person on the plan (who had the same last name as the patient) was listed by the insurer as the patient's spouse.

The billing representative called the patient and asked about the identity of the person on the insurance plan. Initially, the patient said that she didn't know who that was and that it must have been some sort of mistake. When told that the clinic would not see her until this was resolved, the patient said that the person was her brother who was on her plan because of his disabilities. When told that this was inconsistent with what the insurer stated and that it did not make sense, she finally admitted that the person on the plan was her husband, but they were separated.

At this point, the clinic told the patient that no treatment would be provided to the patient because of the deceptive information she had provided. The clinic had potential legal liability if treatment continued because the law in that state indicated that any child born of an existing marriage was presumed to be fathered by the husband and he would have financial responsibility for that child. The husband could sue the clinic for knowingly participating in the care of this patient and subjecting him to possible financial liability.

In this situation, the identity of the patient was not falsified, but the circumstances surrounding the patient's care were grossly mischaracterized. The patient came to the clinic and tacitly implied that she and her boyfriend were legally able to seek fertility treatment. This was fundamentally untrue.

care plan. Is it unethical for a patient to present an insurance card to the health care provider with a good-faith belief that the coverage is in effect, when the patient's spouse failed to tell him that her employer changed the plan? Is it unethical for the patient to be uncooperative and make no effort to learn about his or her health insurance coverage? Or, what if the patient presents an insurance card, believing that the coverage is in effect, when in fact the employer failed to pay the premiums and the coverage is terminated?

At a minimum, the patient has an obligation to be honest about his or her insurance coverage. Moreover, the patient has an ethical obligation not to hide behind a veil of ignorance regarding the coverage. Patients should make an effort to learn the basic details of their insurance coverage, even though it sometimes seems overwhelming and incomprehensible.

The Provider.   Provider offices should realize that, although patients need to be fully aware of their health insurance coverage, they often are not. Therefore, the provider office takes on the responsibility to confirm the patient's coverage and, to the degree possible, educate the patient about his or her coverage. This is frustrating to providers because it is an uncompensated service for which they receive no payment and no credit from patients. However, it is essential to facilitate the reimbursement process as it currently exists.

The Payer.   Payers have an ethical obligation to educate their insured members about their own policy and to publish literature that helps them understand it more clearly. This is always a challenge because insurance coverage, medical billing, and CPT and ICD-9 coding are not easy subjects to grasp. Most payers offer educational programs on site at employer offices to introduce the plan to employees, but they are often poorly attended. A more significant problem is that even if the employee attends, the employee's spouse may be the person attempting to schedule an appointment and the details of the plan may not have ever been communicated between the spouses.

A frustration often communicated by providers is the quality of information received from the payers. The provider office has already determined that the patient may not be an accurate source of information regarding the plan, so they take on the responsibility of learning about the patient's coverage and, accordingly, go to the source for information—the payer. Before speaking to a provider representative, a provider representative may hear an "on hold" message that states that the information that follows is "no guarantee of coverage" and actual benefits payable cannot be determined "until a claim is submitted." This puts the provider in a no-win situation: The patient may not know anything about the coverage and the information provided by the payer representative can't be fully relied on. This places the provider squarely in the middle—if the claim is denied after being told that the service was covered, the provider doesn't get paid and the patient blames the provider for not informing him or her prior to delivering the service.

THE PROVIDER'S INSURANCE PARTICIPATION STATUS

Provider insurance participation status is a challenging aspect of American health insurance coverage. Consider the following example in which the patient is covered by XYZ insurance company's HMO program. The provider participates with XYZ insurance's preferred provider organization (PPO) product, but not the health maintenance organization (HMO) program.

Provider: What insurance coverage do you have?
Patient: I have XYZ insurance.
Provider: Is that the HMO or PPO?
Patient: I don't really know.
Provider: Do you have your insurance card with you?
Patient: No, I left it at home. But my doctor told me that your office participates.
Provider: OK. Well, it must be the PPO then. I'll schedule your appointment.

When the patient comes to the office, she forgets to bring her insurance card. The doctor is made aware that the patient is in the office and while the billing personnel are checking on the insurance coverage, the patient is taken back to the exam room. The billing personnel learn that the patient has HMO coverage and notifies the doctor. The doctor states, "I'm almost done with the patient—let's just file the claim and see what happens." The claim is denied because the provider does not participate with the insurer. A bill is sent to the patient, who strenuously objects, stating "I would never have come to your office if I had known that it wouldn't be covered!"

There is plenty of responsibility to be shared by the parties for this situation and although there was no intention to mislead or deceive, there are ethical problems with nearly every action taken by each party. The patient abdicated her responsibility to be informed about her insurance and, ultimately, her responsibility for payment for services that she received. The provider office provided treatment to the patient without providing full disclosure about its participation status with the patient's insurer.

Although it is a frustrating process and accurate information is sometimes difficult to obtain, providers have an affirmative ethical requirement to ensure that the patient is aware of the provider's participation status. It is completely unethical for a provider to deliver services to a patient when the provider knows that it does not participate with the patient's insurer *and* it does not make a specific effort to ensure that the patient is aware of its nonparticipating status. The patient may still desire to see the provider, but the provider should clearly document that the patient was fully aware of its status—for the benefit of both the patient and the provider.

PAYMENT EXPECTATIONS

Before the patient arrives at the clinic, the provider has the obligation to clarify the patient's financial responsibility for the service. The provider should have some sort of script for its personnel that states as follows:

> You must either complete your intake paperwork on our website or bring it with you at the time of your appointment. We expect you to make payment for your portion of the financial responsibility at the time of service, whether that is your copayment, coinsurance, or the deductible amount, which we will either estimate or calculate for you. We accept cash, checks, and all major credit cards. We will calculate your responsibility based on the information that we receive from your insurer. We will do our best to obtain accurate information, but ultimately it is your responsibility to be aware of what your insurance covers and what you are financially responsible for.

It is not ethical to refuse service to the patient for failure to pay if the expectation of payment is not clearly established *prior* to the patient's arrival in the office. By the same token, it is not ethical for the patient to expect to receive service without paying for his or her portion of the financial liability.

Thinking It Through 9.2

1. If one of the parties in the registration–financial responsibility process fails to act ethically, does that change the responsibility of the other parties regarding their ethical obligation? Why or why not?

2. Some of the ethical issues described in this section are actually illegal or fraudulent acts. Which of the issues are not illegal, per se, but could be considered unethical? In your opinion, does that make them less important than illegal or fraudulent acts?

3. How can the proper defining of expectations eliminate or minimize the effect of ethical issues?

4. In the case study involving the patient and the fertility clinic, why might the clinic choose to overlook the information it obtained and continue with treatment? Without regard to the potential legal issues described, would continuing treatment be ethical? Why or why not?

5. When the provider office sees a patient who has insurance coverage with which the provider does not participate, who is responsible ethically? How can this situation be avoided? If the situation does occur, how can it be equitably resolved?

6. Describe the relationship between the activities that occur prior to the patient's arrival and the billing/coding process. Could unethical actions before the patient's arrival result in unethical billing or coding?

7. Some actions of payers are considered unethical by providers. If they experience these actions, what alternatives do providers have to address and prevent these situations?

9.3 Ethics and Patient Activity in the Facility or Clinic

The interaction between the patient and the provider facility or clinic while the patient is in the office is a critical element in the revenue cycle. The ability to collect funds from a patient will never be any higher than when the patient is face-to-face with a provider staff member. However, the maximum effectiveness is achieved when the patient's expectations are properly established in the first stage of the revenue cycle.

ETHICAL CONSIDERATIONS RELATED TO THE PATIENT

Two specific requirements of patients are related to ethics—provision of accurate information and payment of amounts for which they are responsible. A patient's unethical behavior in relation to these responsibilities can place the provider in the position of having to make decisions with ethical ramifications.

Accurate Information. Because of the dramatic increases in health premiums in the past two decades, employers frequently change insurance plans to keep the costs manageable. Having knowledge of these changes is important to the provider office because claims must be submitted to the insurance policy that was in effect at the time that service was delivered. It is a best practice for the front desk staff to inquire of the patient's insurance coverage each time they check in a patient for service, to ensure that claims are filed to the right company (Figure 9.11). The provider is dependent on the patient to provide accurate information. If inaccurate or false information is provided, the provider may not become aware of this until the claim is denied by

> **BILLING TIP**
>
> The best time to collect money from the patient and shorten the revenue cycle is to do it while they are in the facility or clinic, at the time of the encounter. This also reduces expenses later in the revenue cycle.

> **BILLING TIP**
>
> It is important to phrase questions appropriately so that patients aren't allowed to passively answer questions incorrectly.

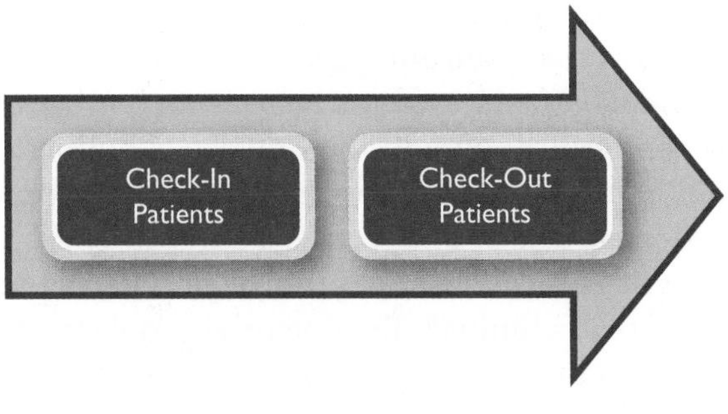

FIGURE 9.11
The component parts of the second stage (steps 3 and 4) of the medical revenue cycle.

Check-In Patients   Check-Out Patients

the patient's previous insurer—insurance coverage that is no longer in effect (Figure 9.14).

A common scenario that occurs in provider facilities or clinics is as follows:

Provider Staff: Any change to your insurance?
Patient: No.
Provider Staff: Okay.

In some cases, the information provided by the patient is inaccurate. The information can be inaccurate for two reasons: (1) a deliberate intent to deceive and (2) ignorance about the status of the coverage

Patients may lose coverage due to the loss of a job or some other circumstance in their life. They feel as though they can't afford treatment without insurance coverage and they don't have the ability to pay for the treatment on the date of service. Therefore, they may either present the old insurance card, knowing the policy is not in effect, or they may be deceptive in a more passive way by stating that there is no change in their coverage when they know change has occurred.

While this unfortunate circumstance occurs, ignorance about their coverage is probably a more common cause of inaccurate information. Often, the person who is seeking treatment is not the person who holds the insurance policy. If the person's spouse does not tell him or her about the change in the insurance coverage, he or she may honestly not know that the policy is no longer effective. Therefore, the individual acts in good faith that the information provided is accurate.

Most would agree that deliberately telling a health care provider that coverage exists when the person knows that it does not is unethical. Sometimes this particular unethical behavior is justified as legitimate because the person requiring treatment is a child and there is concern that the child won't receive the care needed if the provider knows that there is no insurance.

The situation is a little less clear in the case where inaccurate information is provided unintentionally or through the result of ignorance. If the patient's new insurer has a relatively narrow window of time allowed for claim submission (e.g., 90 days) and the provider facility or clinic does not follow up on claim denials effectively (to be discussed later in the chapter), the provider may not be able to obtain payment for the claim. In addition, it may not be able to bill the patient due to the contractual terms between the provider and the insurer. This circumstance would not have occurred if the patient had been knowledgeable about the coverage and provided accurate information at the time of service. Although the patient has no legal or contractual obligation to pay for this service, does the patient have an ethical responsibility for his or her contribution to the circumstance?

Fortunately for providers, technology allows them to be more efficient and proactive in confirming the status of a patient's coverage. Some practice management systems have features that allow for automatic coverage verification and the practice is notified if the stated insurance plan is not in effect. Most insurers now supply online access for providers to check and verify insurance eligibility. Because these tools exist, it is in the best interest of providers to obtain these resources and thereby eliminate the potential problems introduced by both uninformed and unethical patients.

Payment. A great frustration for providers is the seeming unwillingness of some patients to accept responsibility for their financial obligation under the terms of their health insurance contract. Patients will claim that they "forgot" their checkbook or that they "didn't know" that they had a copayment due. Many providers have attempted to remove the obstacle by accepting payment via credit cards or by arranging to have automated teller machines (ATMs) readily accessible. Again, action on the part of the provider has helped mitigate some potential ethical issues on the part of the patient.

ETHICAL CONSIDERATIONS RELATED TO THE PROVIDER

During the second stage of the revenue cycle, the provider has four responsibilities related to the process:

1. Confirming the patient's identity, status, and insurance coverage, if any.
2. Collecting copayments, coinsurance, or other patient due amounts.
3. Providing appropriate medical care.
4. Preliminary coding of services delivered during the encounter.

Patient Nonpayment. Providers are becoming more concerned with the collection of funds at the time of service. The introduction of high-deductible policies has prompted some providers to collect an amount equal to a 99203 or 99204 visit for new patients and a 99214 visit for established patients, prior to the actual delivery of services. If the actual service provided is less than this amount, the provider refunds the patient the excess payment. If the actual service is greater than this amount, the patient is billed for the difference. However, the amount billed is significantly less than it would have been if no amount was collected from the patient.

By making these policies clear and establishing expectations in the first part of the revenue cycle, most ethical issues are avoided. However, the provider must still occasionally deal with the ethical questions, "What are we going to do if the patient can't/won't pay for the service? Does the nature of the patient's condition affect whether or not we turn away the patient? Who makes the decision as to whether we turn away the patient for nonpayment? Does it matter if it is a child?"

Health care is an industry like any other in that it is a business that must have revenue to survive. However, it is somewhat different because of the nature of its services and the inclination of many providers to find turning away sick patients to be undesirable and, perhaps, unacceptable. Therefore, health care providers must decide how they will resolve this difficult ethical issue when it occurs.

Proper Coding and Patient Classification. Of course, proper coding is a key element to revenue cycle, which will be covered at greater length later in the chapter. However, patient classification should occur at the time the patient is in the clinic. Specifically, the provider office must determine whether or not the patient is a "new" or an "established" patient.

According to the CPT code book, a "new" patient is "one who has not received any professional services from the physician or another physician of the same specialty who belongs to the same group

Table 9.4 Relative Value Units for Outpatient E/M Services—New and Established Patients

New Patient	RVUs	Established Patient	RVUs
99201	1.21	99211	0.58
99202	2.09	99212	1.22
99203	3.03	99213	2.03
99204	4.66	99214	3.01
99205	5.80	99215	4.05

Source: Centers for Medicare and Medicaid Services (CMS), 2011.

practice, within the past three years" (AMA, 2010a). In medical coding, "professional services" are those face-to-face services rendered by a physician and reported by a specific CPT code. This can create challenges for the provider staff when certain circumstances occur.

The appropriate assignment of "new" versus "established" patient codes is important because of the higher relative reimbursement for a new patient's services versus that of an established patient (Table 9.4). In addition to the reimbursement, the documentation requirements are significantly higher than for new patients and it is possible that not only would the wrong classification be billed, but the wrong level of service would be billed based on the documentation or lack thereof.

While formalized coding takes place later in the revenue cycle, the framework for incorrect code selection occurs based on the intake information gathered at the front desk during the patient's visit. In some cases, the payer may recognize that the practice has already delivered services to the patient and therefore won't allow a new patient visit code. However, the payer may not notice the billing issue if claims are received out of order or the nature of the initial service is such that it is not recognized by the payer. The ethical issue then becomes, "Should the practice refund the payment to the insurer and refile the claim with

New or Established?

Dr. Cho was on call for his practice over the weekend. He was called to the emergency department at the local hospital to see a patient who was visiting from out of town. Dr. Cho evaluated the patient's condition, made treatment recommendations, and discharged the patient with instructions to follow up in the practice office on Monday morning. Dr. Cho billed for an outpatient consultation for the service he provided over the weekend.

Dr. Cho had Monday off because he was on call over the weekend and the patient saw Dr. Cho's partner, Dr. Craig, in the office on Monday morning. The receptionist asked the patient, "Have you ever been to our office before?" The patient answered no. Therefore, the receptionist indicated on the charge ticket that the patient was new. Based on the information marked on the ticket, Dr. Craig billed 99202 for the patient's service in the office. This was inappropriate because Dr. Cho provided "professional services" to the patient in the emergency department over the weekend. Therefore, since Dr. Craig was Dr. Cho's partner, Dr. Craig must bill the appropriate level of established patient service.

the correct classification and code level when it becomes aware of the codes originally selected?"

Another way in which activity at the front desk can result in improper coding and unethical treatment of patients is related to pre- and postoperative services. For instance, if a patient has a diagnostic laparoscopy (CPT code 49320), all services within the first 10 days following the procedure are included in the procedure and are not separately billable. The CPT code billed for the follow-up service in the 10-day period should be 99024, with a zero charge. However, what if the front desk personnel are instructed to collect a copayment for *every* patient?

The postoperative check is completed and either the patient is billed for an E/M service (99212–99215) or the patient is "billed" for 99024. In either case, the patient has no financial liability because the insurer will deny the billing of an E/M service in postoperative period and there is no charge for 99024.

In the hypothetical case of a copayment collected during the post-operative period for a diagnostic laparoscopy, the billing office may recognize that the copayment should not have been collected when the charge was entered. However, the billing staffperson may choose *not* to refund the money to the patient because there is still an outstanding charge for the surgery and the patient may have some financial liability after the insurer pays. The insurance company adjudicates the claim and the patient has no liability—the insurer pays the full liability for the surgery. The patient continues to have a credit balance on her account. The billing office is shorthanded and, as a result, doesn't have time to process credit balances on patient accounts. The billing office manager has instructed employees not to deal with credit balances, unless the patient calls to inquire about a refund.

This becomes an ethical issue because there is a question about the practice's obligation to refund money to the patient. Does the situation change if the patient is a relatively frequent visitor to the clinic and the amount can just be applied to a future copayment? What if the copayment amount is only $5—does that change the practice's ethical obligation?

CODING TIP

To ensure proper coding and collection of copayments, the front office and billing staff must be aware if the patient has had or will have surgery in the immediate past or future.

Thinking It Through 9.3

1. Discuss how the first elements of the revenue cycle have a specific impact on the subsequent steps of the revenue cycle.

2. What are some ways in which providers can identify and overcome the ethical failures of patients as it relates to collecting the patients' financial obligations?

3. Describe the ethical conflict that exists between the provider's need to collect money to stay in business and the provider's desire or obligation to deliver care to patients.

4. Do you agree with the statement, "It is acceptable to delay refunds to patients or insurers until they ask for the refund"? Why or why not? On what basis do you form your opinion?

5. Discuss the situation described in the chapter in which the enforcement of a reasonable policy can result in unintended consequences that produce an ethical problem.

9.4 Code Assignment, Ethics, and the Revenue Cycle

The ethical considerations of code selection are described in great detail in previous chapters of this book. Therefore, a complete reconsideration of the issues at this point is not necessary. Instead, the focus will be directed toward the place of coding in the revenue cycle and how actions, both before and after the actual act of coding, affect the ethics of coding and success of the cycle (Figure 9.12).

A common truism stated in discussions of psychology is that the greatest predictor of future behavior is past behavior. A person who has demonstrated ethical behavior in the past is more likely to do so in the future than a person who has demonstrated unethical behavior in the past, and vice versa. This principle is also true in the revenue cycle of any health care practice or facility. If unethical actions occur in the early stages of the revenue cycle, it is not surprising that unethical actions take place with regard to the selection of codes, which is the cornerstone of the revenue cycle.

One factor associated with this stage of the revenue cycle that was not included in the previous chapters is the need to properly inform the patient that certain services may not be payable under his or her insurance plan. The Medicare program requires that providers have patients sign an **advance beneficiary notice (ABN)** *prior* to delivering services that may not be covered. The purpose of the ABN is to allow patients the opportunity to decide whether they want to receive a service, even though they may be financially responsible for the service (Figure 9.13).

The ethical issues associated with the ABN fall within two categories:

1. Having *every* patient sign an ABN (commonly known as a "blanket ABN") even though there is no reasonable expectation that the service won't be covered by Medicare.
2. Accepting a patient's ABN even though it is not properly or fully completed.

Providers are required to report on the claim form whether they have a completed ABN in their possession. It is completely inappropriate for a provider to indicate that it has a completed ABN (through the -GA modifier) when it does not.

Other commercial payers may or may not have similar documentation requirements. However, it is definitely in the provider's best

Advance beneficiary notice (ABN) A document that must be signed by patients covered by Medicare whenever they receive services that may not be covered by the Medicare program in circumstances when they are receiving the service more frequently than Medicare allows or they do not have a diagnosis that is required for the service to be covered.

FYI

Ethical issues can occur at any stage of the revenue cycle—not just in association with coding. However, if you are unethical in the early stages of the process, it is very likely that you will be unethical with coding and billing.

FIGURE 9.12

The component parts of the third stage (steps 5 and 6) of the medical revenue cycle.

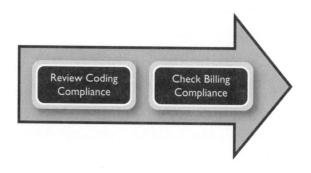

Review Coding Compliance

Check Billing Compliance

FIGURE 9.13
A sample of the Medicare advance beneficiary notice (ABN). It must be fully completed and signed by the patient prior to the delivery of the services in question.

interest to ensure that patients are fully informed of their potential financial obligation *before* the service is provided.

The early stages of the revenue cycle focus on the definition and establishment of the financial responsibility for the potential delivery of medical services. If a provider elects to act unethically regarding its financial relationship with its patients, with whom it has a direct relationship, it would be completely expected that the provider would act unethically toward a relatively anonymous insurance company.

Thinking It Through 9.4

1. Do you agree with the premise that past behavior is the best predictor of future behavior? Why or why not?

2. Discuss how behavior in one element of the revenue cycle can affect and predict behavior in the other elements of the cycle.

3. Who bears the most responsibility for education in the revenue cycle—the payer, the provider, or the patient? Why?

9.5 Ethical Issues in Relation to Third-Party Payers

Once care is provided to the patient, the revenue cycle temporarily changes its focus from the provider–patient relationship to the provider–payer relationship. This in itself develops the opportunity for more ethical issues, with responsibility for those issues originating with both parties in the process (Figure 9.14).

THE PROVIDER'S ROLE IN OBTAINING PAYMENT FROM THIRD-PARTY PAYERS

Potential ethical problems abound in this area of the revenue cycle. The reason is that the objectives of the three parties involved in the health care revenue cycle are not aligned. Providers desire to receive appropriate payment for the services that they deliver. Patients have been conditioned to expect treatment with as little personal financial responsibility as possible. Payers desire to pay their contractual obligations to providers on behalf of the patient, but they want to ensure that they stay financially viable for the benefit of their shareholders (in some cases) and to facilitate being an ongoing concern (Figure 9.15).

Filing a Claim in a Timely Fashion. A primary obligation of the provider, to both the patient and the payer, is to file claims in a timely fashion. "Timely fashion" is usually defined contractually by the payer, but it can also be defined in an unwritten fashion by the patient—particularly if the provider does not participate with the patient's insurer and the patient must file his or her own claim to the

FIGURE 9.14

The component parts of the fourth stage (steps 7 and 8) of the medical revenue cycle.

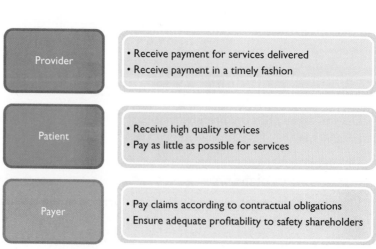

Prepare and Transmit Claims

Monitor Payer Adjudication

FIGURE 9.15

All of the objectives of the parties involved in the revenue cycle are valid and usually reasonable. However, some of them frequently conflict with each other and appear to be impossible to achieve simultaneously.

Provider	• Receive payment for services delivered • Receive payment in a timely fashion
Patient	• Receive high quality services • Pay as little as possible for services
Payer	• Pay claims according to contractual obligations • Ensure adequate profitability to safety shareholders

insurer. The patient, who may have paid the provider for the service, wants to recover his or her money as quickly as possible, but can't do so until the provider prepares a claim form and either submits it to the payer or delivers it to the patient. The patient's unwritten expectations may or may not be based in reality.

On the other hand, payers are explicit concerning the amount of time that a provider has to submit a claim. In the past, that time limit ranged from as little as 30 days to as much as 18 months. However, many providers complained that 30 days was unreasonably short and payers recognized that 18 months was too long for them to be potentially responsible for an unknown amount of liability. Therefore, the majority of insurers require that claims be submitted within 90 to 180 days of the date of service, with a few still allowing submissions up to one year from the date of service.

There is no reasonable advantage for a provider to delay claim submission to the point that it can no longer submit the claim to the insurer or that it severely frustrates the patient. This makes the timing of claim submission *seem* to be free of ethical dilemmas: The main reason that claim submissions are delayed is that there are systemic, operational problems within the practice. However, it can be argued that the practice's problems—incompetence, in some cases—are unnecessarily disruptive to the life or business of others and therefore can be considered a potential ethical problem.

A number of elements can contribute to the delay in preparing and submitting claims. They include:

- An inadequate number of people available to code and post claims.
- A delay by the doctor in completing charge tickets.
- A delay by the doctor in completing medical records to support the billing.
- An unreasonable or inefficient process to confirm the accuracy of claims prior to submission.

Physicians and managers of the health care provider office or facility must ensure that the obstacles that potentially delay the submission of claims are appropriately addressed and/or removed, to facilitate the advancement of the revenue cycle. In most cases, the single factor that delays the correction of these elements is a lack of education. Some practice leaders simply do not understand that the existence of ineffective systems hurts everyone involved in the process, but it hurts no one more than the provider. There is direct economic cost in terms of losing the **time value of money**, but there is also public relations value lost in not operating an efficient billing office.

Properly Following Up on Denied Claims. A certain percentage of claims submitted to third-party payers will be processed in a manner that is unexpected to the provider. The "surprises" can include:

- A claim denied as a noncovered service when the provider believed that it was a covered service (and, in some cases, has an approved preauthorization for the service).
- A claim denied because it is bundled with another service provided on the same day. This happens most frequently when multiple

FYI

Research has consistently shown that the most profitable practices do not necessarily have the smallest number of staff members—in fact, they may have more. The additional cost of the extra staff members is offset by the extra revenue that they bring in and the higher satisfaction level for patients.

Time value of money
The principle that the possession of money now is more valuable than the potential of receiving money in the future.

surgical procedures are done on the same day. The payer will indicate that one (or more) of the services should be included as part of another procedure.

- A claim paid, but at an amount different than what the provider fee schedule indicates.
- A code unilaterally changed by the payer, usually resulting in lower payment to the provider.

The ethical ramifications of these actions on the part of the payer will be addressed later, but there are certainly ethical issues at play on the part of the provider office. Specifically, the billing office personnel are doing a significant disservice to the patient and more so to their employer if they fail to follow up on claim payments from insurers that are not appropriate. Working to obtain proper payment can be difficult work, requiring a significant amount of patience and a high tolerance for frustration. Many of the issues seem to be the same battle over and over again. In addition, the work can be very time-consuming and progress may seem slow or nonexistent.

Accounts receivable (A/R)
The cumulative amount of all balances due to a provider.

This is a substantial ethical issue if this work is not done because it determined to be "not enjoyable" or "too frustrating." A lack of discipline on the part of the employees does not provide them with the

Control the Insurance Accounts Receivable

Elena was thrilled to become the new manager of the billing office. She was told that her first duty was to ensure that the **accounts receivable (A/R)** amount due from insurance companies be reduced, but there were no funds available to hire additional staff—it would have to be done with the staff that she had. If they were successful in reducing the A/R, both she and the staff would be eligible for bonuses.

Elena passed on the news to her staff and emphasized daily how important it was to get the A/R reduced. After three months, she was delighted to see that insurance A/R had been reduced by 15% during her time in the position. She let her staff know the great news.

However, during a conversation with the practice administrator, the administrator expressed concern to Elena that, even though A/R was decreased, revenue to the practice was not increasing—in fact, it had declined 0.5%. She told Elena that a corresponding increase in collections should accompany a decrease in accounts receivable. Elena was told to immediately investigate the situation.

Elena went back to the department and then sat down individually with each member of the team to see how

they had accomplished a significant drop in A/R in a brief period of time. She was alarmed when she learned that:

- The amount paid by insurers was no longer checked against the amount called for by the contract. Those posting payments said that they decided to just assume that the payers were reimbursing the correct amount. In some cases, they were accepting 50% of the contractual amount and writing off the difference.
- When claims were denied as noncovered, they either transferred the balance to "patient due" or wrote it off completely if the insurer said the patient was not responsible.
- When services were bundled by the payer, they simply wrote off the disallowed amount, as indicated by the payer.

Elena was greatly disturbed because this was not what she wanted them to do! She expressed this to one of the members of the billing office and he replied, "You told us to reduce A/R and A/R is down. How else could we do it when the number of denied claims was increasing and we couldn't have any more help?"

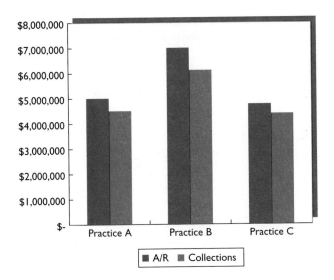

right to choose not to perform or to delay a key element of their job. Management can also unintentionally create ethical issues related to the follow-up of insurance claim denials.

In this case, some of the employees may have understood that the actions they were taking were unethical and not in the best interest of the employer—some employees may not have understood. Either way, management may have created this unethical behavior by requesting a particular activity without full explanation of the real objective. Having a reduction in A/R in itself does not produce benefit to the practice. The real advantage in reducing A/R means that a greater amount of money is being collected by the practice (Figure 9.16).

THE THIRD-PARTY PAYER'S ROLE IN THE REVENUE CYCLE

Many providers and facilities believe that the biggest problem in the revenue cycle is the failure of third-party payers or insurers to pay claims properly or in a timely fashion. In fact, the American Medical Association has established a "Heal the Claim Process" toolkit, which is an effort to reduce the number of claims that are denied by payers. Part of the process is to make the AMA aware of "unfair" practices on the part of payers (AMA, 2011).

In addition, the AMA has also introduced the National Health Insurer Report Card, which measures a number of metrics that quantify the way in which large insurers process claims. Those metrics included accuracy, denials, timeliness, and transparency. A disturbing element of the findings of the report card is that 20% of all health insurance claims are processed improperly, with errors (AMA, 2010b). The report describes that a tremendous amount of unnecessary expense is incurred by providers in attempting to receive payment for these improperly processed claims (Figures 9.17 and 9.18).

It is impossible and imprudent to assign motivation to the actions of others. However, many providers allege that the insurers are

FIGURE 9.17

From 2008 to 2010, all of the major insurers reduced the number of claims that they denied—in some cases, very significantly (AMA, 2010b).

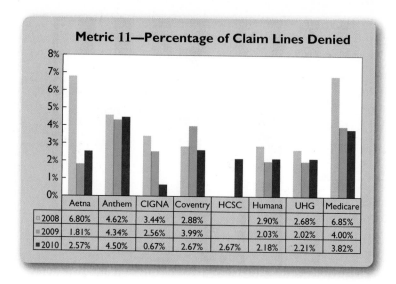

Metric 11—Percentage of Claim Lines Denied

	Aetna	Anthem	CIGNA	Coventry	HCSC	Humana	UHG	Medicare
2008	6.80%	4.62%	3.44%	2.88%		2.90%	2.68%	6.85%
2009	1.81%	4.34%	2.56%	3.99%		2.03%	2.02%	4.00%
2010	2.57%	4.50%	0.67%	2.67%	2.67%	2.18%	2.21%	3.82%

FIGURE 9.18

Since the initiation of the National Health Insurer Report Card, insurers have generally increased the number of times the amount paid on claims is equal to the amount called for in the provider contract (AMA, 2010b).

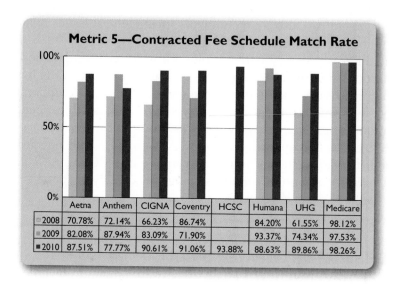

Metric 5—Contracted Fee Schedule Match Rate

	Aetna	Anthem	CIGNA	Coventry	HCSC	Humana	UHG	Medicare
2008	70.78%	72.14%	66.23%	86.74%		84.20%	61.55%	98.12%
2009	82.08%	87.94%	83.09%	71.90%		93.37%	74.34%	97.53%
2010	87.51%	77.77%	90.61%	91.06%	93.88%	88.63%	89.86%	98.26%

inaccurate in their claim payment on purpose to satisfy their shareholders. The position is taken that insurers know that not all providers will thoroughly monitor their claim payments and denials and that they will recognize some benefit in denying or inaccurately paying claims. Another significant issue asked by providers is, "If Medicare (a government-affiliated program) can process claims accurately over 98% of the time, why can't commercial insurance companies come close to this figure?"

A frequent complaint of providers is related to the manner in which customer service representatives of payers respond to patients who dispute the way in which the payer has processed the claim. When the claim is processed differently than the patient would like, the patient calls the payer to complain and/or obtain an explanation for what happened. Whether it is the result of inadequate training for a payer representative or an effort to deflect blame away from the payer, many providers complain that blame is shifted to them. The payer representative may say, "If the provider had coded it 'correctly,' this claim would have been paid." The problem is that this information is often not accurate because in order for the provider to code it differently, it often requires the submission of unethical or false information by the provider.

Whether these statistics are the result of intentional intervention by payers, inadequate systems, or for any other reason, there is a definite ethical question at issue. Correct payments should not be delayed to the detriment of providers and, indirectly, the patients covered by the insurer.

Thinking It Through 9.5

1. Discuss the misalignment of objectives among payers, providers, and patients. What, if anything, can be done to address this issue?

2. Patients frequently complain about the quality of service delivered in medical billing offices—particularly related to insurance claim filing. Why do you believe this occurs?

3. How can practice leadership better achieve its objectives in relation to the revenue cycle without producing unintended consequences?

4. Review the statistics provided from the National Health Insurer Report Card data in Figures 9.17 and 9.18. Does this information surprise you? Why or why not? What are the possible causes for these statistics?

9.6 Ethical Issues in Patient Statements and Collections

The final steps in the medical revenue cycle involve generating statements to patients and following up to ensure that payment is received in response to those statements. Only two parties are involved in this process—the patient and the provider. However, this does not mean that this stage of the process is without ethical difficulties (Figure 9.19).

PATIENTS AND STATEMENTS

In the majority of cases, when a provider sends a statement to a patient, the patient pays the bill. However, to provider billing offices it

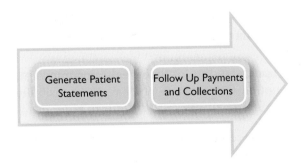

FIGURE 9.19
The component parts of the fifth stage (steps 9 and 10) of the medical revenue cycle.

Secured debt
Debt for which the lender has some means to require repayment, or the option to repossess the item purchased.

Unsecured debt
Debt for which the lender's only recourse if the debt is unpaid is to sue the borrower in civil court.

may feel as if "no one" pays their bill. This false assumption is based on the fact that they spend the largest share of their time working with patients who don't pay or don't want to pay. Very little attention is paid to those who pay their bills without intervention.

The primary reason for patients not paying their bills is based on their prioritization of bills if they do not have unlimited funds available. In fact, many credit counseling agencies place medical bills at the bottom of the list for repayment. The order in which bills should be paid is:

1. Housing.
2. Food.
3. Utilities.
4. Secured debt.
5. Unsecured debt (American Credit Counseling Service, Inc., 2010).

The first three items on the list are understandable. Life without these resources is extraordinarily difficult. **Secured debt** is items that were purchased on credit, without full payment at the time of receipt. However, creditors have a method for obtaining reimbursement for items that are commonly considered to be "secured" debt such as cars, boats, or financial transactions for which the person receiving the money guarantees, in some fashion, the repayment of the debt. If a person fails to make car payments, the creditor has the option of repossessing the car, which helps mitigate the damage it experienced when the payments were not made.

Unsecured debt is debt usually resulting from the provision of services, which cannot be repossessed if the person fails to pay the debt. Credit card debt is generally unsecured, although the credit card agreement allows the company to charge customers interest, which often motivates them to pay the debt. Similarly, medical debt is considered unsecured because there is usually no predefined agreement between the parties as to what will occur if the bill is not paid.

While many patients don't intend to not pay their bills, the prioritization factor unquestionably influences the process. There are several reasons why patients don't pay in response to statements from medical providers:

- The service they received can't be repossessed.
- A relationship usually exists between patient and provider that makes it awkward for the provider to aggressively collect bills.
- Often people with large medical bills have few resources or additional expenses elsewhere in their lives, meaning that they don't have the funds available to pay for the services.
- There is no direct or immediate financial penalty for not paying their bills.
- A lack of understanding of their health insurance provides them the false notion that they do not have responsibility for paying their outstanding balances.

It is unethical to receive service if there is no intent to pay for the service. However, is it unethical if the patient is *unable* to pay his or her bills? What is the provider, which requires income to continue operation, to do in this situation?

PROVIDERS AND STATEMENTS

Because of the requirements of contracts with third-party payers, most providers do not bill patients until the claim has been submitted to the insurer and final adjudication is complete. This can create confusing situations for patients. Table 9.5 shows a sample billing statement.

This statement is relatively straightforward, compared to some statements generated by provider offices. Many patients claim that they don't pay because they don't understand the statements. A factor that complicates these statements is the length of time that can pass between the time the service occurs and the time the payer properly adjudicates the claim. Six to nine months may pass before the patient receives a bill that indicates he or she is responsible for payment. It is for this reason that providers are being more aggressive in attempting to collect the amount the patient owes at the time of service.

However, when statements are sent to the patient and the patient doesn't pay, the provider must make some choices:

1. How many statements will be sent to the patient?
2. Will the provider attempt an internal collection process or will it outsource it to an agency?
3. What type of approach to collections will the provider take— "friendly" or aggressive?
4. Will the patient be **discharged** from the practice for failure to pay the bill? Is there a dollar limit or number of incidents that must occur before this happens?
5. Will any unpaid balance be reported to a credit reporting agency?

Discharged
Released from the practice, no longer able to be seen as a patient.

Another factor complicating this process is the determination of whether or not the provider met its obligation to the patient in obtaining the insurance benefit to which the patient is entitled. Although the insurance belongs to the patient, the patient has no valid way to self-report the services to the payer without the intervention—direct or indirect—of the provider. Many patients claim that they don't owe the balance due on their account because the provider did not follow

Table 9.5 Sample Patient Account Summary

Date of Service	Charge Amount	Paid by Insurance	Amount Due	Amount Due from Patient
1/15/11	$200	**	$200	
1/29/11	100	$80	20	$ 20
2/20/11	500	0	500	500
3/12/11	75	**	75	
Totals	**$875**	**$80**	**$795**	**$520**

**Claim not adjudicated yet by the insurer.

through appropriately in the submission and follow-up of the claim. It does not help when, on occasion, the payer representative falsely accuses the payer of committing an error or otherwise making a mistake.

The primary ethical issues are:

- Did the provider fulfill its obligation to the patient in connection with the claim filing to the payer?
- If the payer paid the claim inappropriately or denied it altogether, is it unethical or illegal for the provider to bill the patient?
- What recourse does the provider have if no one will accept responsibility for the balance due on the patient's account?

Providers are often hesitant to charge patients interest because, if they do so, they are subject to the Federal Fair Credit Reporting Act and any applicable state laws. The penalties for violating these laws are quite severe—much greater than the income lost in not collecting the original bill. To avoid the requirements of these laws, providers are now beginning to charge "statement fees" and other related fees that are not subject to the laws governing interest. The intent of these fees is to encourage the patient to pay the balance due and to discourage slow payment of bills.

Thinking It Through 9.6

1. What are the reasons that patients do not place a high priority on the payment of bills due to medical offices and facilities?

2. What can providers do to help clarify the statements sent to patients?

3. How should a provider determine whether or not a patient is *unable* to pay the account? If it determines that the patient is unable to pay, what should the provider do?

4. What is your opinion about aggressive collection techniques used by health care providers?

CHAPTER REVIEW

Chapter Summary

Learning Outcomes	Key Concepts/Examples

9.1 Identify the five stages of the revenue cycle, their purpose, and their influence on the subsequent stages. Pages 286–295	• The medical revenue cycle is perhaps the longest of any industry because of:
	  1. The third-party payer in the process.
	  2. The complexity of the process.
	• There are five general stages in the medical revenue cycle:
	  1. Scheduling, registration, and determination of financial responsibility.
	  2. Patient encounter at the facility or clinic.
	  3. Coding and billing.
	  4. Filing of claims with the third-party payer.
	  5. Billing of the patient for balances due.

Learning Outcomes	Key Concepts/Examples
9.2 Recognize the possible ethical issues that exist when scheduling patients for appointments, registering them, and assigning financial responsibility. Pages 295–301	• There are four elements to the initial process: 1. Establishing the patient's identity. 2. Obtaining the patient's insurance coverage information. 3. Confirming the provider's status as a participating provider with the patient's insurer. 4. Communicating expectations to the patient concerning payment.
9.3 Discuss the activities related to billing and coding that occur while the patient is receiving treatment. Pages 301–305	• Providers often do not obtain correct information from the patient because of: 1. A deliberate intent by the patient to deceive. 2. Ignorance by the patient regarding their coverage. • Patients are often resistant about making payment for their medical services. • Providers are taking new approaches to collecting funds from patients at the time service is provided. • Activities at the time of service can affect the ethical actions of the provider regarding financial matters.
9.4 Describe the potential ethical issues that can arise in the assignment of codes during the billing process. Pages 306–307	• Unethical behavior during the early stages of communication with the patient can often result in unethical behavior during the coding process. • Each element of the revenue cycle provides information and facilitates the next step of the cycle.
9.5 Evaluate ethical situations that occur in relationships with third-party payers. Pages 308–313	• Ethical dilemmas occur in this portion of the revenue cycle because the objectives of the payer, patient, and provider are not aligned. • Providers have issues with ethics in this area because of: 1. Failure to file claims in a timely fashion. 2. Failure to properly follow up on claims. 3. Unintended consequences associated with managing the billing process. • Payers have issues with ethics in this area because of: 1. A large percentage of claims improperly denied. 2. Inappropriate blame placed on providers by payers for action or inaction.
9.6 Determine the ethical impact of provider behavior and patient response in the patient billing and statementing process. Pages 313–316	• Medical bills are usually one of the last priorities for payment by patients. • Provider statements can be difficult for patients to understand. • Practices must decide what steps they will take to collect unpaid balances from patients.

End-of-Chapter Questions

Multiple Choice

Circle the letter that best completes the statement or answers the question.

1. **LO 9.1** The length and complexity of the revenue cycle can occur as the result of the actions of all of the following *except*

   a. Payer

   b. Provider

   c. Clearinghouse

   d. Patient

2. **LO 9.1** Which of the following statements is *most* true?

   a. Patients usually fully understand their insurance coverage.

   b. There is generally not a large difference in the amount a patient owes when the patient sees a participating versus a nonparticipating provider.

   c. Customers of a retail electronics store usually have more freedom to pick their provider, on an economic basis, than do patients of a health care provider.

   d. Providers are not responsible to notify patients of their participation status with the patient's insurer.

3. **LO 9.1** Which of the following is the easiest for a health care provider to calculate and collect?

   a. Coinsurance

   b. Copayment

   c. Deductible

   d. Balance following insurance payment

4. **LO 9.2** Each of the following is a possible approach to ensuring proper patient identification *except*

   a. No concern or investigation

   b. Reasonable concern and investigation

   c. Dismissal of a patient who provides false information

   d. Detailed confirmation of every patient's identity

5. **LO 9.2** An example of an expectation that should be established with the patient by the provider is

   a. Ensuring that the patient can expect the doctor will resolve his or her concern

   b. Reminding the patient that he or she should not expect the doctor to be able resolve his or her concern

   c. Telling the patient that payment of the amount due is expected at the time of service

   d. Guaranteeing the patient that he or she should expect the insurer to pay the full balance

6. **LO 9.3** Which of the following is *not* a responsibility of the provider, related to the revenue cycle, while the patient is in the office?

   a. Confirming the patient's identity, status, and insurance coverage

   b. Collecting copayments, coinsurance, or other patient due amounts

   c. Providing appropriate medical care

   d. Scheduling the next appointment

7. **LO 9.4** Which of the following is the correct order of the first three stages of the revenue cycle?

   a. Scheduling and registration, patient encounter, coding for the service

   b. Patient encounter, scheduling and registration, coding for the service

   c. Scheduling and registration, patient encounter, patient billing

   d. Patient encounter, scheduling and registration, patient billing

8. **LO 9.5** A primary obligation of the provider, to both the patient and the payer, is

   a. To file claims in a timely fashion

   b. To not bill the patient

   c. To delay billing the patient as long as possible

   d. To code the charges on the date of service

9. **LO 9.5** All of the following are "surprises" that a provider may see after a claim is adjudicated by a payer *except*

   a. A service denied as noncovered when the provider believed it was covered

   b. A claim denied because it is bundled with another service provided on the same date

   c. A code unilaterally changed by the payer, usually resulting in greater payment to the provider

   d. A claim paid, but at an amount different than called for by the payer fee schedule

10. **LO 9.6** Who are the parties involved in the final step of the medical revenue cycle?

   a. Patient, collection agency

   b. Patient, insurance company

   c. Patient, provider

   d. Provider, collection agency

Short Answer

Use your critical thinking skills to answer the following questions.

1. **LO 9.1** Explain why health care in the United States has a relatively long revenue cycle.

2. **LO 9.1** Compare and contrast a transaction at a convenience store versus that at a health care facility.

3. **LO 9.1** Describe how technology has shortened the revenue cycle for health care providers.

4. **LO 9.2** What are the reasons that health care providers need to be more vigilant in ensuring the proper identification of patients?

5. **LO 9.2** Do you believe that it is unethical for a patient to be ignorant about his or her insurance coverage? Why or why not?

6. **LO 9.3** Why is the issue of new versus established patient an ethical matter?

7. **LO 9.5** Describe a better way in which Elena, the manager in the case study, could have achieved reduced accounts receivables.

8. **LO 9.5** Do you believe the National Health Insurer Report Card data is helpful or useful? Why or why not?

9. **LO 9.6** What options are available to health care providers to improve their collections from patients?

10. **LO 9.6** What do you believe is the most important consideration when choosing what to do after a patient doesn't pay his or her bill?

Applying Your Knowledge

At the beginning of this chapter you were introduced to the case of Jason, who was presented with the opportunity join a practice but had concerns regarding some things that he had learned about the practice. Specifically, he was concerned about what he was reading on the Internet about the business practices of the clinic.

In light of what you have learned in this chapter about the medical revenue cycle, consider the following questions about Jason's circumstance.

1. List the questions that you would ask during the interview process that would help you determine if there are problems with this clinic and its revenue cycle. Explain what you would hope to learn from each question.

2. In your opinion, would it be more or less likely for there to be ethical problems with the clinic's business practices if the physicians and administration are aware of these problems?

3. Assume that you are in Jason's position and you choose to join the clinic, knowing there are problems with the business practices. What specific actions would you take in each of the following areas to reduce patient complaints and improve the clinic revenue stream?

    a. Scheduling patients for appointments, registering them, and assigning financial responsibility

    b. Improving activities that occur while the patient is receiving treatment

    c. Assigning codes during the billing process

    d. Working with third-party payers and following up on denied or improper claim

    e. Managing provider behavior and patient response in the patient billing and statementing process

Internet Research

The Internet has dramatically assisted health care providers in the process of managing the revenue cycle. One way in which it has helped is by providing substantial amounts of online information about the patient and the status of claim processing. Instead of calling a payer and waiting in the telephone queue, the provider representative can obtain information almost instantaneously and can retain a written record of what was learned during the inquiry (Figure 9.20).

1. Identify up to five insurers that operate within your geographic area. Look online to find their provider website. To the degree possible, determine which one is the best and which one is the worst. What are the reasons for your opinions?

2. What type of information do you think would be most important for providers to be able to access?

3. In some cases, provider offices must use a username and password to access certain data. Why is this necessary?

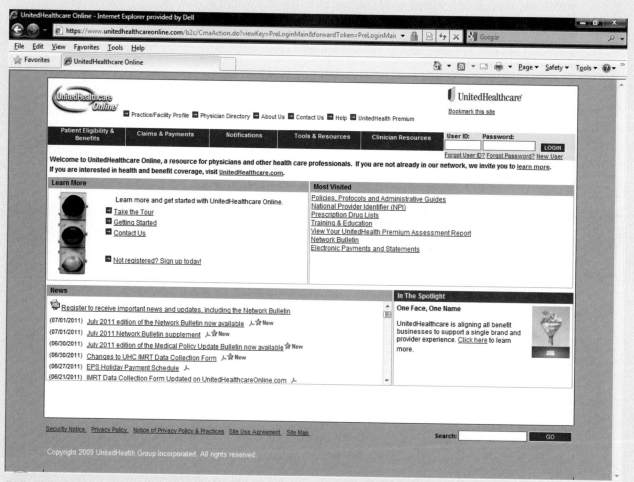

FIGURE 9.20

This website (**www.unitedhealthcareonline.com**) allows the provider the opportunity to gather significant data regarding patients with United Healthcare coverage and their claims.

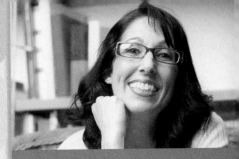

Coding Ethics and Professional Certification

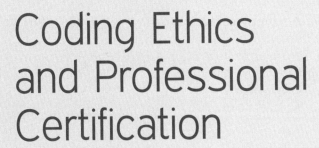

10

LEARNING OUTCOMES

After completing this chapter, you will be able to:

10.1 Describe the benefits to the health care organization in employing certified coders.

10.2 Evaluate the importance of certification in the professional life of a coder.

10.3 Compare and contrast the credentials offered by the two major coding certification entities.

10.4 Describe the process of obtaining certification with the various organizations.

10.5 Analyze the code of ethics published by each of the certification entities.

CASE STUDY

Annie was the manager of the front office staff at a small gastroenterology practice that included an endoscopy center. She recently completed her degree and felt that she was ready to move into a larger administrative role. She began to consult with her network of colleagues and review various job postings. In a relatively short period, she applied for a job as the administrator of a midsized orthopedics practice.

After Annie had been at the practice for three days, the senior billing/coding professional, Charise, who had been at the practice for 20 years, told Annie that she was going to be retiring. Charise provided Annie with two weeks' notice, but now Annie faced the first big challenge in her new job: filling Charise's role.

After reviewing a significant number of resumes, Annie selected three finalists:

- The practice's current receptionist, who has been with the practice for five years. She is reliable and hardworking, and she wants to be "promoted" to the billing/coding department. Her current salary is $12 per hour.

- A candidate with five years of experience in billing/coding in orthopedics. She has no certification and has no evidence of attending formal training classes. She has a desired salary of $15 per hour.

- A candidate with four years of experience in billing/coding, but none in orthopedics. She is a Certified Coding Specialist-Physician (CCS-P) with the American Health Information Management Association (AHIMA). She has a desired salary of $18 per hour.

Annie knew that she would learn a great deal during the actual interview process. However, as she stared at the resumes of these three people, she wondered how their background and experience would affect their ability to contribute to the practice.

1. Based on the information that you have available to you, whom would you select for this position? On what do you base your selection?

2. What additional information would you like to have in order to make a better decision?

Introduction

In the past 20 years, certification for medical billers and coders has become a major topic of conversation. Prior to that time, identifying a certified billing/coding specialist was a relatively rare occurrence. It was not widely sought by employees, nor was it specifically required by employers. However, significant change within the health care environment has prompted a dramatic shift that places certified coders in great demand. The professionalism and expertise required of those in the coding field is now more widely recognized. In addition, the economic pressures affecting health care organizations have increased the importance of efficiency and effectiveness within the billing operation, which certification can help ensure.

The increased focus on coding certification has had a positive influence in a number of different ways. One of these positive influences is the increased emphasis on ethics in coding. To better understand how the emphasis on ethics came about, a greater understanding of the importance and benefits of certification, as well as the various coding entities and their views of ethics, is required.

10.1 The Benefits of Employing Certified Coders

The number of certified medical coders in the United States has exploded in the past 20 years. Today, a substantial number of employers who are seeking billing/coding professionals either require or prefer coders with certification from an **accreditation entity,** which is an organization that gives recognition to an individual or group that meets certain standards. In some cases, depending on the position, a specific credential is required. Why has coding certification become so important to both coders and their employers?

Employers in the health care field often actively seek employees with certification to perform the critical billing/coding role within their practice or institution. They do this because certified coders provide significant benefits to them. The benefits are both financial and operational, resulting in both direct and indirect economic benefit.

Accreditation entity
An organization that gives recognition to an individual or group that meets certain standards, signifying that the recognized person or group has knowledge about a given subject area.

INCREASED EFFICIENCY WITH REDUCED COST

As reflected earlier in this book, the process of medical billing and coding can be complex. A lack of knowledge and understanding of the process can make a challenging endeavor even more difficult. When claims are submitted improperly, payment is delayed and a significant amount of time and expense can be incurred in trying to obtain payment for the claim. At best, claim payment is delayed, which produces an adverse effect on cash flow. At worst, claim payment is never received and/or additional staff is required to research and refile the claims. Submission of an incorrect claim is significantly more expensive than the correct submission of the same claim when done right the first time.

Certified coders are more likely to submit correct claims and, because of their knowledge base, are more likely to be efficient and productive in the submission of those claims. This naturally reduces the net cost of claim submission because money comes in the door more

Midtown Clinic's Coding Problems

Midtown Clinic was located in an economically depressed area of town. The vast majority of its patients were on Medicaid and many did not receive obstetric care on a regular, scheduled basis. As a result, a significant number of its patients had adverse outcomes in their pregnancies, including miscarriages and fetal demises.

It was common for patients who were having miscarriages to come into the office in the morning with symptoms, such as pain and/or bleeding. As a standard of practice, an obstetric ultrasound would be performed to check the status of the fetus. On occasion, the patients would continue to have symptoms later in the day and would return to the office. Another ultrasound would be done—this time, a nonobstetrical ultrasound—because the initial ultrasound did not reveal any evidence of an intrauterine pregnancy.

When this scenario occurred, Medicaid denied the claim for the second ultrasound and the second office visit (evaluation and management [E/M] service) on the same day. Midtown felt that it should be paid for the additional service. The noncertified coder and the physician repeatedly contacted the local Medicaid office to get an explanation as to why the claims were denied, but were unable to obtain a clear answer because it was Medicaid policy not to supply coding advice to providers. The coder had seen information in a coding newsletter that two ultrasounds in the same day should be payable with a −59 modifier (distinct procedural service), but even with this modifier, the claims were denied.

Midtown finally decided to call a certified coder to consult regarding this issue. Within five minutes, the consultant had identified that the National Correct Coding Initiative (NCCI) edits prohibited billing an obstetric and a nonobstetric ultrasound on the same calendar day, whether or not a −59 modifier was used. In addition, the consultant advised Midtown that CPT coding rules prohibit the billing of two E/M services on the same date. The cumulative services provided during the two encounters should have been combined when calculating the level of history, examination, and medical decision making for the one E/M code submitted for that day. She also explained how these ultrasounds should be billed so that proper reimbursement could be received.

quickly and less time and money is spent in refiling claims. Consider the case of Midtown Clinic, an OB/GYN office.

Midtown Clinic lost a great deal of money and expended an unnecessary amount of time trying to be paid for a service that was not billed properly. Even though the coder at Midtown may have had many years of experience in coding, she did not have the training and access to resources that would have supplied the correct information in a short amount of time. Had the coder been certified, the delayed payments and wasted time could have been avoided.

INCREASED COMPETENCE, SKILLS, AND KNOWLEDGE

All of the accreditation entities require that individuals with credentials received through their organization seek ongoing education regarding their field of expertise. These individuals' employers are beneficiaries of this ongoing education because they are up-to-date on the latest coding and compliance information. Whether through attendance at conferences or meetings or through journals and other publications of the accreditation entity, certified coders receive valuable information that will benefit their employers. Consider the case of Meredith Chang, "Failing to Invest."

Failing to Invest

In 2011, managers for a general surgery practice called Meredith Chang, a certified coder, to consult with them regarding problems they were having in cash flow. When she arrived, she went to the billing office and asked to see their coding books. She was handed a 2008 CPT coding book. When Meredith asked if they had a more current book, the lead coder (who was not certified) said, "No, there aren't that many changes each year—the doctor doesn't think that it is worth the investment."

Meredith looked at the billing patterns within the practice and immediately recognized that the surgical code billed most frequently by the practice had been deleted from the CPT book two years ago. She was amazed to find that the dominant insurer in that market had continued to pay this code, but at the payment level of two years ago—no adjustments were made to the reimbursement level. She then looked at the reimbursement level for the new code that replaced the code they had been using—it was 25% higher than the previous code.

Had the surgical practice employed a certified coder, it is highly unlikely that it would have continued to bill a code that had been removed from the CPT code book. Not only would the coder have insisted on the purchase of current coding materials, she would have received training materials from various sources that informed her of this major coding change that affected the bottom line of the practice.

INCREASED PROFESSIONALISM AND REDUCED EXPOSURE TO ACCUSATIONS OF BILLING FRAUD AND ABUSE

The recognition offered by certification raises the level of professionalism of coders. This, in turn, improves the level of their performance and increases the stature of the clinic. Whenever a third-party payer conducts an audit of a clinic in which a certified coder is employed, the odds of **inadvertent** billing errors are dramatically reduced because the certified coder is not going to allow this type of error to happen. Most payers also recognize the professionalism of certified coders, thus the interaction between payer and provider is likely to be more **collegial** and less confrontational, which benefits the provider.

Inadvertent
Unintentional or caused by a lack of care.

Collegial
Friendly and mutually beneficial.

> **COMPLIANCE TIP**
>
> Having a certified coder on staff is a sign that a health care provider is serious about being compliant in its billing and coding. Not only does it improve the quality of the coding, but it lets others (including third-party payers) know that the quality of coding is good.

INCREASED FOCUS ON ETHICS

Virtually all accreditation entities have codes of ethics, to which members are expected to adhere. Not only does the coder have an obligation to the provider as his or her employer, the coder also has an obligation to the professional organization to which he or she belongs. This dual obligation increases the employee's awareness of ethical issues, as well as emphasizing his or her responsibility to behave ethically—which always benefits the employer.

GENERAL AREAS OF BENEFIT

An American Health Information Management Association (AHIMA) study of employers reviewed the opinions of health care employers as it related to coding certification. Figure 10.1 illustrates the employers' positive outlook toward coding certification. The data reflects the

> **CODING TIP**
>
> Although it is difficult to put a specific dollar figure on it, there is great economic value in reducing a provider's exposure to allegations of fraud and abuse.

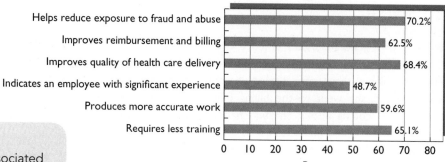

Impact of Credentialed Employees

Statement	Percentage
Helps reduce exposure to fraud and abuse	70.2%
Improves reimbursement and billing	62.5%
Improves quality of health care delivery	68.4%
Indicates an employee with significant experience	48.7%
Produces more accurate work	59.6%
Requires less training	65.1%

FIGURE 10.1

The percentage associated with each statement indicates the number of health care administrators who agreed or strongly agreed with the respective statements.

Source: American Health Information Management Association (AHIMA), 2005.

number of administrators and executives who responded that they agreed or strongly agreed with the statements as applied to hypothetical credentialed employees versus hypothetical noncredentialed employees.

Thinking It Through 10.1

1. Explain the ways in which a certified coder reduces costs for employers.

2. How does having certified coders on staff affect a health care organization's relationship with payers?

3. In Figure 10.1, several benefits are listed for employers that hire certified coders. Which do you believe is the most significant benefit? Why?

10.2 The Importance of Professional Certification for the Coder

Obtaining accreditation as a certified coder is not an easy process. A significant amount of work and study is required to achieve this recognition. However, the benefits and rewards of certification are significant.

HIGHER COMPENSATION

Each year, the American Academy of Professional Coders (AAPC) conducts a survey of its membership concerning salary levels, which is available at the AAPC website (www.aapc.com). In each year of the survey, the results reveal that certified coders make a higher salary than noncertified coders (Figure 10.2). Beyond the higher salary paid to certified coders, the ongoing study shows that certification offers added benefits:

• Certified coder salaries increased at a higher rate than noncertified coders when comparing 2010 to 2009 (1.5 vs. 1.2%).

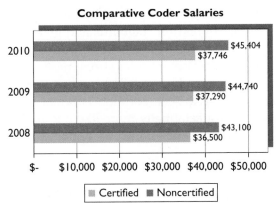

Comparative Coder Salaries

Year	Certified	Noncertified
2010	$45,404	$37,746
2009	$44,740	$37,290
2008	$43,100	$36,500

$- $10,000 $20,000 $30,000 $40,000 $50,000

■ Certified   ■ Noncertified

Source: American Academy of Professional Coders (AAPC), 2010.

FIGURE 10.2
Certified coders make higher salaries than noncertified coders. In addition, their salaries increase at a faster rate than do noncertified coders' salaries.

- Lower unemployment rates for certified coders when compared to the population at large (6.8 vs. 9.6%). In addition, the average period of unemployment for certified coders was only 5.4 months, substantially shorter than the national average.

The variance in salary between certified and noncertified coders can also be seen when comparing education levels, as reflected in Table 10.1.

The benefit of higher salaries for employees would seem to be in opposition to the objectives of the employer, namely the objective of holding down costs. However, most employers are willing to pay more to certified coders because they recognize that paying a higher salary to a coder is actually an investment that will ultimately result in greater **net revenue** for the employer through more quickly paid claims, fewer denied claims, and reduced financial risks associated with payer audits.

FYI

Certified coders make more than noncertified coders, but this actually results in higher net income for providers.

Net revenue
The amount of money that remains after expenses are subtracted from income; also known as profit.

THE OPPORTUNITY FOR CONTINUING EDUCATION

Certification opens doors to opportunities for coders to receive additional education. Education is widely available to noncertified coders, but there is no assurance available regarding the quality of the education. It may be excellent, or it may be substandard. However,

Table 10.1 Comparison of Certified Versus Noncertified Coders' Salaries by Education Level

Education Level	Noncertified Coder Salary	Certified Coder Salary
Some high school	$27,500	$39,167
High school graduate	36,764	41,272
Associate's degree	35,807	43,868
Some college	36,409	45,038
Bachelor's degree	47,421	51,389
Master's degree	50,929	64,807

Source: AAPC, 2010.

education received through or approved by the accreditation organizations meets certain minimum standards and generally is of higher quality than other commercially available education.

Continuing education also provides strong motivation for certified coders to seek additional education. The noncertified coder does not have a similar incentive to seek additional formal education. In addition, employers are substantially more likely to pay for continuing education for a certified professional, as opposed to a noncertified individual.

NETWORKING AND JOB SEARCH OPPORTUNITIES

Certification allows the individual the opportunity to be exposed to large numbers of other professionals with similar interests and career goals. Most organizations offer local, state, and national meeting and networking opportunities, which allow coders to obtain information about career opportunities, gather specific tips and insights from colleagues, and develop relationships with people whom they would never meet without their participation in the organization. The opportunity to meet others and expand their own personal network gives certified coders a head start in a job search process because they are aware of opportunities earlier and develop relationships with people who can assist them in obtaining a new position.

PROVEN KNOWLEDGE BASE AND GREATER FLEXIBILITY IN CAREER OPTIONS

The person with coding certification has an immediate advantage when competing with a noncertified person for a coding position. The certification is third-party confirmation of the fact that the individual has a certain knowledge base. It opens the doors to managerial roles in billing and coding and, as illustrated in some of the earlier case studies, allows coders the opportunity to engage in consulting for practices that do not have certified coders. The credential provides immediate credibility for the consultant and supplies significant opportunities for employment and other positions within the coding industry.

Thinking It Through 10.2

1. Which has a more significant effect on salary—education or certification? Defend your position.
2. Why is continuing education so important? How does certification affect the education process?
3. Why is networking important, even when the coder is not looking for a new position?

10.3 Major Coding Certification Entities

A significant number of coding certifications can be obtained from a variety of different entities. These include the American Academy of Professional Coders (AAPC), the American Health Information

Management Association (AHIMA), the American College of Medical Coding Specialists (ACMCS), the Professional Association of Healthcare Coding Specialists (PAHCS), the American Medical Billing Association (AMBA), the Board of Medical Specialty Coding (BMSC), and others. Because of the number of these entities, a discussion of each organization is not practical. AAPC and AHIMA, the two organizations offering the credentials that are most specifically requested by employers and with the largest number of members, are discussed here.

FYI

Many different entities offer certification in the field of medical billing. The two largest are the American Academy of Professional Coders (AAPC) and the American Health Information Management Association (AHIMA).

AMERICAN ACADEMY OF PROFESSIONAL CODERS

The American Academy of Professional Coders (AAPC) was formed in 1988 with the stated goal of "providing education and professional certification to physician-based medical coders and to elevate the standards of medical coding by providing student training, certification, ongoing education, networking, and job opportunities." AAPC has seen significant growth since its formation. By 2011, it had more than 105,000 members, with more than 70,000 members receiving certification (AAPC, 2011b). In 2009, it had 75,000 members, which was four times the number that it had in 2000 (AAPC, 2009).

Emphasis.   The initial focus of AAPC was based on physician service billing, as opposed to facility billing. The primary base credential offered by the AAPC, Certified Professional Coder (CPC), exclusively demonstrates that the coder has **proficiency** in physician service coding. Specifically, a person with the CPC credential can review and adjudicate coding of services, procedures, and diagnoses on medical claims in the physician office setting, thus improving the finances and operational efficiency of the practice (AAPC, 2011d). The AAPC reports that the CPC has:

Proficiency
Advanced skill or expertise.

- Proficiency in adjudicating claims for accurate medical coding for diagnoses, procedures, and services in physician-based settings.

- Proficiency across a wide range of services, which include evaluation and management, anesthesia, surgical services, radiology, pathology, and medicine.

- Sound knowledge of medical coding rules and regulations including compliance and reimbursement. A trained medical coding professional can better handle issues such as medical necessity, claims denials, bundling issues, and charge capture.

- Knowledge of how to integrate medical coding and reimbursement rule changes into a practice's reimbursement processes.

- Knowledge of anatomy, physiology, and medical terminology necessary to correctly code provider diagnoses and services.

FYI

The primary credentials offered by AAPC are CPC, CPC-H, and CPC-P. Apprentice-level certification is available for those who do not meet the experience requirements. AAPC also offers specialty credentials in 20 different areas.

AAPC later created a second credential that demonstrated knowledge and proficiency in the field of hospital or outpatient facility billing and coding—Certified Professional Coder-Hospital (CPC-H). AAPC reports that a CPC-H has

- Proficiency in assigning accurate medical codes for diagnoses, procedures, and services performed in the outpatient setting.

- Proficiency across a wide range of services, which include evaluation and management, anesthesia, surgical services, radiology, pathology, and medicine.
- Knowledge of coding rules and regulations along with keeping current on issues regarding medical coding, compliance and reimbursement under outpatient grouping systems. A trained coding professional can better handle issues such as medical necessity, claims denials, bundling issues, and charge capture.
- The ability to integrate coding and reimbursement rule changes in a timely manner to include updating the Charge Description Master (CDM), fee updates, and the field locators (FLs) on the UB04.
- A working knowledge of American Hospital Association (AHA) Coding Clinic guidelines in the assignment of ICD-9-CM codes from Volumes 1 and 2.
- The ability to correctly complete a UB04 form, including the appropriate application of modifiers.
- Knowledge of anatomy, physiology, and medical terminology commensurate with ability to correctly code provider services and diagnoses (AAPC, 2011e).

The third credential offered by AAPC was intended for coders who worked for third-party payer organizations and focused on the special needs of that subset of professionals: Certified Professional Coder-Payer (CPC-P). The CPC-P demonstrates a coder's aptitude, proficiency, and knowledge of coding guidelines and reimbursement methodologies (e.g., physician reimbursement, inpatient payment systems, outpatient payment systems, health insurance concepts, and HIPAA) for all types of services from the payer's perspective. The type of medical professionals that would benefit from this credential include

- Claims reviewers.
- Utilization management staff.
- Auditors.
- Benefits administrators.
- Billing service staff.
- Provider relations staff.
- Contracting and customer service staff (AAPC, 2011f).

Conundrum
A puzzling or difficult situation.

As the credentials of AAPC increased in recognition and more employers required certification before hiring a coder, new coders faced a **conundrum.** They could not get a job as a coder without certification, but they could not get certification without at least two years' experience, which was required for the base credentials. To resolve this issue, AAPC created a new credential—the Certified Professional Coder—Apprentice (CPC-A). This credential is given to anyone who passes the CPC exam, but does not have coding experience. The CPC-A credential is upgraded to the CPC credential once the experience requirements are met.

As AAPC continued to develop, it recognized the need to offer a credential that demonstrated a coding professional's knowledge base in a particular specialty. Presently, credentials are offered for 20 different specialties:

- Ambulatory Surgical Center—CASCC
- Anesthesia and Pain Management—CANPC
- Cardiology—CCC
- Cardiovascular and Thoracic Surgery—CCVTC
- Chiropractic—CCPC
- Dermatology—CPCD
- Emergency Department—CEDC
- Evaluation and Management—CEMC
- Family Practice—CFPC
- Gastroenterology—CGIC
- General Surgery—CGSC
- Hematology and Oncology—CHONC
- Internal Medicine—CIMC
- Obstetrics Gynecology—COBGC
- Orthopaedic Surgery—COSC
- Otolaryngology—CENTC
- Pediatrics—CPEDC
- Plastic and Reconstructive Surgery—CPRC
- Rheumatology—CRHC
- Urology—CUC

It is not necessary that a person obtain a CPC credential to obtain these specialty credentials, although many do. The specialty exams are different than the standard CPC exam in that they are almost exclusively based on real-world operative or patient notes. Questions for the exam are based on the coder's review and interpretation of the notes (AAPC, 2011g). There are no specific experience requirements to obtain the specialty credentials, but it would be unlikely that anyone would have sufficient knowledge to pass the specialty exam without experience in that particular specialty.

Organizational Design.   AAPC, based in Salt Lake City, Utah, has an organizational structure that emphasizes interaction between the organization and its individual members. It accomplishes this through advisory boards, on which members serve on a representative basis. Beyond the professional staff in the AAPC office, there are four different AAPC advisory boards.

The most significant element of the interaction between the national office and the individual coder is the local chapter structure. There are more than 450 local chapters throughout the United States and several other countries. Local chapters provide opportunities for coders to receive inexpensive coding education and networking meetings (Figure 10.3).

> **FYI**
>
> The members of all AAPC boards serve on a volunteer basis.

AMERICAN HEALTH INFORMATION MANAGEMENT ASSOCIATION

The predecessor organization of the American Health Information Management Association (AHIMA) was formed in 1928 as the

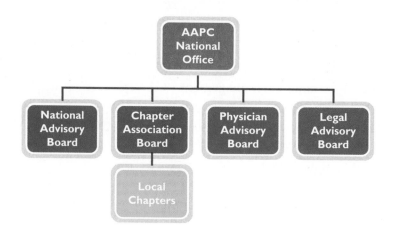

FIGURE 10.3
AAPC's advisory boards serve as a link between the membership and the national office. AAPC places an emphasis on its responsiveness to the needs of its members. It created this advisory-board structure to facilitate the communication.

FYI

AHIMA's scope of interest includes coding, but extends beyond coding. Therefore, some of the credentials that it offers are not specific to the field of coding.

Association of Record Librarians of North America (ARLNA), with the original purpose of improving the quality of medical records. It first credentialed members in 1932. In 1938, it was renamed the American Association of Medical Records Librarians (AAMRL). It was renamed the American Medical Records Association (AMRA) in 1970 and, due to the trend toward electronic records, the name was changed to its current identity in 1991 (AHIMA, 2011b).

Since that time, the organization has expanded its mission into advancing the health information management (HIM) profession through advocacy, education, certification, and lifelong learning, recognizing the dramatic changes that are occurring in health care through electronic health records (AHIMA, 2011a). By 2011, AHIMA had more than 61,000 members.

Emphasis. The original certifications offered by AHIMA focused on medical record management. The reason for this emphasis is that documentation was recognized as a critical function, long before CPT and ICD-9-CM codes existed. Accurate documentation is important because it facilitates

- Evaluation and planning of treatment.
- Communication among providers.
- Accurate claims review and payment.
- Utilization review (UR) and continuous quality improvement (CQI) activities.
- Collection of data.

AHIMA has changed its emphasis over the years to accommodate changes in health care. Its original focus was on an individual paper medical record. As time passed, the emphasis changed to recognize the various venues in which medical records were important, such as hospitals, physician offices, ambulatory care settings, managed care organizations, long-term care facilities, consulting firms, and so on. Most recently, the focus has been placed on the accessibility of records through electronic means, while maintaining the confidentiality that is so essential when working with individuals.

The names of AHIMA's credentials have changed over the years, in recognition of changes in the health care industry. As a result, the base credential offered by AHIMA is currently known as the Registered Health Information Technologist (RHIT). Those who have the RHIT credentials have the ability to ensure the quality of medical records by verifying their completeness, accuracy, and proper entry into computer systems. They may also use computer applications to assemble and analyze patient data to improve patient care or control costs. RHITs often specialize in coding diagnoses and procedures in patient records for reimbursement and research (Commission on Certification for Health Informatics and Information Management [CCHIIM], 2011).

The Registered Health Information Administrator (RHIA) is similar to the RHIT credential, but has a requirement of more advanced education. Unlike any credential offered by AAPC, the RHIA credential replaces the RHIT credential once the candidate has achieved it. AHIMA states that the person with the RHIA credential:

- Is an expert in managing patient health information and medical records.
- Administers computer information systems, collecting and analyzing patient data, and using classification systems and medical terminologies.
- Has expertise and comprehensive knowledge of medical, administrative, ethical, and legal requirements and standards related to health care delivery and the privacy of protected patient information.
- Often manages people and operational units, participates in administrative committees, and prepares budgets.
- Interacts with all levels of an organization—clinical, financial, administrative, and information systems—that employ patient data in decision making and everyday operations (CCHIIM, 2011).

As the issues of documentation and coding began to intersect, AHIMA created certifications that were specific to coding. AHIMA's primary coding certification is the Certified Coding Specialist (CCS). The examination for the CCS credential places an emphasis on coding within the hospital or institutional environment, which is where AHIMA had its initial focus. AHIMA states that a person that has the CCS certification has the following capabilities:

- Skilled in classifying medical data from patient records, generally in the hospital setting.
- Possess expertise in the ICD-9-CM and CPT coding systems, enabling them to submit charges to third-party payers.
- Knowledgeable in medical terminology, disease processes, and pharmacology.

To expand its accreditation services into the physician office setting, AHIMA created the Certified Coding Specialist-Physician (CCS-P) credential. The requirements for obtaining the credential are the same as for the CCS certification, except the individual's experience should be in a variety of physician clinic or other ambulatory care service settings, with knowledge of all sections of the CPT code book, HCPCS Level II codes, and ICD-9-CM codes.

Holding the CCS-P credential means that the person has

- Expertise in physician-based settings such as physician offices, group practices, multispecialty clinics, and specialty centers.

- Skill in reviewing patients' records and assigning numeric codes for each diagnosis and procedure.
- In-depth knowledge of the CPT coding system and familiarity with the ICD-9-CM and HCPCS Level II coding systems.
- Demonstrated expertise in health information documentation, data integrity, and quality.

In 2002, recognizing the increasing integration of inpatient and outpatient coding services, AHIMA created a new entry-level credential—Certified Coding Associate (CCA). Since that time, more than 8,000 people have obtained the credential that, according to AHIMA, demonstrates that the person

- Exhibits a level of commitment, competency, and professional capability that attracts employers.
- Demonstrates a commitment to the coding profession.
- Distinguishes himself or herself from noncredentialed coders and those holding credentials from organizations less demanding of the higher level of expertise required to earn AHIMA certification (CCHIIM, 2011).

Organizational Design. AHIMA has a professional staff at its home office in Chicago, Illinois. In addition to that staff, which includes the chief executive officer, the primary leadership body of AHIMA is the board of directors. The board consists of 13 people—the president, past-president, president-elect, CEO, and nine directors. Each of the nine directors serves a term of three years on the board. This board oversees several groups and committees (Figure 10.4), whose members serve on a volunteer basis.

In addition to the internal groups that exist within AHIMA, affiliated entities also have a specific relationship with AHIMA (Figure 10.5). Those groups include the AHIMA Foundation, the Commission on

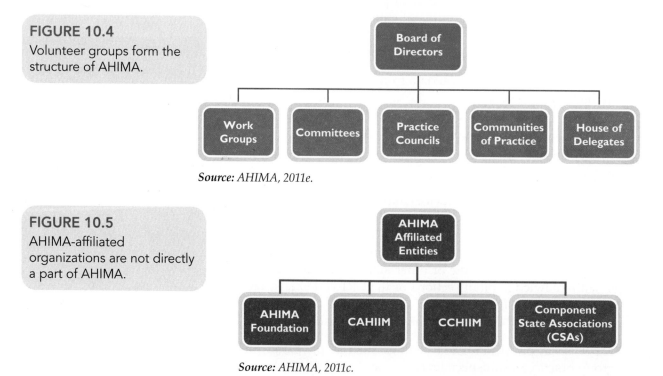

FIGURE 10.4
Volunteer groups form the structure of AHIMA.

Source: AHIMA, 2011e.

FIGURE 10.5
AHIMA-affiliated organizations are not directly a part of AHIMA.

Source: AHIMA, 2011c.

Accreditation for Health Informatics and Information Management (CAHIIM), Commission on Certification for Health Informatics and Information Management (CCHIIM), and the component state associations (CSAs).

The component state associations (CSAs) provide their members with local access to professional education and networking. CSAs also serve as an important forum for communicating national issues and keeping members informed of regional affairs that affect health information management (AHIMA, 2011d).

Thinking It Through 10.3

1. How has the history of each accreditation entity affected the development of the organizations and the certifications they offer?

2. What is your opinion of the fact that AAPC does not require coders who obtain specialty credentials to have a base credential with the organization?

3. Would the location in which a coder worked affect the organization with which he or she would choose to obtain certification? If so, what factors might influence that decision?

10.4 The Certification Process

Coding certification entities have different requirements for obtaining certification and maintaining the respective certifications. The emphasis of each organization influences its requirements.

AMERICAN ACADEMY OF PROFESSIONAL CODERS

AAPC's minimum requirement for issuing its base credentials are based on two factors:

1. Adequate demonstration of the individual's knowledge base.
2. Completion of a minimum of two years' experience as a biller/coder.

CPC Credential. The CPC examination consists of 150 multiple-choice questions. Those taking the test have 5 hours and 40 minutes to complete the exam, which focuses on the correct application of CPT, ICD-9-CM, and HCPCS Level II codes. It is a broad-based exam that covers all types of coding that occur within a physician practice setting, including medical terminology, anatomy and physiology, practice management, and coding guidelines. It is an open-book examination, but test-takers are allowed to use only books that list the codes from the three relevant code sets. If a person fails to pass the examination on the first attempt, he or she is able to retake the exam one time, without any additional fees.

To be able to take the CPC examination and receive the CPC credential, the person must meet the following four requirements:

1. Two years' experience in billing/coding, as indicated by two letters of verification of job experience, with one letter on letterhead from an employer.

2. Current membership in AAPC.

3. A passing score on the examination.
4. AAPC recommends that the person has an associate's degree, but it is not a requirement.

To maintain this certification, the CPC must renew his or her AAPC membership annually and must submit proof of attending 36 hours of **continuing education units (CEUs)** every two years. The purpose of the CEUs is to verify and authenticate expertise on the part of the coder (AAPC, 2011d).

CPC-H and CPC-P Credentials.   The requirements for taking the examination and maintaining the certification are the same as those of the CPC. The only difference between the exams is the subject areas on which the exams focus. Table 10.2 illustrates the topics covered on the exams.

If a person has two credentials (e.g., both CPC and CPC-H), he or she is required to obtain 48 CEUs every two years. Each additional base credential requires an additional 12 hours of continuing education every two years. If the person holds the CPC designation *and* a specialty credential, at least 16 hours of the total must be specialty-specific.

CPC-A, CPC-H-A, and CPC-P-A Credentials.   If a person passes the respective examination but does not have two years of experience as a coder, he or she will be designated as an **"apprentice"** until accomplishing one of the following:

- Supply two letters of verification of at least two years' experience, including one from an employer.
- Supply one letter from an employer verifying one year of coding experience *and* documentation of 80 hours of approved coding education.
- Completion of an online coding exercise. The exercise consists of 800 actual progress or operative notes, which must be coded with 90% accuracy. If the person fails to achieve the 90% accuracy, he or she will be given two additional opportunities to correct the erroneous questions. If the accuracy requirement is not met after three attempts, the person must restart the process with 800 new notes.

Table 10.2 Comparison of Topics in the CPC-H and CPC-P Examinations

CPC-H Examination	CPC-P Examination
Outpatient facility/hospital services	Coding accuracy and reimbursement methodologies
Anatomy and medical terminology	Anatomy and medical terminology
Coding guidelines	CPT
Payment methodologies	ICD-9-CM
CPT	HCPCS Level II
ICD-9-CM	Physician reimbursement
HCPCS Level II	Inpatient and outpatient payment systems
Surgery and modifiers	Health insurance concepts
Compliance	HIPAA

AMERICAN HEALTH INFORMATION MANAGEMENT ASSOCIATION

RHIT Certification. A person taking the RHIT exam is not required to be an AHIMA member. The RHIT examination is 150 multiple-choice questions, which the candidate has 3.5 hours to complete. One hundred thirty questions are used in calculating the candidate's score—the other 20 questions are categorized as pretest questions, which may be used in future RHIT exams.

Before being eligible to take the RHIT exam, the candidate must successfully complete the academic requirements, at an associate's degree level, of an HIM program accredited by CAHIIM. If he or she achieves a passing score on the examination, the individual will have achieved the RHIT designation. To maintain the RHIT credential, the person must document proof of participating in 20 CEUs during the previous two-year period and pay the recertification fee.

RHIA Certification. A person taking the RHIA exam is not required to be an AHIMA member. The RHIA examination consists of 180 multiple-choice questions, which the candidate has four hours to complete. One hundred sixty questions are used in calculating the candidate's score—the other 20 questions are categorized as pretest questions, which may be used in future RHIA exams.

A person with the RHIA credential must meet the requirements of the RHIT credential, but must also have a bachelor's degree in HIM from an approved institution. To maintain the RHIA credential, the person must document proof of participating in 30 CEUs during the previous two-year period and pay the recertification fee.

CCS Certification. To qualify for the CCS exam, the candidate

- Must have a high school diploma or GED.
- Is recommended, but not required, to have
  - Three years' experience in hospital-based inpatient coding for multiple case types.
  - Three years' experience in hospital-based ambulatory/outpatient care coding for multiple case types.
  - Completed coursework in anatomy and physiology, pathophysiology, and pharmacology, or demonstrated proficiency in these areas.

The examination consists of two parts. The first part is 60 multiple-choice questions (50 of which are scored), which the candidate has 60 minutes to answer. This portion of the test is *not* open-book and no additional materials can be used by the test-taker. The second part of the test is based on six inpatient coding scenarios, which encompass ICD-9-CM codes in Volumes 1 to 3, and seven outpatient coding scenarios, which encompass both ICD-9-CM and CPT codes. The candidate has three hours to complete the exam and can use the various code books for this part of the exam. However, this portion is fill-in-the-blank and candidates are not provided any recommended options for code selection.

To maintain the credential, the coder must have proof of completing 20 CEUs in the previous two-year period. Of those units, 10 must have been accomplished through mandatory annual self-assessments— 5 units each year.

> **FYI**
>
> The CCS and CCS-P examinations include both multiple-choice and fill-in-the-blank questions. The multiple-choice questions are not "open-book" and must be answered without any assistance. The second part of the exam allows candidates to use the coding books, but does not offer suggested answers—like a real-life coding scenario.

CCS-P Certification. The requirements for the CCS-P exam are the same as for the CCS test, except that the recommended experience should occur in the outpatient/physician setting. The pattern of the examination is the same, except the second part of the test consists of 16 outpatient cases encompassing ICD-9-CM Volumes 1 and 2, CPT, and HCPCS Level II. The standards for recertification are the same as for the CCS credential. If a person has more than one AHIMA credential, he or she must obtain 10 additional CEUs for each credential per two-year period.

CCA Certification. To take the CCA exam, the following standards must be met:

- High school diploma or GED.
- It is recommended, but not required, that the person have *one* of the following:
  - Six months' experience in a health care setting that uses ICD-9-CM and CPT codes.
  - An AHIMA-approved coding certificate program.
  - Completion of another formal coding training program.

The CCA exam consists of 100 multiple-choice questions (90 of which are scored). The candidate has two hours to complete the exam. Persons taking the exam can use the CPT, ICD-9-CM, and HCPCS Level II books. CCA certification is maintained in the same way as the CCS and CCS-P credentials.

Table 10.3 illustrates the requirements, examinations, and maintenance needed for the coding credentials offered by AAPC and AHIMA.

Table 10.3 Comparison of Credential Requirements and Examinations

	AAPC			AHIMA				
	CPC	CPC-H	CPC-A	RHIT	RHIA	CCS	CCS-P	CCA
Qualifications								
High school diploma				X	X	X	X	X
Associate's degree				X				
Bachelor's degree					X			
6 months' experience								R
2 years' experience	X	X						
3 years' experience						R	R	
Examination								
Multiple choice	X	X	X	X	X			X
Multiple choice/fill-in-the-blank						X	X	
Questions	150	150	150	150	180	60/13	60/16	100
Time (minutes)	340	340	340	210	240	60/180	60/180	120
Maintenance of Certification								
CEUs (per 2 years)	36	36	36	20	30	20	20	20
Extra CEUs for multiple certifications	12	12	12	10	10	10	10	N/A

X = required; R = recommended, but not required.

1. AAPC has experienced massive growth in the past few years. What elements of the certification/recertification process may have contributed to that growth?

2. Which of the exam formats do you believe is most challenging? What is the basis for your answer?

3. Imagine you had two coders applying for a position in an internal medicine clinic—one a CPC and one a CCS-P. Both had held their certification for 10 years. Based on this information alone, which do you believe is the best prepared for the position?

10.5 Certification Entity Codes of Ethics

Ethics are fundamental to the purpose of both AAPC and AHIMA. Both organizations use a code of ethics to define ethical behavior and encourage their members to engage consistently in ethical behavior as it relates to their coding duties. Each code of ethics has a similar purpose and objective, but slightly different approaches in communicating expectations to members.

Exemplary
Commendable and worthy of imitation.

AAPC CODE OF ETHICS

Compared to the AHIMA Standards of Ethical Coding, the AAPC Code of Ethics is relatively brief. However, in its brevity, AAPC clearly indicates that its ethical principles are based on a combination of deontological (duty) ethics and rights theory. The AAPC Code of Ethics is stated as follows:

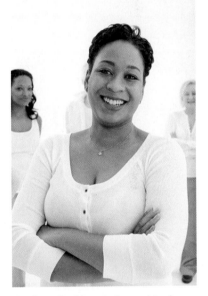

> Members of AAPC shall be dedicated to providing the highest standard of professional service for the betterment of healthcare to employers, clients, vendors, and patients. Professional and personal behavior of AAPC members must be **exemplary**.
>
> AAPC members shall:
>
> - Strive to maintain and enhance the dignity, status, competence, and standards of the healthcare industry.
> - Maintain the highest standard of personal and professional conduct. Members shall respect the rights of patients, clients, employers and all other colleagues.
> - Use only legal and ethical means in all professional dealings and shall refuse to cooperate with, or condone by silence, the actions of those who engage in fraudulent, deceptive or illegal acts.
> - Respect and adhere to the laws and regulations of the land.
> - Pursue excellence through continuing education in all areas applicable to our profession.
> - Ensure that professional relationships with patients, employees, clients, or employers are not exploited for personal gain.
>
> Adherence to these standards assures public confidence in the integrity and service of medical coding, auditing, compliance, and practice management professionals who are AAPC members.

Codes of ethics define ethical behavior and encourage professionals to make ethical choices. In professional organizations like AAPC and AHIMA, the existence of a formal code of ethics shows that the organization is dedicated to promoting ethical behavior. Codes of ethics, and the networks behind them, have the added benefit of showing coders that they are not alone when they are faced with ethical challenges.

Failure to adhere to these standards, as determined by AAPC's Ethics Committee, will result in the loss of credentials and membership with AAPC (AAPC, 2011a).

The complete AAPC Code of Ethics appears in Appendix A.

AHIMA CODE OF ETHICS

AHIMA has a Code of Ethics that applies to all of its members (Appendix B). In addition, AHIMA outlines its Standards of Ethical Coding in a separate document. This document is specific to coding, whereas the general AHIMA Code of Ethics applies to other areas of health information management. The two documents are consistent with AHIMA's mission and focus related to health information management, with coding being a component part of that mission.

The AHIMA Standards of Ethical Coding are exclusively deontological in their basis. In other words, the standards are based on the premise that coders have a duty to a number of objectives and entities in the performance of their job. The standards elaborate on those duties. The AHIMA Standards of Ethical Coding are stated as follows:

Coding professionals should:

1. Apply accurate, complete, and consistent coding practices for the production of high-quality healthcare data.
2. Report all healthcare data elements (e.g., diagnosis and procedure codes, present on admission indicator, discharge status) required for external reporting purposes (e.g., reimbursement and other administrative uses, population health, quality, and patient safety measurement, and research) completely and accurately, in accordance with regulatory and documentation standards and requirements and applicable official coding conventions, rules, and guidelines.
3. Assign and report only the codes and data that are clearly and consistently supported by health record documentation in accordance with applicable code set and abstraction conventions, rules, and guidelines.
4. Query provider (physician or other qualified healthcare practitioner) for clarification and additional documentation prior to code assignment when there is conflicting, incomplete, or ambiguous information in the health record regarding a significant reportable condition or procedure or other reportable data element dependent on health record documentation (e.g., present on admission indicator).
5. Refuse to change reported codes or the narratives of codes so that meanings are misrepresented.
6. Refuse to participate in or support coding or documentation practices intended to inappropriately increase payment, qualify for insurance policy coverage, or skew data by means that do not comply with federal and state statutes, regulations and official rules and guidelines.
7. Facilitate interdisciplinary collaboration in situations supporting proper coding practices.
8. Advance coding knowledge and practice through continuing education.
9. Refuse to participate in or conceal unethical coding or abstraction practices or procedures.

10. Protect the confidentiality of the health record at all times and refuse to access protected health information not required for coding-related activities (examples of coding-related activities include completion of code assignment, other health record data abstraction, coding audits, and educational purposes).

11. Demonstrate behavior that reflects integrity, shows a commitment to ethical and legal coding practices, and fosters trust in professional activities (AHIMA House of Delegates, 2008).

In addition to the Standards of Ethical Coding, AHIMA published an accompanying guide that explicitly outlines instructions related to each of the 11 points of the standards (see Appendix C of this textbook). Some of these instructions provide specific examples of what coders should and should not do.

AAPC CODE OF ETHICS VERSUS AHIMA STANDARDS OF ETHICAL CODING

Both codes of ethics promote the same general principles; however, they approach the issue in two different ways. The AAPC Code of Ethics is an **aspirational** document that describes, in theory, the way that coders should think and defines the goals for which they should strive. There are two primary principles that emerge in this document:

Aspirational
Establishing an objective or goal to be achieved.

- Coders should strive for the highest possible level of professionalism in all that they do.
- Coders should respect the rights of all people associated with the process, including patients, clients, employers, colleagues, and anyone else involved in the coding process.

On the other hand, the AHIMA Standards of Ethical Coding are more **prescriptive** in nature. This document is very practical and directive in describing the expected behavior of coders. Each of the 11 points elaborates on a specific behavior that the coder should or should not do. The primary principle is that coders should always conduct themselves in a specific, appropriate manner.

Prescriptive
Giving direction or instruction.

Similarities. Although the two documents are different in both their format and approach, nothing in the two documents conflicts in any way. Examples of the similar principles are listed in Table 10.4.

Differences. As indicated previously, the two documents are essentially identical in their objective—encourage and/or instruct regarding ethical conduct in the field of coding. However, two differences are significant.

1. *The AHIMA document encourages interdisciplinary collaboration in situations supporting proper coding practices—the AAPC document does not address the topic.* There is nothing in the AAPC document that suggests that this is not important—it simply does not address it. This is not surprising, given that AHIMA, as an organization, is multidisciplinary. On the other hand, AAPC has a singular focus on coding.

2. *The AHIMA document specifically requires the protection of the confidentiality of the health record at all times—the AAPC document is silent*

Table 10.4 Comparison of the AAPC Code of Ethics and the AHIMA Standards of Ethical Coding

AAPC Code of Ethics	AHIMA Standards of Ethical Coding
Strive to maintain and enhance the dignity, status, competence, and standards of the healthcare industry.	1. Apply accurate, complete, and consistent coding practices. 2. Report all healthcare data elements . . . required for external reporting purposes . . . completely and accurately. 3. Assign and report only the codes and data that are clearly and consistently supported by health record documentation. 4. Query provider . . . for clarification and additional documentation prior to code assignment when there is conflicting, incomplete, or ambiguous information in the health record.
Use only legal and ethical means in all professional dealings and shall refuse to cooperate with, or condone by silence, the actions of those who engage in fraudulent, deceptive, or illegal acts.	5. Refuse to change reported codes or the narratives of codes so that meanings are misrepresented. 6. Refuse to participate in or support coding or documentation practices intended to inappropriately increase payment, qualify for health insurance policy coverage or skew data. 9. Refuse to participate in or conceal unethical coding or abstraction practices or procedures.
Respect and adhere to the laws and regulations of the land.	6. Refuse to participate in or support coding or documentation practices . . . that do not comply with federal and state statutes, regulations, and official rules and guidelines.
Pursue excellence through continuing education in all areas applicable to our profession.	8. Advance coding knowledge and practice through continuing education.
Adherence to these standards assures public confidence in the integrity and service of medical coding.	11. Demonstrate behavior that reflects integrity, shows a commitment to ethical and legal coding practices, and fosters trust in professional activities.

on this issue. Again, the AAPC document's silence does not suggest that it is not important. AAPC's statement regarding the protection of the rights of patients would certainly encompass this concept because patients have a right, under the HIPAA laws and general principle, to have their records be confidential.

Examples of Ethical Behavior. The AHIMA document titled *How to Interpret the Standards of Ethical Coding,* which is available on the AHIMA website, includes a number of specific examples of ethical behavior that is expected or unethical behavior that is unacceptable. Samples of these examples include the following:

- "Code assignment resulting in misrepresentation of facts carries significant consequences." (Comprehensive coding guidelines—including systems of enforcement—should be in place.)
- "Failure to research or confirm the appropriate code for a clinical condition not indexed in the classification, or reporting a code for the sake of convenience or to affect report for a desired effect on the results, is considered unethical."
- "Policies regarding the circumstances when clinicians should be queried are designed to promote complete and accurate coding and complete documentation."
- "The description of a code is altered in the encoding software, resulting in incorrect reporting of this code." (Incorrect information [intentional or unintentional] entered in computer software is not an excuse for improper coding.)

- "A patient has a health plan that excludes reimbursement for reproductive management or contraception; so rather than report the correct code for admission for tubal ligation, it is reported as a medically necessary condition with performance of a salpingectomy. The narrative descriptions of both the diagnosis and procedures reflect an admission for tubal ligation and the procedure (tubal ligation) is displayed on the record."
- "Following a surgical procedure, a patient acquired an infection due to a break in sterile procedure; the appropriate code for the surgical complication is omitted from the claims submission to avoid any adverse outcome to the institution."
- "Failure to advocate for ethical practices that seek to represent the truth in events as expressed by the associated code sets when needed is considered an intentional disregard of these standards" (AHIMA House of Delegates, 2008).

Thinking It Through 10.5

1. Which of the two codes of ethics do you believe would be the most helpful to coders? Why?
2. Why do you think both organizations constructed their codes of ethics in the manner that they did?
3. Why do you think these codes of ethics are important?

CHAPTER REVIEW

Chapter Summary

Learning Outcomes	Key Concepts/Examples
10.1 Describe the benefits to the health care organization in employing certified coders. Pages 323–326	• There are significant benefits to the employer to hire certified coders. They include: 1. Increased efficiency with reduced cost. 2. Increased competence, skills, and knowledge. 3. Increased professionalism and reduced exposure to accusations of billing fraud and abuse. 4. Increased focus on ethics. 5. A variety of other areas of benefit.
10.2 Evaluate the importance of certification in the professional life of a coder. Pages 326–328	• Certification is important to the coder and brings substantial personal benefits, which include: 1. Higher compensation. 2. The opportunity for continuing education. 3. Networking/job search opportunities. 4. Proven knowledge base/greater flexibility in career options.

Learning Outcomes	Key Concepts/Examples

10.3 Compare and contrast the credentials offered by the two major coding certification entities. Pages 328–335	• The American Academy of Professional Coders (AAPC) certification features include the following:
	   1. The primary emphasis is physician service billing, as opposed to facility billing. The base credential is the Certified Professional Coder (CPC) designation, although additional credentials have since been created.
	   2. AAPC created a group of specialty credentials to recognize coders with demonstrated expertise in specific specialty coding.
	 • AAPC organizational design includes:
	   1. AAPC national office.
	   2. AAPC local chapter system.
	 • The American Health Information Management Association (AHIMA) certification features include the following:
	   1. Emphasis was on the management of medical records and other health information, with initial certifications of Registered Health Information Technician (RHIT) and Registered Health Information Administrator (RHIA).
	   2. AHIMA coding credentials are Certified Coding Specialist (CCS) credential, which focused on facility-based coding, and Certified Coding Specialist-Physician (CCS-P) credential, which focused on physician office coding.
	 • AHIMA organizational design includes a formalized structure, with a board of directors. There are several affiliated entities that are not part of AHIMA, but are closely related.

10.4 Describe the process of obtaining certification with the various organizations. Pages 335–339	• American Academy of Professional Coders (AAPC) certification requirements:
	   1. To obtain the Certified Professional Coder (CPC), CPC-H, or CPC-P credential, the person must pass a 150-question multiple-choice exam and have proof of two years' experience in the coding field.
	   2. To maintain the credentials, the certified coder must obtain 36 continuing education units (CEUs) every two years.
	   3. The Certified Professional Coder—Apprentice (CPC-A) credential is available for those who pass the exam but do not have documented experience.
	 • American Health Information Management Association (AHIMA) certification requirements:
	   1. To become a Registered Health Information Technician (RHIT) or Registered Health Information Administrator (RHIA), the person must pass a multiple-choice exam and hold an appropriate degree from an approved educational institution.
	   2. To become a Certified Coding Specialist (CCS) or Certified Coding Specialist-Physician (CCS-P), the coder must pass a two-part exam consisting of multiple-choice and fill-in-the-blank questions.
	   3. To maintain the credentials, the person certified by AHIMA must obtain 20 continuing education units (CEUs) every two years (30 for the RHIA credential).

10.5 Analyze the code of ethics published by each of the certification entities. Pages 339–343	• The AAPC Code of Ethics is relatively brief and is based on a combination of deontological ethics and rights theory.
	 • AHIMA has a Code of Ethics, which applies to all members. In addition, it has a Standards of Ethical Coding document, which is specific to the field of coding. It is exclusively deontological in its basis.
	 • The AAPC document is aspirational while the AHIMA document is prescriptive.
	 • Each document has the same objectives and many of the principles are very similar.
	 • There are two minor variances between the two documents:
	   1. AHIMA encourages interdisciplinary collaboration, while AAPC does not address the issue.
	   2. AHIMA explicitly requires the maintenance of confidentiality of the health record, while AAPC does not specifically mention the issue.

Multiple Choice

Circle the letter that best completes the statement or answers the question.

1. **LO 10.1** In recent years, the number of certified coders has
   a. Increased slightly
   b. Increased dramatically
   c. Decreased
   d. Remained essentially unchanged

2. **LO 10.1** The following are benefits of certification for employers *except*
   a. Increased efficiency
   b. Reduced cost
   c. Higher salaries
   d. Increased competence

3. **LO 10.2** The following are benefits of certification for the coder *except*
   a. Higher salary
   b. Continuing education
   c. Networking opportunities
   d. Improved reimbursement and billing

4. **LO 10.3** Which of the following statements is *not* true about AAPC?
   a. It was formed in 1988.
   b. It is based in Salt Lake City, Utah.
   c. It does not offer a credential for facility-based coders.
   d. It has more than 100,000 members.

5. **LO 10.3** Which AHIMA certification does *not* specifically apply to coders?
   a. CCS
   b. CCS-P
   c. CCA
   d. RHIA

6. **LO 10.3** Which of the following is *not* an AHIMA "affiliated entity"?
   a. AHIMA Foundation
   b. AHIMA Board of Directors
   c. CAHIIM
   d. CCHIIM

7. **LO 10.4** Which of the following is required to obtain the CCS credential?
   a. A high school diploma
   b. Two years' experience as a coder
   c. Membership in AHIMA
   d. Membership in AAPC

8. **LO 10.4** A CPC-A can have the apprentice designation removed from his or her credential before earning two full years of experience if
   a. The person passes the CPC exam
   b. The person supplies two letters of recommendation indicating that his or her employer is satisfied with the person's skill level

c. The person attends a coding training course

d. The person achieves 90% accuracy on the online coding exercise

9. **LO 10.5** The AAPC Code of Ethics is based on

a. Deonotological ethics

b. Rights theory

c. Both deontological ethics and rights theory

d. Teleological ethics

10. **LO 10.5** The AHIMA Code of Ethics is

a. Aspirational

b. Prescriptive

c. Theoretical

d. Authored by the board of directors

Short Answer

Use your critical thinking skills to answer the following questions.

1. **LO 10.1** Does the history or background of a certification/accreditation entity matter when seeking credentials? Why or why not?

2. **LO 10.1** How can a certified coder result in reduced costs for an organization, given that certified coders usually have higher salaries?

3. **LO 10.2** Which of the benefits of certification from the perspective of the coder do you think is most important? Why?

4. **LO 10.3** Why do you believe the AAPC's primary focus was initially on physician-based coding?

5. **LO 10.3** What influence does the offering of the CPC-P credential by the AAPC have on the United States' health care system?

6. **LO 10.3** How important do you believe is AAPC's focus on the local chapter? Would this affect your decision to affiliate with this organization?

7. **LO 10.4** Do you believe that the requirements for taking the CCS examination are sufficient? Why or why not?

8. **LO 10.4** Explain the benefits of required continuing education units (CEUs).

9. **LO 10.5** What may be the possible reasons that the AAPC Code of Ethics is relatively brief?

10. **LO 10.5** There are two elements in the AHIMA Standards of Ethical Coding that do not appear in the AAPC Code of Ethics. Why do you believe this is the case? Does it make sense? Why or why not?

Applying Your Knowledge

At the beginning of this chapter, you were introduced to Annie, the new manager of a midsized orthopedics practice. Charise, the practice's longtime billing/coding person, announced that she was retiring and Annie had to select a replacement. Annie had three candidates—the practice's current receptionist, who had no coding experience; an experienced orthopedics coder with no certification; and a certified coder who did not have any specific experience in orthopedics.

Annie had hoped that the solution would become clearer following the interview process. Unfortunately, the interviews had not achieved what she had desired. Each of the candidates seemed excellent in her own right. The strengths that Annie had identified for each of them on paper were confirmed during the interview. The candidates each explained how they would address the weaknesses about which she was concerned. Annie could not find any obvious personality issues that would keep them from fitting in at the practice and the references offered by each candidate were very strong. Annie felt like she was in a tough spot and was not sure which one to select.

Following your study of this chapter:

1. Which candidate would you select? Why? Was your answer different than the answer you provided when you first read the case? If so, what changed your answer? If not, what factor most supported your original answer?

2. During the interview process, the certified coder asked Annie if the practice would cover his expenses for recertification and travel expenses to obtain CEUs. The previous person in the job was not certified and did not ask for this benefit. Annie did not know what to say. Would you agree to this or not? How would you decide? What are the arguments for and against offering this benefit?

3. List the pros and the cons for hiring each candidate. If necessary, assign traits to the candidates that would affect your decision. (If you assign traits, list them prior to your answer.)

4. What questions would you ask these candidates to elicit answers that would help you decide?

Internet Research

AHIMA offers an unusually large number of resources on its website concerning ethics, ethics training, and ethical self-assessment. Each of these tools can be valuable in spreading the message of ethics throughout a health care organization and encouraging individual employees to follow ethical standards.

Download the AHIMA Ethical Self-Assessment, which can be located at www.ahima.org within the Ethics section. Complete the self-assessment.

1. Did your answers surprise you?

2. Did you find an element of ethics that you had not previously considered? If so, what was it?

3. Did you find the self-assessment helpful? Why or why not?

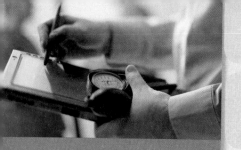

11

Current Trends in Coding Ethics

LEARNING OUTCOMES

After completing this chapter, you will be able to:

11.1   Summarize the current environment in health care related to electronic health records (EHRs).

11.2   Describe the potential ethical issues associated with selection and installation of an EHR system.

11.3   Evaluate the specific ethical issues associated with coding within the context of the use of an EHR.

11.4   Discuss how elements of health care reform may create ethical problems in medical coding.

11.5   Analyze how the mandatory compliance component of the Patient Protection and Affordable Care Act (PPACA) could influence medical coding in the future.

CASE STUDY

Russell was an experienced, certified coder who had worked for six years at the Family Practice clinic operated by Arthur Parker, MD. Dr. Parker was a solo practitioner who had been in practice for 35 years. He notified Russell and the rest of his staff that he was retiring in six months and that they were free to begin looking for a new job.

Because of the length of time he had been in practice at the same location and the fact that he knew he would not practice much longer, Dr. Parker had not implemented an electronic health record (EHR), nor was he planning to do so. All of his medical records were found in paper charts, stored in a file room. The only electronic element of his practice was his billing, which was accomplished through a basic, inexpensive practice management system. The physician relied on Russell to ensure his practice's billing was appropriate and compliant.

Russell was nervous about facing the job market, but he was excited at the potential opportunity to work in a larger setting that had an EHR and was more electronically sophisticated. He found what he was looking for at Fancourt Springs Internal Medicine, a practice in the suburbs with six physicians and three nurse practitioners. The practice had implemented a new EHR three months prior to Russell's arrival. During the interview process, the practice administrator showed Russell an example of an evaluation and management (E/M) note produced by the EHR. Russell was impressed because it was legible (which he was not used to) and highly detailed (something with which he was not familiar).

After a month at the new practice, Russell noticed that there were an unusual number of Level 4 and 5 established patient visits being billed at Fancourt Springs. He was aware of the usual or average distribution of E/M service levels billed, and Fancourt Springs's billings were skewed heavily toward Level 4 and 5 services.

Russell asked the billing manager about this billing pattern. She told him that this was a significant change for the practice. Before the installation of the EHR, most established patient visits were billed as a Level 2 or 3 encounter. She mentioned that a major selling point with the physicians concerning this particular EHR was the fact that the software sales representative guaranteed it would pay for itself through higher levels of E/M coding. Russell had heard that this could be the case because of the frequent occurrence of undercoding, but it still bothered him that they used this as a marketing tool.

About a month later, a representative from the EHR company came to Fancourt Springs to check on the installation. She provided lunch for the physicians and staff, and during that time, Russell asked her about the system—particularly the E/M coding function. He asked her, "What is the **algorithm** used to assign code levels?"

The representative looked confused. He asked again, "How does the system select the codes?"

"I don't know," she replied, "But that type of information is **proprietary**. I can tell you that our clients have been very happy with how it works."

Russell asked, "Were there any certified coders involved in programming the system?"

Algorithm
A computational procedure that arrives at the correct solution through a step-by-step process.

Proprietary
Privately owned and controlled.

"I don't know—I'm sure there were," replied the representative.

Russell did not feel very good about that answer. However, being new at the practice, he was not sure what to do next.

1. Do you think that Russell's experience at the solo practitioner's office was unusual?
2. What might be the reasons that a physician would not install an EHR, given the benefits it provides?
3. Do you think there is an ethical problem with the way the software company marketed this product? Why or why not?
4. Is Russell's question about certified coder involvement in the software design process relevant? Why or why not?

Introduction

The common saying that "the only constant in life is change" certainly applies to the U.S. health care system. As indicated in Chapter 4, the health care system as a whole has undergone tremendous transformation in the past century, the pace of which has quickened dramatically in the past 30 years.

In the last 30 years, the transformation of health care has had a dual-tracked emphasis. Not only have there been major advances in diagnostic and treatment medical services, but there has been dramatic change in administrative services—the business of medicine. Several of these changes have created the current environment of continuous transformation for the health care industry. These changes have both direct and indirect influence on the process of medical coding, and the ethics that accompany that process. The three particular areas we will focus on in this chapter are electronic health records (EHRs), health care reform, and compliance program development.

11.1 The Health Care Environment: Electronic Health Records

DEFINITIONS

To discuss accurately the issue of technology implementation in the U.S. health care system, it is necessary to define the terms that are frequently used in the process.

Electronic Medical Record.   The definition of an *electronic medical record (EMR)* has evolved over time as it has become significantly more sophisticated. When EMRs are discussed, they generally refer to a digitized version of the traditional paper-based medical record for an individual (Figure 11.1).

Electronic Health Record.   The use of the term *electronic health record (EHR)* has gained in popularity in recent years. Some have assumed that EMR and EHR are interchangeable terms, while others believe that EHR is just the next step in the progression from the EMR terminology. The EMR designation emerged from the original term

The Change in Terminology

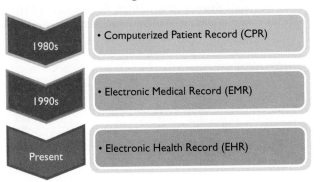

1980s	• Computerized Patient Record (CPR)
1990s	• Electronic Medical Record (EMR)
Present	• Electronic Health Record (EHR)

FIGURE 11.1

Over time, the terminology used concerning the technology of patient record management has changed. Some believe that the concepts are the same, but only the terminology has changed.

from the 1980s—computerized patient record (CPR). On the other hand, some that believe that the terms are not interchangeable and that an EHR is a completely separate concept from an EMR (Figure 11.1).

However, not all parties agree on a precise definition. Some focus on the EHR's ability to facilitate sharing of medical information among stakeholders and to have the patients' information follow them throughout their care. Others focus on the EHR's ability to automate and streamline the clinician's workflow and to produce a detailed and legible record.

For the purpose of this discussion, the system illustrated in Figure 11.2 will serve as the definition of EMR and EHR. The terms *EMR* and *EHR* are not directly interchangeable, although every EHR has an EMR as a primary component. The primary difference is that EHRs facilitate communication with other entities and have more advanced connectivity than EMRs.

THE HISTORY OF TECHNOLOGY ADOPTION IN HEALTH CARE

The health care industry has been slow to adopt technology that is not directly associated with patient care. Other industries, such as banking, finance, travel, and retailers, have spent enormous sums of money in advancing the infrastructure necessary to take advantage of the opportunities that technology offers in building their business.

The Technology Transition

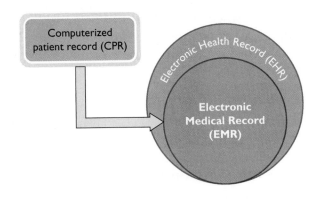

Computerized patient record (CPR)

Electronic Health Record (EHR)

Electronic Medical Record (EMR)

FIGURE 11.2

As technology has evolved, concepts of patient record management have changed and grown. The initial concept was that of the computerized patient record (CPR). It grew and evolved into the electronic medical record (EMR). As networking technology has expanded, the focus has been on interoperability and communication between health care organizations, to benefit the patient's health.

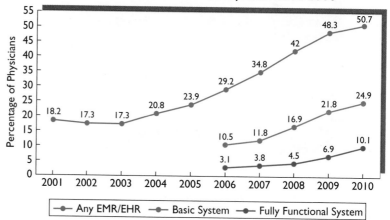

% of Office-Based Physicians with EMRs/EHRs: United States 2001–2009; Estimated 2010

Source: Hsiao, Hing, Socey, and Cai, 2010.

Technology has allowed some to dramatically change their business model, transferring the responsibility for much of the transaction to the customer. In many cases, this is seen as a positive for the customer because it is significantly more convenient. Once the investment has been made by the company, it is beneficial to them because ongoing costs are substantially reduced in terms of payroll and per-transaction expenses (greater efficiency), and customer satisfaction increases because there is greater standardization in the customer experience and greater convenience.

Why has health care been slow to adopt technology (Figure 11.3)? There are several reasons.

First, *technology is expensive.* All industries that have advanced in their use of technology have invested substantial sums of money in the technology. After implementation, tremendous cost savings are available, but prior to implementation, there is substantial financial outlay without any immediate financial return.

A second reason for not adopting technology is that *health care economics and realities are not conducive to the implementation process.* The health care industry's tradition as a **cottage industry** still has influence on the decision-making processes concerning purchases. Most other industries have substantial capital resources available to them because of their status as a publicly traded company. On the other hand, the majority of health care provider organizations are either physician-owned or hospital-owned, the majority of which are nonprofit entities. Therefore, capital investment is far more difficult because the funds must either come from operating income or directly from the physicians' pockets.

Moreover, the U.S. tax law and the corporate structure of many physician practices actually provide a disincentive for saving and investing in the business. To avoid paying corporate taxes on profits, many practices ensure that they have no profit at the end of the year—usually accomplished through payouts to the physician owners. This, of course, leaves no money to invest in technology.

Third, *physicians are not knowledgeable about technology that is not directly related to patient care.* Although there is a new generation of physicians coming that is more open to the use of technology, many of them

Cottage industry
A small-scale, loosely organized industry.

FYI

The economic structure of practices and current tax law are often roadblocks to the implementation of technology and other capital expense.

desire practice opportunities that do not include ownership. They are satisfied with being employees, which dramatically reduces financial risk and substantially improves their quality of life. This leaves the previous generation, which has practiced for many years without administrative technology, in control of the money needed to incorporate technology within the medical practice setting. Most physicians did not go to medical school because they were interested in administrative technology implementation. In addition, the software industry has not done a particularly good job in making the case for technology to physicians by adequately explaining the benefits.

A fourth reason for the health care industry's slow adoption of technology is that *the history of technology implementation in health care settings has not been strong.* For a variety of reasons, technology installations historically have not gone well. Whether it was because of inadequate investment of money, inadequate investment of time, inadequate psychological commitment to the project, technology that was not ready for "primetime," or some combination thereof, an unacceptable number of installations have failed. According to the April 1, 2006, issue of *CIO* magazine, "The [Health and Human Services] department itself has acknowledged that the failure rate for EHR system implementation is 30 to 50 percent. Some health care network providers claim it is as high as 70 percent" (Grider, Linker, Thurston, & Levinson, 2009).

Finally, *a positive return on investment (ROI) has not been consistently demonstrated from the use of health care technology.* Whenever a major purchase is contemplated, an analysis of the **return on investment (ROI)** should be conducted. The return on investment is a calculation of how long it will take the business to realize savings from the purchase that is sufficient to cover the cost of that purchase. For example, if a program was purchased for $100,000 and $20,000 would be saved per year because of the system, the ROI would be five years. The problems associated with ROI calculations are as follows:

Return on investment (ROI)
A calculation that defines the length of time needed to recover the expenditure associated with a project and make the project financially advantageous.

- The total cost of the systems can been underestimated.
- The total savings realized from the system can be overstated.
- Providers are hesitant to let go of previous systems and continue to operate redundant systems, which reduce or eliminate any possible savings.

LEGISLATIVE INFLUENCE ON EMR/EHR INSTALLATIONS

The federal government has recognized for some time that the delay in implementation of technology in the health care industry is not in the best interest of patients or the government. The use of EHRs will result in dramatic improvement in health care in a number of different ways:

- *Reduced cost to the government and third-party payers because of reduced numbers of diagnostic tests performed.* Frequently, tests are done repeatedly simply because previous results are not available. EHRs that facilitate obtaining records from other sources make repeat tests unnecessary.
- *Improved quality of care.* EMRs are generally more complete and legible than handwritten notes. Physicians who are reviewing electronic records from the past will have more information than they would otherwise.

> **FYI**
>
> EHRs will improve quality of patient care and reduce cost because of the ordering of fewer unnecessary tests and fewer errors due to computerized physician order entry (CPOE).

Table 11.1A Funds Available to Non-Hospital-Based Physicians Through the HITECH Act

Year	2011	2012	2013	2014	2015	2016	Total
2011	$18,000	$12,000	$ 8,000	$ 4,000	$2,000	-	$44,000
2012	-	18,000	12,000	8,000	4,000	$2,000	44,000
2013	-	-	15,000	12,000	8,000	4,000	39,000
2014	-	-	-	12,000	8,000	4,000	24,000
2015	-	-	-	-	-	-	-

Source: Woodcock, 2010.

Table 11.1B Penalties for Failure to Implement an EHR

Year	Penalty
2015	1%
2016	2
2017	3
Afterward	<5

- *Fewer medical errors.* Illegibility of medical records is the cause of numerous medical errors and adverse events for patients. One specific area in which these errors occur is prescription errors due to illegible physician writing. Electronic communication from the patient's EHR in the physician office directly to the pharmacy (CPOE) is faster and *dramatically* reduces the opportunity for errors.

The government has an interest in promoting the implementation of EHRs. To help facilitate this interest, Congress passed the American Recovery and Reinvestment Act (ARRA) of 2009—commonly known as the 2009 Stimulus Package. One element of that package was the Health Information Technology for Economic and Clinical Health (HITECH) Act, which allocated $19 billion to encourage the implementation of EHRs (Table 11.1A and 11.1B).

The process is not as easy as simply purchasing a product and using it in some fashion. To receive the stimulus funds from the government, the provider must demonstrate that it is engaging in "meaningful use" of the EHR. *Meaningful use* was defined by the Centers for Medicare and Medicaid Services (CMS) on July 13, 2010, and many providers have installed or are installing EHRs that meet these guidelines to receive the available funds. In addition, the package requires providers that participate in the Medicare and Medicaid programs to have an acceptable EHR in place by 2015, or they will be penalized in their payment levels (Figure 11.4).

Due to the positive incentive (funds to help pay for the acquisition of an EHR) and negative incentive (penalties in reimbursement from Medicare/Medicaid), the percentage of providers who use an EHR will climb significantly through 2015. It will substantially influence the practice of medicine and will affect the way in which coding occurs in the United States.

FYI

The Stimulus Package of 2009 has had an enormous impact on the expansion of EHRs in the United States, through incentive payments to practices that install EHRs that meet certain standards.

CMS Medicare and Medicaid
EHR Incentive Programs
Milestone Timeline

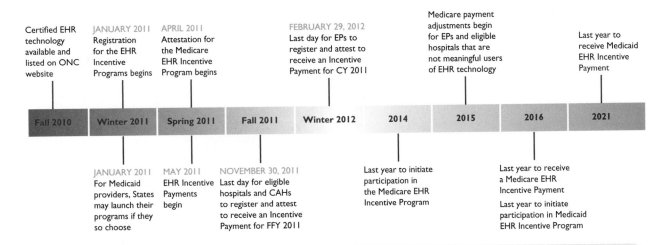

FIGURE 11.4

This timeline created by Medicare illustrates some of the key dates that providers must meet to receive funds through the HITECH Act.

Source: Centers for Medicare and Medicaid Services, 2011.

Thinking It Through 11.1

1. Do you believe that the size of an organization will affect whether it installs an EMR or an EHR? Why or why not? Does the definition of EMR or EHR make a difference in your answer? Why or why not?

2. What do you think is the most significant factor that has slowed the implementation of electronic records in the U.S. health care system? Why?

3. What is your opinion regarding the government's investment in EHRs? How should the government measure its return on investment (ROI)?

11.2 Ethical Issues Associated with Selection and Installation of Electronic Health Records

Within this complex context, the widespread implementation of EHRs continues and grows. The process of coding within the EHR supplies opportunities for ethical issues, as will be discussed later in this chapter. However, some of those issues have their origin in the selection and installation process because a complete review of the ethical considerations often does not occur at the time.

THE PARTIES INVOLVED

Most ethical dilemmas occur because of problems in relationships between individuals, groups, or organizations. This is the case in

FIGURE 11.5
The three parties involved in the EHR process all relate to one another.

EHR Relationships

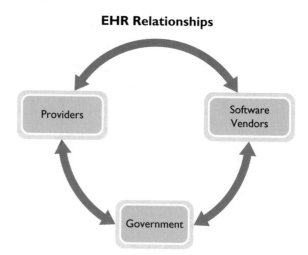

WARNING

Providers are at the greatest disadvantage in the EHR implementation and use process because they do not have expertise in the field of software, there is enormous expense involved, and many don't realize that systems and processes may require revision.

connection with EHR implementation and use, primarily because the interests of the other parties in the process are not considered and the potential influence of one party's actions are not fully reviewed and addressed. Before specific coding concerns are discussed, identifying the parties and their ethical responsibilities is required (Figure 11.5).

Providers. Providers, which include both physician practices and other institutional providers, are perhaps the most disadvantaged party in the EHR implementation and use process. Most EHRs are highly complex software programs in which the vast majority of providers do not have expertise. They are required to identify and obtain software that dramatically influences their practice of medicine and has the potential to affect the coding submitted—either for good or for bad.

As a result, providers are largely reliant on the software vendors to explain the product and assist in the installation/implementation process. The providers must trust that the software does what the vendor says it will do and that the vendor will provide the necessary support to use the product effectively.

This need to rely on others for information, however, does not relieve the providers of responsibility in the process. The providers must perform due diligence in selecting a company and evaluating their capability to make the installation a success. This due diligence must take a minimum of two forms:

1. *Providers must review the product and analyze how it works.* Most importantly, providers need to determine if the product will work within the context of the provider setting. In conjunction with this step, providers must perform reference checks, to talk with others who are using the program.

2. *Providers must make site visits to facilities that use the product to see how it operates in a clinical setting.* Ideally, the site will be similar in size, type, and specialty to enable the most accurate evaluation of how the product functions.

CODING TIP

When selecting an EHR that has a coding component, do not select the software unless a coder participated in the development of the software, or the system supplies the provider with the capability of controlling the code selection process.

Of the three parties involved in the process, providers probably are the least knowledgeable about the software but this actually increases their responsibility because they know or should know of their knowledge deficiency.

Software Vendors. The stimulus package that provided government funding for the purchase of EHRs was a tremendous benefit for the software vendors that develop that product. The marketplace opened dramatically because providers that were previously hesitant to invest in the software suddenly had strong incentive to make the purchase. The number of software vendors increased substantially due to the growth in available funding. This increased the competition between vendors, which makes the selection process more challenging for providers.

A major controversy within this process is the **operability** of the system—both clinically and as it relates to coding function. Some software sales representatives encourage providers to buy their software because it will enhance their revenue through improved coding. However, there are documented cases where no certified coder participated in the development of the software. The company developed its coding function by reading the Documentation Guidelines published by Medicare, but did not include anyone in the process who could practically interpret those guidelines.

The Federal Government. Because the federal government is providing money to fund the acquisition of EHR software and systems, it also has the ability to define the requirements for the system and what functionality they must have to qualify for funds. The government's interest in EHRs includes the desire to improve the quality of care, to reduce the cost of care, and to improve the documentation that exists for services provided to Medicare beneficiaries and Medicaid recipients.

The government's influence extends to both providers and software vendors because it, in large part, is defining what the systems must do and prescribing how providers must use them. The government's involvement in funding EHRs is an expansion of its previous presence in health care, through the funding of care.

ETHICAL DILEMMAS IN EHR IMPLEMENTATION

Providers. There are specific ethical considerations that providers must review prior to acquiring an EHR system. First, although it may not seem on the surface to be an ethical issue, providers must be committed to modifying their method of practice to accommodate all the benefits that the technology provides. This is an ethical issue because, if a provider is going to accept government funding for the system, it is unethical for the provider to use the system to less than its full advantage. Technology changes systems in every industry in which it is implemented. To insist that the systems of clinical practice remain the same after the EHR is installed is to be wasteful and inefficient. In fact, the failure of many EHR installations can be attributed to the inability or failure of the provider to consider the necessity of adjusting its thinking. Using the EHR in the same fashion as a paper chart is the same as trying to fit a square peg in a round hole—the EHR is the square peg and the practice pattern is the round hole.

For the same reason, providers have the obligation to ensure that they can use the system they are purchasing in the context of their organization. In other words, if the organization purchases a system that is a square peg, it needs to ensure that the organization is ready to receive that square peg.

Operability
The ability of a product to function according to its stated capabilities.

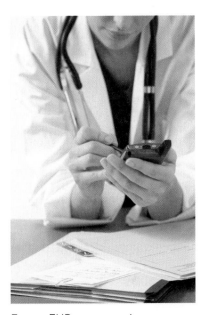

For an EHR system to improve a provider's efficiency and delivery of health care, the provider must often adjust the way it thinks about documentation, history taking, and other basics of health care. Attempting to use an EHR system like a paper chart fails to capture the benefits of the system.

WARNING

Providers that are receiving government funds to facilitate installation of an EHR have an ethical obligation to use the software to its maximum benefit.

Second, the provider must ensure that the EHR produces coding output that is accurate and is consistent with coding guidelines—particularly evaluation and management (E/M) guidelines). Systems whose coding functions were designed in conjunction with certified coders should get primary attention. Even if coders were not involved in the system design, providers have the obligation to ensure that they have the ability to modify and tailor the system so that inappropriate coding is not produced.

Software Vendors. Software vendors have often pointed to the fact that, to receive accreditation as a program that meets the **meaningful use** requirements established by the government, their software has to meet certain minimum standards. The accreditation, which is provided by the nonprofit Certification Commission for Health Information Technology (CCHIT), lists 330 separate criteria or standards that the software must possess. However, of these 330 standards, only 6 address issues such as the capturing of data for the electronic history and physical (H&P), ease of data entry, and E/M compliance (Grider et al., 2009). The remaining elements focus on key issues such as interoperability and security, but have nothing to do with the promotion of correct coding.

Software vendors have a special ethical obligation to ensure several key features in their programs:

Does the program facilitate appropriate collection of H&P and examination elements? If the process is too difficult or time-consuming, providers will be tempted to copy data from previous encounters, which may or may not be relevant to the visit at hand. If the process is too easy (e.g., facilitating prefilled fields or automatic copying), documentation may be overstated, resulting in overcoding.

Does the program adequately take into account the role of medical decision making in assigning code levels? The Medicare Carrier Manual indicates the following:

- *Medical necessity* of a service is the overarching criterion for payment in addition to the individual requirements of a CPT code. Medical decision making is the primary factor involved in quantifying medical necessity.

- The *volume of documentation* should *not* be the primary influence on which a specific level of service is billed (American Congress of Obstetricians and Gynecologists, 2011).

If the software solely calculates elements checked in the areas of history, examination, and medical decision making, it might be possible for a system to calculate a Level 4 or 5 established patient visit (on the basis of history and examination documentation) without regard to the medical necessity of the service (e.g., a common cold without any systemic or other complicating factors). While automation of some elements of the medical record is beneficial at times, it provides an enormous opportunity for improper and unethical billing.

Does the software vendor take any responsibility for documentation and coding compliance? Most contracts between vendors and providers specifically state that the vendor does not have responsibility for coding compliance. Some have questioned the fairness of this clause in the contracts because the coding function is often used as a marketing tool to promote the product. Yet, the vendor usually does not take responsibility when the product allows or leads clinicians into creating noncompliant documentation (Grider et al., 2009).

Meaningful use
Federal guidelines that encourage openness and improvements in health care by setting standards for EHR software.

WARNING

"Hold harmless" clauses in contracts with software vendors that relieve them of all liability for faulty coding produced by the system must be addressed before signing the contract.

Federal Government. A number of individuals in the coding community have expressed concern about the federal government's role in the publication of the Documentation Guidelines while simultaneously promoting EHR implementation. The claim is that the government has a serious conflict of interest because it benefits from penalties and fines it collects from providers because of fraudulent and abusive claims but, at the same time, it promotes the implementation of EHRs that facilitate the creation of fraudulent and abusive claims (Grider et al., 2009).

It is not the government's intention to trap providers in creating improper medical record documentation. However, the question remains, "Is it doing enough to ensure that the 'government-approved' EHRs adequately assist providers in doing their job?" Those that question the government's role point to the fact that improper E/M coding is actually a profit center for the government. In fiscal year 2010, the Justice Department recovered $4.02 billion in fraudulent and abusive billing through the Health Care Fraud and Abuse Control (HCFAC) Program. From 1997 through 2010, the program collected $4.80 for every dollar spent on enforcement. From 2008 through 2010, the program averaged $6.80 in collections for every dollar spent (U.S. Department of Justice, 2011).

On the other hand, the Department of Health and Human Services (HHS) requires only that "an audit version of the EHR that shows the tools used and the individuals who used them [to] enable retroactive detection of patterns of abuse or fraud." It would be more advantageous if the government required features that identified improper billing *before* claims were submitted and providers were subject to potential criminal prosecution (Grider et al., 2009).

> **FYI**
>
> The federal government's requirements for EHR funding do not place a significant emphasis on the coding function or its accuracy.

Thinking It Through 11.2

1. Do you agree that providers are the most disadvantaged party in the EHR selection and implementation process? Why or why not?

2. Based on the information supplied in this chapter, who do you believe is most responsible for EHR installation failures? Support your opinion.

3. Do you agree that the failure of some EHR installations is an ethical issue? Why or why not?

4. Summarize the government's place in the current environment as it relates to EHRs and code selection. Is the government's involvement too much, too little, or about right? Support your position.

11.3 Ethical Problems Associated with EHR Use

EHRs are a major step forward in advancing the use of technology within the administrative function of the medical setting. The use of an EHR makes previously illegible medical documentation easy to read and has the capability of improving health care because important information concerning past care is available (Figure 11.6).

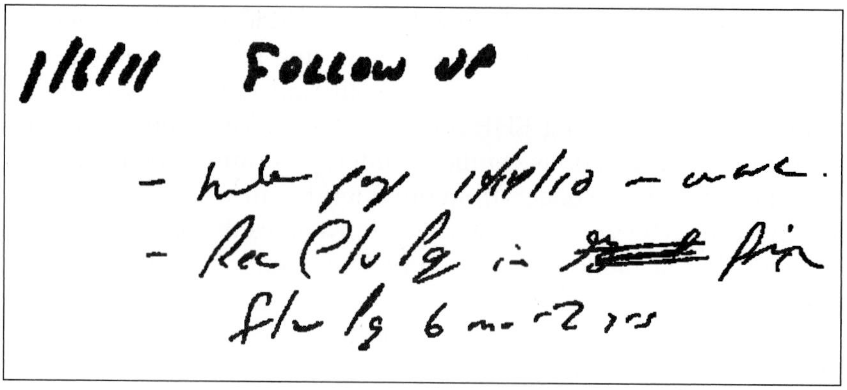

FIGURE 11.6

This sample of an actual medical record is virtually illegible and less than thorough. This is the complete documentation that was used in support of billing a 99214 established patient E/M service. Had this provider been using the coding function of an EHR, he or she either would have been prompted for more information or would have received a suggested code at a significantly lower level.

BILLING TIP

Before a claim is submitted to a third-party payer, the provider must ensure that there is adequate documentation to support the service being billed. Some practices do this on a prospective basis prior to the submission of the claim—others do it on a retrospective basis after the claim is submitted.

However, one of the most significant benefits that using an EHR offers—legible and complete documentation—is also one of the most troubling elements. The automation and time savings offered by templates can easily result in overstated documentation, inaccurate information, and a major disruption to the normal flow of patient care. Some EHRs force providers to document in a fashion that is not consistent with the manner in which they were trained, making the encounter unnatural and the documentation of questionable integrity. Extreme examples of inaccurate automated documentation include cases in which females had received prostate exams and males had negative Pap smears (Grider et al., 2009).

Although these may seem to be silly or humorous mistakes, they raise doubt about the legitimacy of the document, which then causes doubt about the quality of the codes assigned to the given service. Figure 11.7 demonstrates some of the major concerns about EHR documentation. The EHR assigned a code of 99214—Established Patient E/M service, Level 4, along with a procedure code of 58100—Endometrial Biopsy and 76856—Non-OB Pelvic Ultrasound. The concerns with this documentation include:

- The patient came to the office because of irregular, but heavy uterine bleeding and some menopausal symptoms. A pelvic ultrasound revealed a very large uterine fibroid. However, in the review of systems (ROS), it says, "Patient denies any fever, chills, or malaise. Feeling generally well." This is not consistent with the reason that the patient presented to the office on that date. In addition, in the personal medical history (PMH) section, it states, "Cycles: Regular, monthly."

- The physical examination information is clearly automated because the third and fourth lines are identical to the first and second lines. The phrase "Gait is WNL" (within normal limits) is odd because it does not seem applicable to the patient's condition. It is highly probable that this information is automatically plugged into every medical record, unless the physician specifically changes it.

- The patient was billed for both an E/M service and a procedure. However, the notes for the procedure are comingled with the notes for the physical examination. For the person reviewing this chart, it is difficult to determine where the E/M exam ends and where the normal preoperative services for an endometrial biopsy begin.

- The reference to the pelvic ultrasound is inadequate documentation to support the billing of the ultrasound. The CPT book specifically states, "Use of ultrasound, without thorough evaluation

```
PUBLIC, JANE          PATIENT: 23434        DOS: 11/29/2011
Age: 44

CC:  Fibroids

HPI: G5P4
     LMP 10/5/11:  Periods irregular, but heavy
     Hot flashes 6-7 times per day; sweats @ night, worse in last two
     months
     Pelvic ultrasound results: 14.1 cm leiomyomatous uterus with 2.6
     cm endometrium and 3.8 cm cystic left ovary

ENDOMETRIAL BIOPSY TODAY

ROS: Patient denies fever, chills or malaise.  Feeling generally well

PMH: No significant history or surgical procedures
     GYN-menarche at 13 years.  Cycles:  Regular, monthly
     Last Pap: 24 months ago-normal
     Denies STDs
     Contraception: Birth control

SH:  Marital: Married
     Occupation: RN
     Denies tobacco, recreational drugs, occasional ETOH

FH:  Mother-deceased at age 64; bone cancer
     Father-deceased at age 68; emphysema (non-smoker)
     Siblings: 1 sister with diabetes; 1 brother, 3 sisters all well

Vitals:  BP 121/71

PE:  Well nourished and well developed in no acute distress.  Affect
     is normal and appropriate.  Mucosa pink and moist.  Chest is CTA.
     Heart is RRR without murmers.  Gait is WNL.  Well nourished and
     well developed in no acute distress.  Affect is normal and
     appropriate.  Mucosa pink and moist.  Chest is CTA.  Heart is RRR
     without murmers.  Gait is WNL.  Normal female external genitalia.
     Herniation of rt lateral vaginal wall into vaginal canal.  No
     discharge.  Cervix normal, without discharge.  No cervical motion
     or tenderness.  Uterus, 12-14 weeks size, mobile, non-tender,
     anteverted.  No adnexal or ovarian masses noted.  No adnexal
     tenderness.  Cervix cleaned with betadine.  EMB device passed to 6
     cm in cavity and aspiration sampling performed.  Adequate sample
     obtained.  No pelvic tenderness with bimanual examination after
     procedure

A/P: Uterine leiomyoma
     F/U in two weeks with EMB results
     Consider hysterectomy, possibly laparoscopic
```

FIGURE 11.7
An example of a medical record created in an EHR. There are a number of troubling elements associated with this record.

of organs(s) or anatomic region, image documentation, and final, written report, is not separately reportable" (American Medical Association, 2011).

- The diagnosis reported as part of the medical decision making (218.9—Uterine fibroid, unspecified) is incomplete. The record also reflected the following diagnoses:
  - 626.2—Menometrorrhagia (excessive or frequent menstruation)
  - 627.2—Symptomatic menopausal or female climacteric states
  - 618.00—Unspecified prolapse of vaginal walls

In summary, although the electronic record in Figure 11.7 is highly legible and appears to be quite detailed, there are major flaws in its documentation and, as a result, significant flaws in the coding. Technically, the documentation meets the requirements for billing 99214. However, serious doubt exists as to whether the examination elements really occurred because the documentation is inconsistent within itself (e.g., irregular *and* regular periods, generally feeling well *and* hot flashes eight to nine times a day with night sweats). These inconsistencies call into question the **veracity** of the entire record.

Veracity
Correctness or accuracy.

PUBLIC, JANE   PATIENT: 23434   DOS: 12/15/2011
Age: 44

CC: Fibroids

HPI: G5P4

LMP 12/4/11: "It came gushing down. It is so bad. Can I have the surgery before the next one?"

Hot flashes 6-7 times per day: sweats @ night, worse in last two months
Pelvic ultrasound results: 14.1 cm leiomyomatous uterus with 2.6 cm endometrium and 3.8 cm cystic left ovary

ENDOMETRIAL BIOPSY TODAY

ROS: Patient denies fever, chills or malaise. Feeling generally well

PMH: No significant history or surgical procedures
GYN-menarche at 13 years. Cycles: Regular, monthly
Last Pap: 24 months ago-normal
Denies STDs
Contraception: Birth control

SH: Marital: Married
Occupation: RN
Denies tobacco, recreational drugs, occasional ETOH

FH: Mother-deceased at age 64: bone cancer
Father-deceased at age 68: emphysema (non-smoker)
Siblings: 1 sister with diabetes: 1 brother, 3 sisters all well

Vitals: BP 124/79

PE: Well nourished and well developed in no acute distress. Affect is normal and appropriate. Mucosa pink and moist. Chest is CTA. Heart is RRR without murmers. Gait is WNL.

A/P: Uterine leiomyoma
Prolapse of vaginal walls

F/U for pre-op

Requesting TVH/BSO/A-P Repair

The situation worsens when the record for the same patient for a visit two weeks later, on December 15, is examined (see Figure 11.8). Multiple examples of chart duplication and questionable data entry exist in this record. Some of the examples include:

- Everything from the third paragraph of the history of present illness (HPI) is identical to the February 1 record through the medications, except the addition of information concerning her previous deliveries, which did not exist in the previous record. This is problematic because:
  - The patient was in "For an endometrial biopsy today." This is unlikely, given that she had a biopsy two weeks earlier.
  - In the personal medical history (PMH), it states that she has had "no significant history or surgical procedures," even though she had an endometrial biopsy two weeks ago.
  - In PMH it states cycles are "regular, monthly"; under ROS it says, "Feeling generally well"; while under HPI it states, "It came gushing down. It is so bad. Can I have the surgery before the next one?" This is seriously inconsistent.
- The documentation of the physical examination is word-for-word identical to the first visit but is not particularly relevant to the

patient's condition. There is no mention of a genitourinary exam, although that is the primary system of complaint.

- There is no documentation regarding the medical decision making that occurred for this visit. It appears that the patient is going to return for a preoperative visit prior to the surgery (a total vaginal hysterectomy and anterior/posterior repair).

- There is no documentation regarding the results of the endometrial biopsy from the first visit. This, presumably, was the reason for this encounter, but there is no mention of it.

- The EHR selected a code of 99214 for this service, which could be supported based on the written documentation that exists. However, there is serious doubt as to whether these issues were pertinent to the visit or were simply copied from the visit (or perhaps a visit prior to that one).

EHRs have numerous benefits, including the ability to improve the legibility of documentation, the facilitation of more complete documentation, and better connectivity with other health care providers, which benefits the patient and the health care system as a whole. Greater efficiency and fewer errors are achieved through electronic orders and electronic prescribing.

However, serious ethical problems can be created through the improper use of EHRs. These problems include:

- Improper copying of previous history and physical information, which can result in inaccurate records.

- Improper use of encoding systems within the EHR which does not take into consideration some of the more subtle and complex elements of coding, such as the place of medical necessity in the selection of codes.

- Voluminous, but irrelevant, notes, created through the copying process, that do not contribute to the appropriate care of the patient. In some cases they can cause harm to the patient because important or relevant information is missed due to the quantity of documentation.

- Overcoding caused by the copying of previous information or the simple clicking of a box that automatically populates substantial data within the record. This opens the door to substantial financial penalties if audits reveal that the records are misstated or inaccurate.

Because of the government's incentive to providers to install EHRs, they are here to stay. However, users must be aware of the potential problems and ethical issues that the product can create.

Thinking It Through 11.3

1. In your opinion, is the benefit of legibility in EHR documentation sufficient to outweigh the potential ethical issues associated with EHR use? Why or why not?

2. In Figures 11.7 and 11.8, which of the errors pointed out is the most significant? Why?

3. How can EHRs adequately consider the place of medical necessity and medical decision making in the E/M code selection process?

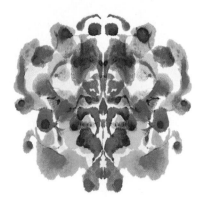

FIGURE 11.9

An inkblot similar to the type used in the Rorschach test.

Rorschach test
A psychological test in which participants explain what they think an inkblot looks like, used to gain insight into the participant's mindset and assumptions.

11.4 Health Care Reform and Coding Ethics

For the past several years, health care reform has been a major part of the national conversation. Beyond the political realm, nearly every person in America has an opinion regarding health care reform. This is not surprising because nearly every person in America has a stake in the outcome of whatever does or does not happen if and when health care is reformed. However, before there can be meaningful discussion concerning this reform, a significant clarification about definitions must occur.

WHAT IS HEALTH CARE REFORM?

Some say that health care reform is a **Rorschach test** for America. Developed by psychologist Hermann Rorschach, the test (often known as the "inkblot" test) supplies insight into how an individual interprets the factors in his or her world. People are asked to look at the inkblot and describe what they see. Their answer is thought to explain how they think and what is at the forefront of their mind—that which is important to them (Figure 11.9).

When people speak of health care reform, they are often using the same terminology but are thinking of substantially different concepts (Figure 11.10). They are thinking about three primary issues:

1. *The provision of and/or opportunity for increased, if not universal, access to health care at a reasonable cost for a greater number of people.* When the conversation began in the late 1990s, 44 million people did not have health insurance and a large number of people in the country felt that this number was unacceptably high. The primary objective should be to reduce that number—the issue is one of human rights.

2. *The ever-increasing cost of health care must be controlled. Costs have increased at a rate far in excess of the rate of inflation* (Figure 11.11).

FIGURE 11.10

The emphasis of health care reform has changed over time. Different stakeholders have also tried to emphasize the area of greatest interest to them.

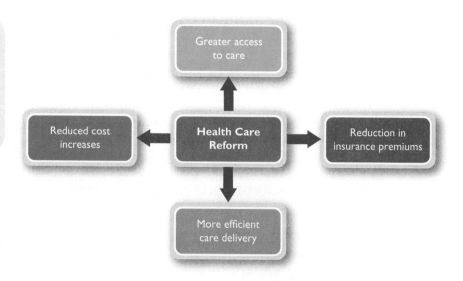

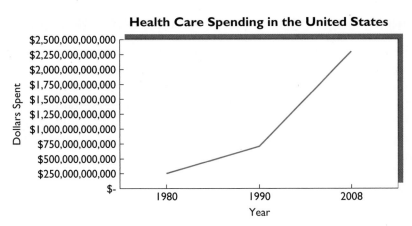

Health Care Spending in the United States

Dollars Spent	
$2,500,000,000,000	
$2,250,000,000,000	
$2,000,000,000,000	
$1,750,000,000,000	
$1,500,000,000,000	
$1,250,000,000,000	
$1,000,000,000,000	
$750,000,000,000	
$500,000,000,000	
$250,000,000,000	
$-	

Year: 1980   1990   2008

FIGURE 11.11

The dramatic increase in health care spending in the United States.

Source: Kaiser Health Care, 2010.

Because the situation is so complex and so many variables contribute to the cost of health care, some have changed the discussion to "health insurance reform." The key principle of health insurance reform is that the cost of obtaining and maintaining health insurance coverage should be controlled and health insurers should be prevented from excluding certain people from coverage because of any preexisting conditions they may have.

3. *To some, health care reform will be a combination of the first two objectives*—increasing the availability of coverage while reducing the cost of coverage to the individual.

A number of factors make these objectives more difficult than they already appear:

1. *The economics of health care have been skewed because the user of the health care services (the patient) has been largely shielded from the actual cost of service.* Patients think of health care costs in terms of copayment and deductible amounts—not the total cost of service. Many patients are unhappy with any outcome that will require them to pay more than they have paid in the past.

2. *Reductions in available funds to pay for publicly financed health care services have reduced the reimbursement levels given to providers for the services they deliver.* This has led to a trend of shrinking reimbursements for other third-party payers. This is occurring in an atmosphere of increased costs and increased debt incurred by students who are entering medical school, while practice expenses are also increasing. Providers are spending more to become a doctor, paying more to run their practice, but receiving less payment. Expenses can be reduced only to a certain degree, so providers are seeing a reduction in their income, which provides a disincentive for prospective students to enter the medical field.

3. *The number of physicians, especially primary care physicians, is declining.* This is problematic because the proposed number of people insured will increase, which is expected to increase the number of people seeking health care. Many expect the increase in utilization, combined with the decrease in the number of providers, to stress the existing health care system further.

WHERE DOES CODING FIT IN HEALTH CARE REFORM?

The objectives of the various parties in the health care reform debate are mutually exclusive. Without a total overhaul of the health care system, including both financing and delivery of care, achieving only one objective is not possible, let alone more than one. The difficulty is that there are very few parties who are willing to adjust their health care **paradigm** needed to effect the reform and achieve the results.

The easiest solution for providers is to increase the average revenue per patient. This can be accomplished by increasing the level of E/M services that they bill. In a perfect storm of sorts, the widespread implementation of EHRs makes this easier to do—high-quality documentation that supports higher levels of billing, even if the billed level of service was not actually supplied. Moreover, the fact that patients are insulated from the costs of health care contributes to the provider's ability to overbill the insurer without the knowledge or interest of the patient.

The government's attempt to control costs by auditing for fraud and abuse does help control the damage caused by unethical billing by recovering a portion of improperly paid claims and causing providers to think twice about engaging in inappropriate billing. Unfortunately, it can add cost to the system by forcing ethical providers to incur substantial expense in establishing and maintaining compliance programs and defending themselves against accusations of fraud and abuse in claim submission.

Paradigm
A model, pattern, or way of thinking.

CODING TIP

Do not use unethical overcoding as a means by which to increase revenue. Overcoding is sometimes justified by the fact that the provider does not feel that it receives adequate reimbursement from the payer. If that is true, it is an issue to be solved through contract negotiation—not overcoding.

Thinking It Through 11.4

1. What do you think should be the highest priority in health care reform? Why?

2. Do you agree that the objectives of health care reform are, in many respects, mutually exclusive? Why or why not?

3. Is it appropriate to use coding to address the issues that health care reform hopes to address? Why or why not?

11.5 Mandatory Compliance Programs and the Patient Protection and Affordable Care Act

Compliance programs are helpful in encouraging ethical behavior by

- Establishing expectations for appropriate behavior.
- Providing monitoring systems to ensure that ethical behavior occurs and identifying circumstances in which standards are violated.
- Creating discipline and corrective systems to address occurrences of unethical behavior.
- Supplying resources to employees who wish to report improper conduct or activity.

To date, all compliance programs prescribed by the federal government have been voluntary in nature. No provider of any type has been required to implement a compliance program, unless they are subject to a specific **corporate integrity agreement (CIA)**, as required in response to some finding of fraudulent or abusive billing. Any other organization that has a compliance program has done so because it elected to do so.

THE PATIENT PROTECTION AND AFFORDABLE CARE ACT

The Patient Protection and Affordable Care Act (PPACA), more commonly known in the media as the "Affordable Care Act," was signed into law on March 23, 2010. The overwhelming focus of the media concerning this legislation has been on the expansion of the availability of health insurance and other government programs, which will allow people to receive medical care who cannot currently access health care because they are unable to afford it. However, within the legislation, two specific sections mandate required compliance programs, if a provider intends to participate in Medicare, Medicaid, or the Children's Health Insurance Program (CHIP).

The two relevant sections of the PPACA are Sections 6102 and 6401. Section 6102 (Accountability Requirements for Skilled Nursing Facilities and Nursing Facilities) applies to long-term care facilities and is substantially more detailed than Section 6401, which applies to all other participants in the government insurance programs. Here is a brief summary of this section of the legislation:

- Within 36 months of the enactment of the section (March 23, 2013), facilities are to have a compliance and ethics program in place that is "effective in preventing and detecting criminal, civil, and administrative violations."

- Regulations for effective compliance and ethics programs shall be issued by the secretary of the Department of Health and Human Services (HHS) and the inspector general of HHS, no later than two years after the enactment of the law (March 23, 2012).

- Within three years after the issuance of regulations, the secretary of HHS shall do an evaluation of the compliance and ethics programs to determine their effectiveness. Specifically, they are tasked with determining if the number of deficiency citations decreased, whether quality improved, and whether other changes in various quality metrics can be identified. The secretary of HHS shall make a report to Congress regarding the findings.

- The compliance and ethics programs must be reasonably designed, implemented, and enforced so that it generally will be effective in preventing and detecting criminal, civil, and administrative violations and in promoting quality of care.

The required components of the program specifically include:

a. The organization must have established compliance standards and procedures to be followed by its employees and other agents that are reasonably capable of reducing the prospect of criminal, civil, and administrative violations under this Act.

b. Specific individuals within high-level personnel of the organization must have been assigned overall responsibility to oversee

Corporate integrity agreement (CIA) A program often required by the federal government when a provider or institution is found to be noncompliant in its billing/coding practices. The purpose is to facilitate monitoring of future billing and ensure corrective action on the part of the provider.

FYI

Very few people recognize that the PPACA discusses mandatory compliance programs and may have an effect on coding practice.

compliance with such standards and procedures and have sufficient resources and authority to assure such compliance.

c. The organization must have used due care not to delegate substantial discretionary authority to individuals whom the organization knew, or should have known through the exercise of due diligence, had a propensity to engage in criminal, civil, and administrative violations under this Act.

d. The organization must have taken steps to communicate effectively its standards and procedures to all employees and other agents, such as by requiring participation in training programs or by disseminating publications that explain in a practical manner what is required.

e. The organization must have taken reasonable steps to achieve compliance with its standards, such as by utilizing monitoring and auditing systems reasonably designed to detect criminal, civil, and administrative violations under this Act by its employees and other agents and by having in place and publicizing a reporting system whereby employees and other agents could report violations by others within the organization without fear of retribution.

f. The standards must have been consistently enforced through appropriate disciplinary mechanisms, including, as appropriate, discipline of individuals responsible for the failure to detect an offense.

g. After an offense has been detected, the organization must have taken all reasonable steps to respond appropriately to the offense and to prevent further similar offenses, including any necessary modification to its program to prevent and detect criminal, civil, and administrative violations under this Act.

h. The organization must periodically undertake reassessment of its compliance program to identify changes necessary to reflect changes within the organization and its facilities.

When compared with the compliance programs currently published by HHS and CMS, the requirements of PPACA are not substantially different than the previous recommendations. The primary difference is that these are now mandatory, although PPACA does not spell out the specific penalty for failing to comply with this law. The prescribing and assignment of discipline and penalties has been assigned to the secretary of HHS, who will make these determinations at some future date.

It is important to note that the required components of the program are specific to certain long-term care facilities. Section 6401 covers all other providers under the heading, "Provider Screening and Other Enrollment Requirements under Medicare, Medicaid, and CHIP." The subparagraph under this heading, titled "Compliance Programs," states:

a. IN GENERAL.—On or after the date of implementation determined by the Secretary under subparagraph (C), a provider of medical or other items or services or supplier within a particular industry sector or category shall, as a condition of enrollment in the program under this title,

b. title XIX, or title XXI, establish a compliance program that contains the core elements established under subparagraph (B) with respect to that provider or supplier and industry or category.

c. ESTABLISHMENT OF CORE ELEMENTS.—The Secretary, in consultation with the Inspector General of the Department of Health and Human Services, shall establish core elements for a compliance program under subparagraph (A) for providers or suppliers within a particular industry or category.

d. TIMELINE FOR IMPLEMENTATION.—The Secretary shall determine the timeline for the establishment of the core elements under subparagraph (B) and the date of the implementation of subparagraph (A) for providers or suppliers within a particular industry or category. The Secretary shall, in determining such date of implementation, consider the extent to which the adoption of compliance programs by a provider of medical or other items or services or supplier is widespread in a particular industry sector or with respect to a particular provider or supplier category.

There is substantially less information supplied in the law for providers that are not long-term care facilities. In addition, there are no dates established as to when enforcement of these requirements will go into effect. It is reasonable to presume that the requirements will not be substantially different than those for providers of long-term care. However, it will be necessary to wait until the administrative rules are published by HHS before additional information is available.

MANDATORY COMPLIANCE AND CODING

Until more details are known about the specific requirements of compliance programs, it will be difficult to know what effect these programs will have on the practice of coding and the incidence of unethical coding behaviors. However, it is certain that compliance and ethics will become an even bigger topic in the field of health care and health care administration as compliance programs become required of all providers that participate in government-funded health programs.

The question remains: "Will making compliance programs mandatory reduce the quantity and scope of unethical coding behavior?" There are two schools of thought regarding this question (Table 11.2).

1. **Yes, making compliance programs mandatory will reduce the quantity and scope of unethical coding behavior.** Raising the visibility of compliance programs increases the awareness of the issue. Those who may not have considered a particular coding pattern unethical will be forced to think at greater length about

> **COMPLIANCE TIP**
>
> The implementation of a mandatory compliance program is not a guarantee of ethical behavior.

Table 11.2 The Effectiveness of Mandatory Compliance Programs

Yes, They Are Effective	No, They Are Not Effective
There is increased awareness.	Voluntary programs are more effective than mandatory programs.
Individuals are forced to more deeply consider their actions.	There are always ways to circumvent ethics programs.
Penalties may become more well known, providing disincentive to unethical behavior.	Ethics is a personal decision and commitment that is not easily influenced by education or instruction.
Preventive elements of programs will dissuade people from attempting unethical actions.	

their actions. The penalties associated with unethical coding will become better known, which may provide a disincentive to engage in that behavior. More preventive actions, as part of the compliance programs, may be put in place, making unethical coding more difficult to execute.

2. **No, making compliance programs mandatory will not reduce the quantity and scope of unethical coding behavior.** The most significant advances in promoting ethical behavior have already been gained because those that are implemented voluntarily are more effective than those that are done out of obligation. There is significant historical evidence that those inclined to circumvent ethics programs and applicable laws will always find ways to do so. Ultimately, the person who chooses to behave unethically has made that decision without regard to the risk of detection or the potential penalty that he or she may face.

Thinking It Through 11.5

1. Were you previously aware of the mandatory compliance element of PPACA? Why do you think it is not a significantly publicized element of the legislation?

2. Why do you think there are more detailed compliance programs associated with long-term care facilities than for all other health care providers?

3. Discuss the possible influences of mandatory compliance programs on coding practice in the United States. How will it be different than the current state of coding?

CHAPTER REVIEW

Chapter Summary

Learning Outcomes	Key Concepts/Examples
11.1 Summarize the current environment in health care related to electronic health records (EHRs). Pages 350–355	• Terminology concerning administrative health care technology needs to be clarified because many use the terms *EMR* and *EHR* interchangeably. However, best practice makes a distinction between the terms: 1. EMR—a digitized version of the patient's paper chart, usually used exclusively within a single practice or organization 2. EHR—every EHR has an EMR as a primary component. The primary difference is that EHRs facilitate communication with other entities and have more advanced connectivity than EMRs. • Health care as an industry has been slow to adopt technology for a variety of reasons. • The federal government has enacted legislation that promotes the implementation of EHRs by supplying funding for systems that meet certain criteria.

Learning Outcomes	Key Concepts/Examples
11.2 Describe the potential ethical issues associated with selection and installation of an EHR system. Pages 355–359	• There are usually three parties involved in the transaction that facilitates an EHR implementation: 1. Providers 2. Software vendors 3. Federal government • Each of the parties has ethical concerns related to the transaction: 1. Provider 2. Software vendors 3. Federal government
11.3 Evaluate the specific ethical issues associated with coding within the context of the EHR system. Pages 359–363	• Serious ethical problems can result from the use of the EHR: 1. Improper copying of previous history and physical information, which can result in inaccurate records. 2. Improper use of encoding systems within the EHR which does not take into consideration some of the more subtle and complex elements of coding. 3. Voluminous, but irrelevant, notes created through the copying process, which do not contribute to the appropriate care of the patient. 4. Overcoding caused by the copying of previous information or the simple clicking of a box that automatically populates substantial data within the record.
11.4 Discuss how certain elements of health care reform may create ethical problems in medical coding. Pages 364–366	• When discussing health care reform, many people are confused by exactly what is meant. The discussion generally means: 1. Providing affordable access to health care for a larger number of people by providing a form of health insurance. 2. Reducing the total cost of health care. 3. Achieving both objectives. • Without substantial change in the health care paradigm, achieving these objectives is not possible. One solution for providers in addressing declining revenues is to increase their E/M coding levels. The use of EHRs has the potential to facilitate improved, increased documentation that may not necessarily support the actual service that was provided.
11.5 Analyze how the mandatory compliance component of the Patient Protection and Affordable Care Act (PPACA) could influence medical coding in the future. Pages 366–370	• Compliance programs are helpful in encouraging ethical behavior in a number of ways. • Until the passage of the PPACA, compliance programs were voluntary. The PPACA makes them mandatory for all providers that participate in government health care programs. • There is significant controversy as to whether making compliance programs mandatory will increase the ethical conduct within the health care community concerning coding.

End-of-Chapter Questions

Multiple Choice

Circle the letter that best completes the statement or answers the question.

1. **LO 11.1** Which of the following concepts was introduced first?

   a. Electronic medical records.

   b. Computerized patient records.

   c. Electronic health records.

   d. They were all introduced simultaneously.

2. **LO 11.1** Technology has not been adopted easily in health care for all of the following reasons *except*
   a. It is expensive.
   b. The economics of health care do not facilitate this type of investment.
   c. Most physicians are well versed in administrative technology.
   d. There have been a significant number of failures in implementation attempts.

3. **LO 11.1** *ROI* stands for
   a. Results of implementation
   b. Results of investment
   c. Return on implementation
   d. Return on investment

4. **LO 11.2** The government stimulus package had what effect on EHR software vendors?
   a. It had no significant effect.
   b. It opened up the marketplace significantly.
   c. It made selling their product more difficult.
   d. It reduced the number of requirements that EHRs must have.

5. **LO 11.3** Which of the following is *not* an ethical problem associated with the improper use of EHRs?
   a. Excessive copying and pasting of history and examination information
   b. Creation of voluminous, but irrelevant, notes
   c. Overcoding
   d. Precise calculation of the medical necessity of a service when selecting E/M codes

6. **LO 11.4** When discussing health care reform, people are discussing all of the following *except*
   a. Increasing access to affordable health care
   b. Increasing payments to physicians and other providers
   c. Reducing the total, aggregate cost of health care
   d. Reducing the cost of health insurance premiums

7. **LO 11.4** The easiest solution for providers to address the issue of shrinking revenue is to
   a. Increase per-patient revenue
   b. Install an EHR
   c. Use the coding function of an EHR to assign E/M codes
   d. Lay off long-term employees

8. **LO 11.4** What is a key principle of health insurance reform?
   a. The number of insurers should be reduced.
   b. Insurers can restrict coverage on a larger number of people.
   c. The cost of health insurance should be controlled.
   d. Insurers should pay claims more quickly.

9. **LO 11.5** A corporate integrity agreement is
   a. Usually a voluntary part of a compliance program established by large health care entities
   b. Implemented when an organization is found to have unsatisfactory levels of customer service
   c. Implemented and enforced by the government when there has been evidence of billing fraud and abuse
   d. An alternative name for a compliance program

10. **LO 11.5** Which of the following is *not* a way in which compliance programs are helpful in encouraging ethical behavior?
    a. Establishing expectations for appropriate behavior
    b. Supplying a monitoring system to ensure ethical behavior occurs
    c. Creating discipline systems when unethical behavior does occur
    d. Changing the fundamental moral system of a person

Short Answer

Use your critical thinking skills to answer the following questions.

1. **LO 11.1** Do you agree that there is a distinction between an EMR and an EHR? Why or why not?

2. **LO 11.1** Discuss the responsibility that EHR software vendors have for the current environment. Has the government's involvement in the transaction complicated the ethics of the situation? If so, how?

3. **LO 11.2** What action (or lack thereof) on the part of providers contributes most to poor outcomes in EHR installations? Explain your answer.

4. **LO 11.2** Do you believe the CCHIT criteria adequately address the issue of correct coding? Why or why not?

5. **LO 11.3** In your opinion, what is the most troubling element of the sample notes provided in Figures 11.7 and 11.8? Why?

6. **LO 11.3** If you encountered the handwritten note shown in Figure 11.6, with a billing of 99214 associated with that documentation, what action, if any, would you take as a coder?

7. **LO 11.4** Explain what is meant by the statement, "Healthcare reform is a Rorschach test for America."

8. **LO 11.4** Why do you believe that health care costs have increased at a rate greater than the rate of inflation?

9. **LO 11.5** Examine the section titles for Section 6102 and 6401 of the PPACA. What influence, if any, do you believe these titles have on the way the law was written?

10. **LO 11.5** Review the statements in Table 11.2. With which position do you most agree? Why?

Applying Your Knowledge

At the beginning of this chapter you were introduced to Russell, an experienced coder who had worked in a practice that had no electronic records of any kind, who was recently hired at a practice that had just installed an EHR. He was disturbed by some of the things that he learned and saw in relation to the billing that was generated from the EHR's billing function.

In an attempt to understand the billing patterns at the practice, Russell selected 10 random established patients who had been seen in the past month. He printed a copy of the medical record documentation for those visits. He then went to the paper charts of the same patients and selected the documentation of a previous visit (prior to the EHR installation). He made a copy of those records and returned to his desk to compare them with the accompanying service billings.

Generally, Russell's findings were as he had been told. Most of the handwritten charts were billed at a level of 99212 or 99213. The documentation was hard to read, very limited, and, in some cases, did not support the 99213 level of service. The documentation from the EHR for follow-up visits, with the same chief complaints, was substantially different. The documentation was highly thorough and very complete. The services were consistently billed as 99214 or 99215, and the documentation seemed to support those levels of service.

In light of this information, answer the following questions:

1. Do you have any concerns regarding Russell's investigation? Why or why not?

2. How do you interpret his findings? Can you tell from the information whether the previous billings were undercoded or if the EHR billings were overcoded—or both? What additional information would make answering this question easier?

3. If Russell determines that overcoding is currently occurring, what action should he take if there is a compliance plan in place? What should he do if the practice does not have a compliance plan?

Internet Research

One of the elements that has significantly delayed the implementation of EHRs is the high cost—particularly to small providers. There is substantial entry cost to the process, regardless of provider size. Generally, larger provider organizations are more easily able to absorb that startup cost.

One advance that has made the process somewhat more affordable is the introduction of the application service provider (ASP) model of software access. Advances in the technology have allowed even more flexibility and power, which is commonly known as "cloud computing." A provider using a cloud-based EHR does not have a server in the office and, therefore, does not need to incur the expense of the computer server hardware, nor does it have to be concerned about the maintenance and repair of the server. A growing number of providers are selecting this model (Figure 11.12).

1. Perform an Internet search regarding the ASP/cloud model of EHR software. Create a table, listing the advantages of the ASP/cloud model in the left column and the disadvantages in the right column.

2. What are the most important factors on your list that would influence your decision for or against choosing cloud-based software?

3. Is the following statement true or false: "Two identical practices, operated in the same way, but in different geographic locations, could make opposite decisions regarding the selection of a cloud-based EHR." If it is true, why would it be true? If it is false, on what do you base your answer?

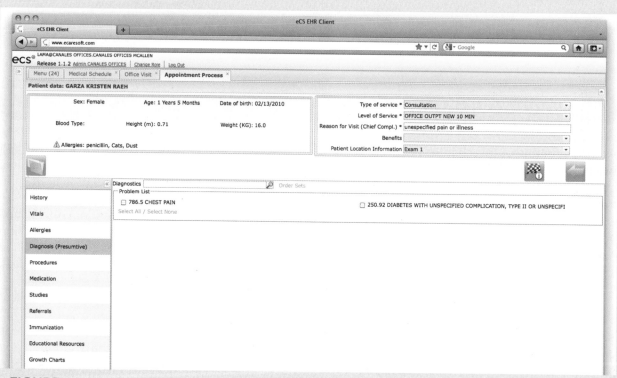

FIGURE 11.12

Many software vendors, such as eCareSoft, now provide cloud-based models for their EHR software (www.ecaresoft.com).

PART THREE

Applying Ethical Principles

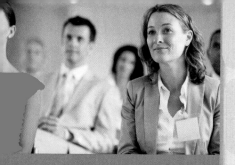

12

Avoiding Ethical Problems

LEARNING OUTCOMES

After completing this chapter, you will be able to:

12.1   Describe key strategies for avoiding ethical problems in medical billing and coding.

12.2   Identify the purpose and characteristics of effective ethics policies in the health care arena.

12.3   Explain how billing department protocols can help effectively avoid ethical problems.

12.4   Construct strategies for communicating with patients that reduce the opportunity for ethical dilemmas to occur.

CASE STUDY

Everyone in town was aware of Downtown Internal Medicine—but for all of the wrong reasons. Two years ago, a report was published on the front page of the local newspaper concerning serious charges of Medicare fraud and abuse against the practice. Based on a combination of data accumulated by the **Medicare carrier** in the area and a random chart audit, the government alleged that Downtown Internal Medicine had billed and collected more than $250,000 to which it was not entitled.

The practice's attorneys negotiated with the Department of Health and Human Services (HHS)—the government agency responsible for the Medicare program—regarding the actual amount due, what penalties were payable, and the repayment schedule for the improper billings. The negotiations regarding this matter concluded just before Melvin, the current administrator, arrived, so he did not know much about the details.

When the negotiations were complete, the attorneys told Melvin that the clinic had to pay approximately $125,000 in overpayments and penalties within the next year. While Melvin was still attempting to comprehend how he would be able to repay that amount out of practice revenues, the attorneys also mentioned that the practice was subject to a corporate integrity agreement (CIA). He had never heard of this before and assumed that the attorneys would take care of that matter. There was no further discussion about the topic because the practice owners did not like the outcome and fired the clinic's attorneys.

Early on a Monday morning, the receptionist called Melvin and said nervously, "There are two gentlemen here to see our compliance officer. Whom should I call?"

Melvin responded, "I guess I'm the compliance officer—I'll be right up."

"Hurry," the receptionist whispered. "They have badges."

Melvin introduced himself to the men, who showed their badges and gave him their cards. They were from the **Office of Inspector General (OIG)** of the Department of Health and Human Services. Melvin took them back to his office.

The men indicated that the practice had fulfilled its obligation to repay overpayments and pay the penalties for their past offenses, but no reports had ever been filed, as required by the corporate integrity agreement. In addition, complaints had been filed regarding the clinic's billing practices by a number of Medicare beneficiaries who were patients of the clinic. To make matters worse, the OIG had received a complaint from a practice employee, indicating that she had been instructed by the practice's billing manager to submit fraudulent claims to the Medicare program.

As the officers continued to list the serious issues at hand, Melvin's mind began to spin. "What is going on here? How are we going to survive this? How am *I* going to survive this?" Melvin soon realized that this was not going to be a good Monday.

1. How might the practice have been so noncompliant with the OIG corporate integrity agreement?

2. What might have Melvin done differently to avoid the current situation?

Medicare carrier
A company that contracts with the federal government to process Medicare claims from physicians and other providers in a given state or region.

Office of Inspector General (OIG)
An arm of the federal government responsible for investigation and enforcement of the rules and regulations of a given governmental department.

Introduction

Finding an enforcement officer from a government agency at the reception desk of the clinic or facility can be one of the most terrifying experiences for anyone involved in medical practice management. In a best-case scenario, some inconvenience will be involved as the officers perform their review of whatever information they seek to obtain. In a worst-case scenario, this review can result in significant financial liability and penalties, and can place the continuing viability of the practice in doubt.

Ideally, whenever an insurer or government entity visits a clinic to audit its billing records, the results of the audit will indicate that the billing is appropriate and fully supported by accurate and complete medical records that support the medical necessity of the services provided and billed. In addition, the only visits from insurers or government entities would be routine or random audits and there never would be a visit for the purpose of investigating an allegation of wrongdoing. For this idyllic situation to occur, preparation and planning must take place—it never happens accidentally.

The best way to deal with an ethical problem is to ensure that the circumstances that allow it to occur are avoided to the greatest degree possible. It is not possible to avoid the incidence of ethical dilemmas completely. However, key strategies can and should be implemented to reduce the occurrence of ethical problems.

12.1 Creating Strategies for Avoiding Ethical Problems in Medical Billing and Coding

When classifying improper behavior related to medical billing and coding, the U.S. federal government places the behavior in one of three categories (Figure 12.1):

- **Waste** includes incurring unnecessary costs as a result of deficient management, practices, or controls.
- **Abuse** includes excessively or improperly using government resources.
- Fraud includes obtaining a benefit through intentional misrepresentation or concealment of material facts (Office of Inspector General, 2009).

Each of these elements is a step further down the continuum of wrongdoing. In other words, waste is less severe than abuse, which

Waste
Unnecessary costs as a result of deficient management, practices, or controls.

Abuse
Excessively or improperly using government resources.

FIGURE 12.1

When engaging in unethical behavior related to medical billing, there are three levels—waste, abuse, and fraud. While none of them is good, fraud is the most serious offense.

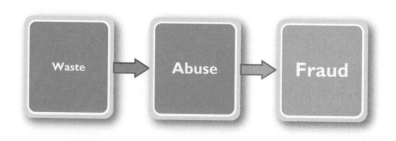

is less severe than fraud. The degree of severity is determined by the level of intent associated with the action. When wasteful action occurs, it may be the result of inattention to or ineffective performance of tasks, but there is no specific desire to do something that is improper or illegal. In the case of abuse, there is likely no specific intent to commit illegal acts, but the nature of the behavior is so negligent that financial liability may be imposed on the persons engaged in the behavior. Those who engage in "abuse" in medical billing and coding are often guilty of violating rules that they "knew or should have known," and clearly made no effort to educate themselves regarding their obligations to insurers and/or government entities. Fraud is the *intentional* decision to *mislead* or *misrepresent* the services for which billing occurs. Those who are convicted of fraud are guilty of criminal activity.

EXAMPLES OF WASTE, ABUSE, AND FRAUD

Sometimes, the line between waste, abuse, and fraud is not obvious. There could be differences of opinion regarding into which category a particular activity falls. However, Table 12.1 presents some examples of behavior that could be construed to fall within each of the categories.

Waste generally does not originate within the realm of medical billing and coding—it is usually the result of inappropriate medical care, for which billing then occurs. Those in the billing office may or may not

Table 12.1 Examples of the Differences Between Waste, Abuse, and Fraud

Type of Behavior	Examples
Waste	• A physician writes prescriptions for more expensive brand-name medications instead of a suitable generic medication. This is done out of habit and not because of a good-faith belief that the brand-name medication is superior. • A physician does not want to wait to obtain the results of expensive laboratory tests that were done last month. Since there is no cost to the patient under the terms of the patient's health care plan, she orders the tests again. • A physician, who was recently sued for malpractice following a dilation and curettage (D&C) procedure, now exercises extreme care for all patients who have this procedure. This includes billing for three follow-up visits outside of the standard 10-day global surgical follow-up period.
Abuse	• A technician mistakenly takes an x-ray of a patient's left leg, then takes a second x-ray when he discovers his error. The hospital bills Medicare for both x-rays. • A physician admits a patient to a hospital to ensure that drugs are paid for that would not otherwise be covered under Medicare (Van de Water, 1995). • A provider bills for services or supplies in excess of the actual cost of delivering the service. • A provider submits claims for services that are not medically necessary. • A provider bills Medicare patients at a higher fee schedule rate than non-Medicare patients, or submits bills to Medicare where Medicare is not the beneficiary's primary insurer (Kansas Department on Aging, 2010).
Fraud	• A provider bills for services or supplies that were not provided. • A provider intentionally bills twice for the same service or item. • A provider bills separately for services that should be included in a single service fee. • A provider misrepresents the diagnosis to justify payment. • A provider bills for rental equipment after date of return. • A provider bills "noncovered" services or items as "covered" services. • A provider uses unethical or unfair marketing strategies, such as offering beneficiaries free groceries or transportation, to switch doctors, pharmacies, insurance, and so on. • A provider bills social activities as psychotherapy. • A provider bills group services as individual service for each patient in the group.

FIGURE 12.2

If the root behavior of an individual or organization is based in ethics, they will not advance to the more serious conduct of waste, fraud, and abuse.

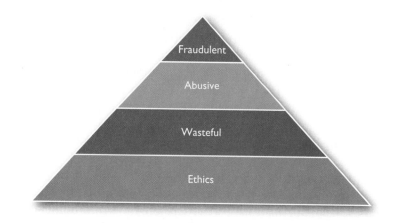

ever be aware of the wasteful nature of the service provided. Abuse and fraud are, unfortunately, more in the domain of the billing function.

ALLEGATIONS OF UNETHICAL BEHAVIOR

The best way to avoid allegations and the occurrence of waste, abuse, and fraud in medical billing and coding is to engage in ethical behavior consistently, thereby avoiding the occurrence of unethical behavior (Figure 12.2). Ethical behavior is a higher standard that goes beyond simply fulfilling the "letter of the law." If the higher standard is consistently followed, then the risk of engaging in wasteful, abusive, or fraudulent behavior is dramatically reduced (Figure 12.3). In fact, the benefit of acting ethically goes beyond avoiding the negative effects of unethical actions. There are significant benefits to the morale of the organization, the reputation of the organization, and the financial standing of the organization.

Avoidance of ethical dilemmas occurs when ethics are intentionally infused throughout the organization—from top to bottom and from theoretical, philosophical activities to nitty-gritty, deeply practical activities. Whereas a practice may behave ethically in theory and unethically in practice (and vice versa), the odds of consistency in ethics occurs when ethics resides in all areas of the organization.

Ethics in the Big Picture. For ethical behavior to exist within an organization, it is essential that the organization makes it clear that ethical behavior is not only acceptable, but expected. One way in which this occurs is through a corporate ethics policy in which billing and coding is a key part. The purpose of the corporate ethics policy is

FIGURE 12.3

Without a base of ethics, there is nothing that mitigates the potential for engaging in wasteful, abusive, or fraudulent behavior.

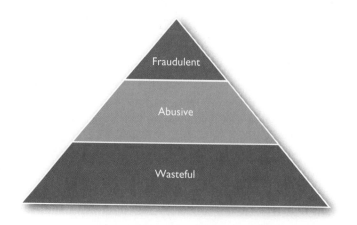

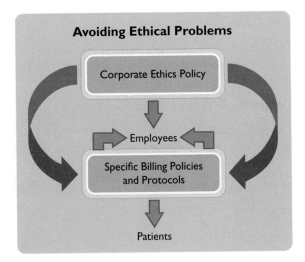

Avoiding Ethical Problems

Corporate Ethics Policy

↓

→ Employees ←

Specific Billing Policies
and Protocols

↓

Patients

FIGURE 12.4
The corporate ethics policy tells employees what is expected of them, as do the specific billing policies and protocols. While the patients are generally aware only of the specific billing policies and protocols, they benefit from the corporate ethics policy because it establishes the atmosphere in which all transactions take place.

to establish a general atmosphere of expectations concerning the behavior of the employees throughout the company (Figure 12.4).

Specific Billing and Coding Policies and Protocols.

A general corporate ethics policy is not sufficient to resolve all ethical issues that a health care provider might face. There are a variety of possible interpretations of what is or is not "ethical," and the situations may be "gray" in nature, which require more detailed analysis of possible alternatives that can be encompassed within a general ethics policy.

An effective billing and coding policy will include general principles, as well as specific direction as to what will occur in the event of certain circumstances. Each medical practice will have its own "trouble" spots and it is wise for the practice to think through the process of dealing with the situation before it is in the middle of it.

Communication with Patients.

Discussions of ethics in medical billing and coding can't occur without the inclusion of the patient.

Most of the issues related to fraud and abuse focus on the relationship between the provider and payer because they are the parties directly involved in the transactions most likely to produce this type of behavior. However, the patient can feel the effect of fraud and abuse by providers and payers. They can also be the initiator of ethical problems by requesting unethical and inappropriate conduct to be performed by the other parties in health care financial transactions (Figure 12.5).

Ethics and Relationships

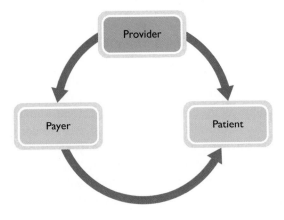

Provider

Payer   Patient

FIGURE 12.5
The provider is in the center of the ethical relationships involved in the health care system in the United States.

Thinking It Through 12.1

1. Describe the range of ethical behavior as it pertains to medical billing and coding. Do you believe that all the elements are equally wrong, or is one worse than the others? Why?

2. Do you agree that the majority of ethical issues occur in the relationship between payer and provider? Why or why not?

3. Do you believe that the majority of ethical problems created by patients are done intentionally or unintentionally? Why?

12.2 Implementing Effective Corporate Ethics Policies

Ethics policies are sometimes considered interchangeably with compliance programs (which are discussed at length in Chapter 11), because many elements of compliance programs and ethics policies overlap. However, while there is some overlap in their final objective—appropriate conduct—compliance plans and ethics policies have different purposes and it is advisable that most health care organizations of all sizes and types have both.

THE PURPOSE OF ETHICS POLICIES

Ethics policies are needed to define several key items for the employees of the health care organization.

Establish the Meaning of Ethical Behavior—a Values Statement. The *values statement* of an organization can provide great insight into the things that are most important to the organization. Without a values statement, there can be conflicted understanding of what the organization desires. Individuals can make ethical decisions on their own that are inconsistent with each other, leaving significant confusion among the employees as to what is and is not acceptable behavior.

Values statements can take a variety of different forms. In part, the nature of the statements will be governed by the corporate culture and personality. Some examples follow.

- **Merck, Inc.** "To preserve and improve human life. At Merck, corporate conduct is inseparable from the conduct of individual employees in the performance of their work. Every Merck employee is responsible for adhering to business practices that are in accordance with the letter and spirit of the applicable laws and with ethical principles that reflect the highest standards of corporate and individual behavior. . . . At Merck, we are committed to the highest standards of ethics and integrity. We are responsible to our customers, to Merck employees and their families, to the environments we inhabit, and to the societies we serve worldwide. In discharging our responsibilities, we do not take professional or ethical shortcuts. Our interactions with all segments of society must reflect the high standards we profess" (Merck, Inc., 2010).

- **Google.** "'Don't be evil.' Googlers generally apply those words to how we serve our users. But "Don't be evil" is much more than that. Yes, it's about providing our users unbiased access to information, focusing on their needs and giving them the best products and services that we can. But it's also about doing the right thing more generally—following the law, acting honorably and treating each other with respect" (Google, 2009).

- **Ministry Health Care System (Wisconsin).** "Faithful to the Values of our Founding Sisters, which guide our actions,
  - "We provide holistic SERVICE that meets people's needs while considering the good of society. We involve people in decisions that are important to them.
  - "Our Christian beliefs shape our VISION of social responsibility. We enable risk-taking and reward creativity that improves people's quality of life.
  - "Wherever we are, our PRESENCE is marked by compassion, integrity, collaboration and accountability. We set future direction that assures the dignity and development of people above all else.
  - "We stand with the poor. JUSTICE calls us to confront conditions of oppression and to help change structures that violate people's dignity" (Ministry Health Care, Inc., 2010).

The values statement is a critical part of the ethics policy because it sets the tone for the organization. It provides guidance to the employees as to what is important to the organization. In addition, it can provide significant assistance to the leadership of the organization in remembering their primary objectives, which can influence choices and behaviors in both good and difficult times.

Provide a Detailed Guide to Acceptable Behavior.   Some ethics policies are philosophical and provide only high-level theoretical guidance. The policies of other companies go into more detail, because the marketplace is growing increasingly complex and demanding.

In the health care marketplace, the complexity of the ethical environment is high (Figure 12.6). The customers (patients) rightfully expect high-quality service, but sometimes are not interested in learning about their insurance or personally paying for their services.

The Need for Ethical Guidance

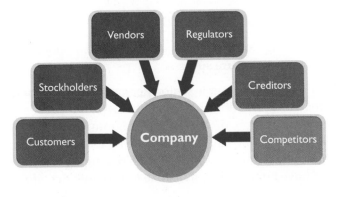

FIGURE 12.6
Like most other companies in the United States, health care providers feel pressure from a variety of sources. All of these sources challenge their ethical frameworks and, therefore, the employees of these companies need detailed guidance as to how to conduct themselves appropriately.

Stockholders, who can range from traditional investors to physician owners, expect the largest possible return on their investment in the company, regardless of the economic realities. Vendors are becoming increasingly aggressive in their desire to sell medical supplies, medical equipment, and financial services. Sometimes they offer to frame the deals in such a manner that is ethically questionable.

Regulators are not directly encouraging providers to behave unethically—the alternative is true. However, some entities believe that the only way to satisfy these regulators is to manipulate the circumstances to achieve the appearance of compliance, but actually engaging in improper behavior. Creditors are seeking repayment of their loans, while providers are seeing revenue dropping. Finally, health care is becoming an increasingly competitive environment, where peaceful coexistence has been replaced with cut-throat marketing—which comes at a fairly high price.

Faced with all of these challenges, provider-specific guidelines are needed to let employees know their behavioral boundaries. These guidelines must be consistent with the company's values statement so that the staff knows the objectives of the company, as well as how the company would like them to achieve those objectives in light of the marketplace realities.

THE AUDIENCE FOR AN ETHICS POLICY

The audience for an ethics policy is every stakeholder in the organization, which can include:

- Investors
- Customers/patients
- Suppliers
- Employees (Ghillyer, 2010)

The primary purpose is to put everyone on notice that the provider is serious about ethical performance. Ideally, publishing a code of ethics would discourage stakeholders of the company from even considering unethical behavior because they know that unethical proposals will be rebuffed. The code of ethics also makes the line very clear for employees. In fact, one entity—Ministry Health Care, which operates a number of hospitals and clinics and provides home-based care in the state of Wisconsin—requires of job seekers at its website (Figure 12.7) to acknowledge that they understand the organization's mission and values statement before they can see the available positions (Ministry Health Care, Inc., 2010).

EFFECTIVE CODES OF ETHICS

For a code of ethics to be effective, several basic, nonnegotiable steps must be followed to ensure success.

1. *Find a champion.* Unless a senior person within the organization (e.g., the CEO, a senior physician, etc.) is willing and able to lead the implementation of the ethics program, it will not succeed. The employees who must live under the terms of the ethics code will not view it as important if the leadership of the organization doesn't have enough time available to promote the effort.

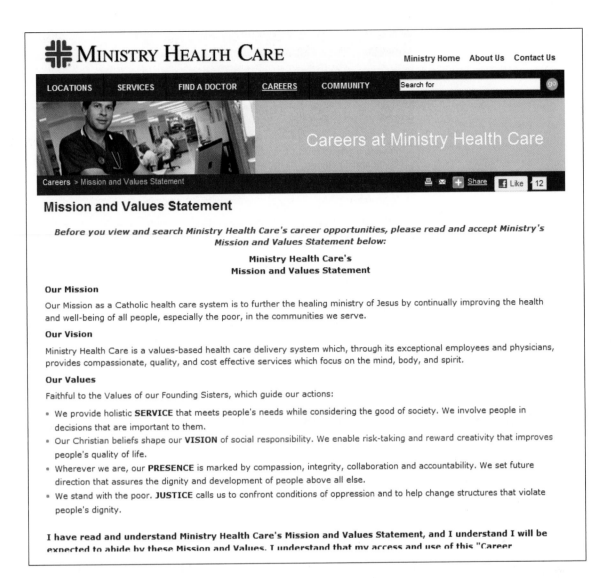

Before you view and search Ministry Health Care's career opportunities, please read and accept Ministry's Mission and Values Statement below:

Ministry Health Care's Mission and Values Statement

Our Mission

Our Mission as a Catholic health care system is to further the healing ministry of Jesus by continually improving the health and well-being of all people, especially the poor, in the communities we serve.

Our Vision

Ministry Health Care is a values-based health care delivery system which, through its exceptional employees and physicians, provides compassionate, quality, and cost effective services which focus on the mind, body, and spirit.

Our Values

Faithful to the Values of our Founding Sisters, which guide our actions:

• We provide holistic **SERVICE** that meets people's needs while considering the good of society. We involve people in decisions that are important to them.
• Our Christian beliefs shape our **VISION** of social responsibility. We enable risk-taking and reward creativity that improves people's quality of life.
• Wherever we are, our **PRESENCE** is marked by compassion, integrity, collaboration and accountability. We set future direction that assures the dignity and development of people above all else.
• We stand with the poor. **JUSTICE** calls us to confront conditions of oppression and to help change structures that violate people's dignity.

I have read and understand Ministry Health Care's Mission and Values Statement, and I understand I will be expected to abide by these Mission and Values. I understand that my access and use of this "Career

2. *Get "buy-in" from the board of directors, owners, or other responsible parties.* The values of an organization must be consistent throughout and are a matter of governance. If the highest governing body within an organization does not participate, there will be no influence on other members of the organization to follow through on its requirements.

3. *Identify the issues that matter to those in the company.* Simply copying the ethics code of another organization is not effective, because the organizations may have two different personalities and greatly differing ethical struggles. It is acceptable to look at the ethics codes of other organizations for guidance, but they must be tailored specifically for the individual practice or facility.

4. *Make the code widely available.* It should be distributed throughout the company to ensure maximum exposure. In addition, appropriate forms of the policy should be distributed to various stakeholders, including vendors and stockholders (if applicable). The code should be placed on the website in a prominent location so that patients, payers, and competitors can also see the company's commitment to ethical behavior (Ghillyer, 2010).

Table 12.2 describes ways to correctly and incorrectly implement a corporate ethics policy.

> **FIGURE 12.7**
> Ministry Health Care, which operates clinics and hospitals in northern Wisconsin, requires visitors to the jobs section of its website to read and acknowledge their understanding of the mission and values statement of the entity.

Table 12.2 Implementing a Corporate Ethics Policy

Doing It Right	Doing It Poorly
Root the code in core ethical values.	Pin the code to the notice board.
Give a copy to all staff.	Fail to obtain board commitment to the code.
Provide a way to report breaches in a confidential manner.	Leave responsibility for its effectiveness to HR or any other department.
Include ethical issues in corporate training programs.	Fail to find out what concerns the staff at different levels.
Set up a board committee to monitor the effectiveness of the code.	Do not feature the code in induction training and management development activities.
Report on the code's use in the annual report.	Do not have a procedure for revising the code regularly.
Make conformity to the code part of a contract of employment.	Make exceptions to the code's application.
Make copies of the code available to business partners, including suppliers.	Fail to follow up breaches of the code's standards.
Review the code in light of changing business challenges.	Fail to set a good example by corporate leaders.
Make sure senior staff "walk the talk."	Treat the code as confidential or a purely internal document.
	Make it difficult for staff to have direct access to the code.

Source: Adapted from the Institute of Business Ethics, 2011.

PRACTICAL TIPS FOR POLICY IMPLEMENTATION

There are two different schools of thought regarding ethics policies:

1. They are a genuine effort to encourage and facilitate ethical behavior.

2. They are a thinly veiled attempt to mislead others into believing that the company really cares about ethical behavior (Mallor, Barnes, Bowers, & Langvardt, 2010).

The reason for the cynicism regarding ethics policies is based on the massive failures of some companies related to their ethical behavior. Some of the most notorious names in corporate greed and ethical failure had excellent codes of ethics. For example, Enron's code of ethics began as follows under the heading of "Values: Respect":

> We treat others as we would like to be treated ourselves. We do not tolerate abusive or disrespectful treatment. Ruthlessness, callousness and arrogance don't belong here.
>
> *Integrity.* We work with customers and prospects openly, honestly and sincerely. When we say we will do something, we will do it; when we say we cannot or will not do something, then we won't do it.
>
> *Communication.* We have an obligation to communicate. Here, we take the time to talk with one another ... and to listen. We believe that information is meant to move and that information moves people.

Excellence. We are satisfied with nothing less than the very best in everything we do. We will continue to raise the bar for everyone. The great fun here will be for all of us to discover just how good we can really be. (Ghillyer, 2010)

This would be a highly impressive beginning to a code of ethics if you didn't know that the leadership of Enron violated nearly every aspect of their policy with wanton disregard for the well-being of its shareholders, employees, and the law. Failure of this type causes observers to doubt the effectiveness of a policy in any setting.

Having an ethics policy does not automatically produce ethical behavior. However, there are some key tips that, if implemented, will improve the opportunity for success.

- Talk about ethics and the ethics code continuously. Holding an "ethics" class once per year does not place sufficient emphasis on the issue to make the stakeholders take the matter seriously.
- Name an **ethics officer.** This person must have real authority to address occasions in which the ethics policy may have been violated. It is best for the officer not to be a senior executive, but it must be someone who has the ear of the senior executive and who can discuss difficult issues at that level.
- Celebrate and reward ethical behavior when it is demonstrated by employees. Rewarding the desired behavior is a fundamental means of producing additional behavior of the same type. This truth is the same for ethics.
- Executive-level administrators, physicians, and other leaders must model ethical behavior *consistently.* One incident of unethical behavior by a respected member of the leadership team can seriously undermine the effort of any organization to maintain its ethical standards on an ongoing basis.

COMPLIANCE TIP

Writing an ethics policy is only the first step in ensuring that ethical behavior occurs within your organization. Stopping at that point will usually result in failure.

Ethics officer
A designated person within an organization with the responsibility to ensure that the ethics policies of the organization are followed consistently.

FYI

Ethical behavior produces more behavior that is ethical. When employees are publicly rewarded for their ethical actions, other employees will take note and desire similar recognition.

Thinking It Through 12.2

1. Can a business have a high ethical culture without a formal code of ethics? Why or why not?
2. Describe how the marketplace is growing increasingly complex, related to the issue of ethics.
3. In your opinion, which of the four steps in making a code of ethics effective is the most important? Why?
4. How can society regain trust in corporations if major incidents of ethical violations continue to occur?

12.3 Avoiding Ethical Dilemmas by Developing Business Department Protocols

Ethics policies are highly effective in that they create a general atmosphere in which doing the right thing is the norm and is expected of each employee. However, these broad, sweeping concepts and theories—even though they are essential to facilitating ethics—are not enough to make ethical behavior a reality. Beyond the general principles, health care providers must also establish specific business department policies and protocols to address potential ethical dilemmas.

Every situation may appear to be unique, which would make it difficult to prepare a policy in advance of the problem. Further investigation of the common ethical problems that occur will reveal that there are some features of each circumstance that are consistent. These consistencies make it possible to establish consistent responses to the problem.

EMPOWER EMPLOYEES TO RESOLVE ISSUES

As indicated in Chapter 4, many of the ethical issues that occur are the result of conflict in the relationships that exist in the medical billing/coding process. For example, patients can ask providers to modify codes to facilitate payment. While the ethics policy is often developed by the leadership of the practice, the employees "on the ground" in working with the patients are the people that must be prepared to respond to requests that challenge the ethics of the individual and the organization (Figure 12.8).

Since these people are the ones who "touch" the customer, the quality of customer service has to be of concern. One critical element of customer service is the timeliness in which a problem is resolved. Some research regarding the timeliness of problem resolution reveals that

- A dissatisfied consumer will tell between 9 and 15 people about his or her experience. About 13% of dissatisfied customers tell more than 20 people.
- 91% of unhappy customers will not willingly do business with your organization again. However, if their complaint is resolved quickly, 82% of them will return.
- Previously dissatisfied customers who get their issue resolved tell about 4 to 6 people about their experience (Zaibak, 2010).

The matter of customer service is addressed in this discussion of ethics because there is ample opportunity for patient dissatisfaction as it relates to medical service. When patient dissatisfaction occurs,

FIGURE 12.8
Ethical problems can exist in relationships between the various parties in the health care financing process. Specific ethics policies governing certain situations can help—particularly in the relationship between the patient and provider.

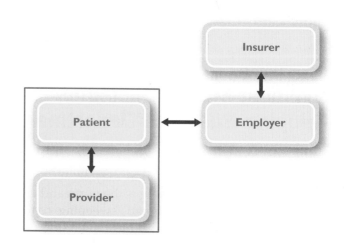

Just Change the Billing

An enraged patient calls the billing department of Jordan Beach Internal Medicine. "I am never coming back there again! The entire experience from start to finish was horrible! And now you idiots are billing me in error and I will not pay the bill!"

The unfortunate representative who received this call reviewed the account and saw that the payer denied the claim for the patient's annual physical because it allows only one "wellness" visit per year, CPT codes 99384 to 99387 or 99394 to 99397. This apparently was the patient's second wellness visit processed by the payer during the current year. "Did you happen to see your OB/GYN for your annual exam recently?" asked the representative. "Yes, I did—three months ago," said the patient. "That's the problem," responded the representative. "Your payer will pay for only one wellness visit a year and it counted your visit to the gynecologist as your one visit per year."

"I called the insurance company and they said that the problem was that you billed it wrong. If you called it something other than a wellness visit, then it would be paid." The representative accessed the EHR and found the patient's record for the date in question. There was no doubt—it was a wellness visit. "I'm sorry; we can't make that sort of change," said the provider's representative. "The insurer said you could," said the patient. "Well, I need to have you speak with my supervisor. Unfortunately, she's out until next week, but I will give her a message to call you back when she returns," said the representative. "She'd better!" exclaimed the patient, who then proceeded to hang up on the bewildered representative.

1. What sort of ethical responsibility does the payer have in this situation?

2. What circumstances might cause the representative simply to change the code, even if she knew it was not correct?

3. Is satisfying this patient possible, without submitting an inaccurate or false insurance claim?

---

opportunities for ethical dilemmas can arise. Some of these issues include

- Excessive waits in the reception area.
- Delays in the examination room, waiting for the doctor.
- Real or perceived rude behavior on the part of the staff.
- Improper claim processing on the part of the payer.
- Improper claim filing on the part of the provider.
- Mailing of an incorrect or inaccurate billing statement to the patient.
- Patient confusion about responsibility for payment for services.

Because dissatisfied customers are so harmful to the practice and quick resolution of the issue is in the best interest of the patient and the practice, often the provider will do whatever it takes to satisfy the patient—even if the action is potentially unethical.

Conventional wisdom states that, to satisfy the customer, the philosophy of the "customer is always right" must be followed. Taken literally, this means that in the health care setting the patients must always get what they want. For that to occur, ethical shortcuts must take place on the part of someone in the process.

Regardless of the misconception associated with this common belief about customer service, the general principle of customer satisfaction is critical. The fact is that businesses, including all health care providers, desire to have satisfied customers—but the customers are *not* always right. In some cases, they are flat out wrong. The provider cannot accommodate a patient who insists that the provider submit

> **FYI**
>
> Giving the customers what they want every time is not a best practice—either for customer service or for ethics. Sometimes customer service requires some creativity and strong listening skills to find out what they really want.

a fraudulent claim to an insurance company. What does the ethical health care provider do?

"The customer is always right" should be restated to be *The customer should always feel as though he or she has been heard."

A common temptation when faced with an angry person is to become defensive and to think more about the response than to actually make an effort to hear the person's complaint. This does not happen automatically and, in fact, feels quite unnatural for most people. To maintain ethical standards and not be tempted to compromise them, the staff must be specifically trained to communicate that they are hearing the person's point of view. This cannot be done well while attempting to formulate the perfect defense.

"The customer should have their concerns addressed in a timely fashion" does not mean that they necessarily get what they want, but there is no circumstance in which delaying the customer's answer produces a more positive result than if the matter is addressed immediately. In addition, forcing the provider representative to seek advice from a person at a higher level (e.g., a supervisor) is harmful for the following reasons:

- *It may promote unethical behavior.* By asking for a supervisor's assistance in escalating an issue, the employee is effectively admitting that he or she cannot solve a problem. If the employee's job performance is already in question, the employee will have a disincentive to seek out assistance. The employee can "solve" the problem by writing off the charge or "correcting" the diagnosis. In this manner, the patient gets what he or she wants and the employee's performance appears good—but only through the occurrence of unethical behavior.

- *It is demeaning to the employee.* The implicit message communicated to all parties is that the employee cannot solve the problem—he or she needs further help. If the supervisor overrules the original position of the provider representative, the problem has only been made worse. If the supervisor supports the original position of the provider representative, nothing has been gained.

- *It does not produce a timely response for the patient.* Unless the supervisor is immediately available, further communication is required later. There may be the exchange of phone calls, voice mails, and so on, none of which produce a resolution for the patient's problem. Even if the final resolution is exactly what the patient wanted, the benefit of solving the problem quickly is lost in the time wasted by delaying the answer.

Hearing the customer and addressing his or her needs in a timely fashion sounds like an easy and reasonable objective. If it is so easy, then why do so many businesses (including medical providers) *not* do it? First, the ability to listen without being defensive is not a trait commonly found in most individuals. Therefore, the right people must be hired for these positions. Once hired, these employees need a significant amount of training so that they respond to customers/patients in the manner that the provider desires. This time and effort expended on finding and training the "right" employees requires a significant financial investment on the part of the business. However, supplying the key staff with the ability to resolve issues in a timely fashion produces results that dramatically improve customer service and reduce the opportunities for ethical dilemmas.

CREATE SPECIFIC POLICIES AND PROCEDURES

In many medical settings, it is often said that the job is always exciting because no two days are the same. The impression is that many things happen randomly and that there is a low degree of predictability in terms of events and the ability to respond to those events. Management research, however, seems to indicate that there is very little randomness in the events that occur within an organization, if enough study and attention is given to the contributing elements. That which seems random and chaotic really is not if the entire process is understood.

This is the case with regard to the circumstances that create ethical dilemmas in the health care field. When patients call with complaints about their bills, there may appear to be an infinite number of issues. Yet, when analyzed and categorized, very few unique circumstances actually occur—the variations are only in the details. Similarly, with regard to insurance claim denials, although there may seem to be a hundred different reasons for a claim to be denied, in reality, the fundamental issues are relatively few. When this is recognized, it makes dealing with the apparent chaos much more manageable.

The best way to avoid ethical issues regarding patient interactions and denied insurance claims is to formulate specific policies that guide and instruct the appropriate personnel in resolving these issues. If the same problem occurs frequently (with minor variations), the employees can be empowered to resolve the issue by using clear policies and protocols. The clarity of understanding on the part of the employees reduces the temptation to behave unethically.

Each health care entity will have a different set of problems that occur frequently. A problem encountered daily at one facility may never be encountered at another facility. Therefore, the policies must be tailored specifically for the issues that are unique to the facility. A particular **policy** and **protocol** should be established at Jordan Beach Internal Medicine, the practice in the earlier case study, to guide the staff whenever a claim is denied because a second "wellness" visit is billed within the same calendar year. OB/GYN practices should have a similar policy because they are usually the practice on the other end of the situation faced by Jordan Beach Internal Medicine. Fertility practices should have a specific policy that clearly defines the difference between "diagnosis" and "treatment."[1] Plastic/reconstructive surgery practices should have policies and protocols for dealing with circumstances when there is a lack of clarity when defining reconstructive procedures and elective cosmetic procedures. Every practice has some

Policy
A course of action adopted and followed by an organization to provide guidance in future conduct.

Protocol
Formal rules, guidelines, and regulations adopted by an organization to ensure specific, consistent conduct in the future.

CODING TIP

Every health care entity should establish a policy and protocol for the "after-the-fact" changing of diagnosis codes. In some cases, it is appropriate to make the change—but the circumstances and the procedure should be clearly defined to avoid abuse and unethical or illegal conduct.

---

[1]Many insurance policies make a distinction between "diagnosis" and "treatment" for payment purposes. The majority of insurance companies will pay for diagnosis of fertility-related problems (because of possible serious systemic issues, for which infertility is a symptom). However, a far smaller number will pay for the *treatment* of fertility issues.

issues of this nature that require guidance to avoid unethical conduct when challenged with a difficult circumstance.

One policy and protocol that every practice should establish is defining how and when diagnosis codes can or should be changed. It would be incorrect to assume that every diagnosis code assigned by every practice is correct 100% of the time. Some of these incorrect diagnoses will result in claim denials. It would be ethically inappropriate for the practice to insist that an incorrect diagnosis *cannot* be corrected and the patient will just have to pay the bill. However, the policy would need to be carefully crafted to ensure that it is not abused. All denials for which the diagnosis is causing an issue for claim payment should not automatically be an "error" and changed without some sort of care and guidance. Consider the case of Sonoma Hills Family Practice.

Example

A patient visited Sonoma Hills Family Practice. The patient came to the office with a complaint of vaginal itching. Dr. Fernandez assigned a diagnosis of 698.1—Pruritis of genital organs. However, Melanie, the office coder, mistyped the diagnosis as 798.1—Instantaneous death. The insurance company denied the claim, indicating on the EOB a reason of "Inappropriate clinical setting for this diagnosis."

Would changing this diagnosis code and resubmitting the claim be unethical?

Of course, changing this diagnosis is not unethical—it is simply the correction of an error. However, guidelines must exist to ensure that the staff has the ability to make these corrections *and* handle circumstances that are not as clear-cut as this example, ensuring that they are operating within the context of carefully designed and fully understood protocols.

ESTABLISH POLICIES BEFORE PROBLEMS OCCUR

A third particular emphasis in avoiding ethical dilemmas is to establish the policies prior to the actual occurrence of the event, as opposed to doing it in response to the event. When a policy is written in the absence of a specific complaint, intense emotion, or anger, the outcome will be more rational and helpful than it would be otherwise. It is very difficult to assess all elements and viewpoints of a situation fairly and accurately when intense emotion is present or an emotional attachment to a particular person exists. A patient with a strong personality who is in disagreement with the clinic's handling of his or her account may cause the physician or clinic personnel to take the course of least resistance, which may be an unethical action.

Table 12.3 illustrates how various factors in the Jordan Beach Internal Medicine case influence decisions when the decisions are made in the middle of the controversy, as opposed to having the decisions made in advance.

Table 12.3 Ramifications of Avoiding Ethical Problems by Preparing Policies in Advance

Issue	Policy Determined in Response to Present Issue	Policy Established in Advance
Patient's anger	Explosive and threatening	Not an issue
Employee's defensiveness	Greatly heightened	Not an issue
Duty to insurance company	Unchanged	Unchanged
Physician intervention	Wants to avoid conflict/ keep patient happy, regardless of methodology	Takes ownership of policy/has understanding of ramifications of acting unethically

Thinking It Through 12.3

1. Explain the relationship between corporate ethics policies and specific billing policies and protocols. Why are both necessary?

2. Have you previously considered the relationship between customer satisfaction and the potential for ethical problems? Do you believe that there is a connection? Why or why not?

3. Restate the principle "The customer is always right" in a concise way that takes ethical considerations into account. Explain why you stated it the way that you did.

4. How does the timeliness of responding to patient complaints affect the potential for ethical problems?

12.4 Constructing Strategies for Communicating with Patients to Avoid Ethical Problems

The patient's role in creating ethical dilemmas in the billing and coding process was discussed in detail in Chapter 4. In large part, patients and ethical dilemmas intersect because patients do not understand the billing/coding process and do not consider what they are asking the provider to do. The primary method to avoid ethical dilemmas related to patients is to provide them with as much knowledge as possible.

> **FYI**
>
> It is much more difficult to accuse someone of behaving unethically when a person (1) knows the other person (or organization), and (2) understands the motivation of the other person.

COMMUNICATE THE PROVIDER'S OBJECTIVES

In any conflict or circumstance that generates strong emotion, there is the tendency to focus only on one's own feelings, opinions, and concerns. The position of the other party takes a back seat to the perceived needs and desires of the aggrieved party. It is a great challenge to attempt to communicate a particular position when the other persons are committed to their position and are focused only on ensuring that they get adequate attention for their position (Figure 12.9).

If one knows that the potential for conflict exists and wants to ensure that a message is communicated, the message should be transmitted in advance—before the conflict begins. The message is received

Communication in Conflict

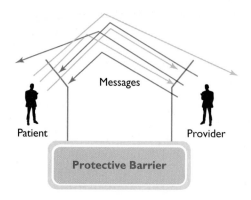

FIGURE 12.9
When conflict exists, communication is difficult because each party establishes a protective barrier. The position of the other party either is blocked or sails over the head of the other person.

FIGURE 12.9
When conflict exists, communication is difficult because each party establishes a protective barrier. The position of the other party either is blocked or sails over the head of the other person.

Communication in Conflict

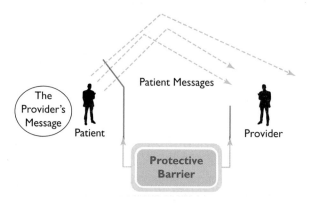

FIGURE 12.10
When the provider has communicated the message to the patient before conflict occurs, the provider does not have to make extra effort to communicate the message because the patient already has it. It also reduces the provider's potential defensiveness because it does not have to "overcome" the messages communicated by the patient.

by the patient before the protective barrier is established, allowing the provider to make the point known clearly (Figure 12.10).

When the provider's message is "precommunicated," there is little or no temptation on the part of the provider to cut ethical corners to satisfy the patient—it is able to point to and stand behind its policy, which was provided in advance of the conflict. Therefore, the patient must understand that the determination regarding the handling of this case is not a random or vindictive reaction to the patient—it is simply the adherence to the policy.

The ethical standard is strengthened when the patient understands the provider's intentions related to the matter. If the provider states that the intent is to behave ethically toward all parties (patients and payers), it becomes difficult for the patient to argue with that position. Unless the patient is so cavalier that he or she is disinterested in any form of ethical behavior, it provides significant support to the provider's position.

REMOVE THE MYSTERY FROM THE PROCESS

A second major advantage of communicating the provider's position to the patient in advance of any potential conflict is that the patient is aware of the potential sequence of events that may occur. Therefore, when certain events occur that might be perceived by the patient as negative or adverse, the patient knows what to expect. The provider may respond in exactly the same fashion as it would have otherwise—the difference is that the patient knows what the provider is going to do in advance, which removes the element of surprise and mystery from the process. The following sample policy illustrates how this type of communication may appear, for a practice that sometimes receives payments that are inconsistent with the benefit quote issued by the payer prior to supplying service.

Example

In this process, it is our objective and mission to be ethical in its dealings with both our patients and insurers. Therefore, we have established the following protocol for determining benefits and payment requirements for our patients.

- As soon as we are notified of a patient's intent to receive services, we will contact the patient's insurer(s) to obtain a benefit quote.

- Based on that benefit quote, we will determine the patient's financial responsibility, whether that be copayments, deductibles, or payment for the full amount if benefits do not exist for the services provided. Payment of the amount determined is due prior to the beginning of treatment.

- We will bill insurers for all services provided. If the insurer makes payment for services that are not consistent with the benefit quote originally received, we will contact the insurer to be certain that the benefit payment is correct. If it is correct (and the benefit quote was incorrect), we will promptly refund any patient overpayment. If the payment is not correct, we will return the payment to the insurer.

- Our objective is for you to obtain every penny of benefit to which you are entitled, but we have a contractual obligation with the insurers to not accept incorrect benefit payments.

> **FYI**
>
> Communication, or lack thereof, can be a source of ethical problems. When an organization makes a specific effort to communicate effectively with its key stakeholders (e.g., patients, employees, etc.), there is a positive effect on ethics.

"OVERCOMMUNICATE" WITH THE PATIENT

To ensure the most effective possible communication with the patient, the provider must **overcommunicate** with the patient. This means that the provider communicates appropriate information more frequently and in more formats than it might think is necessary. The reason for this is that patients are not necessarily attuned to issues of medical billing and coding prior to receiving care. Therefore, they may not pay attention to the message the first or second time that they receive it. In addition, they may not necessarily receive the message via one method, so multiple methods may be necessary and appropriate. Some possible alternatives include the following:

- In written materials, such as brochures, financial counseling materials, etc.
- On the website.
- In group educational sessions.
- In individual financial counseling.
- In "on hold" messages.

Overcommunicate
To provide more communication than is normally considered necessary, with the goal of ensuring that the message reaches its intended audience with an appropriate level of effect.

FIGURE 12.11

Medical practices can use their websites, such as the one for this fictitious practice, to communicate with their patients regarding how they will respond to improperly paid claims. The purpose of the materials is to help avoid ethical dilemmas by telling patients in advance how certain situations related to claim payment will be handled.

process.

INSURANCE CAN BE COMPLICATED AND CONFUSING

At ___ we recognize that working with insurance coverage can be a complicated and confusing issue. In most business transactions, there are only two parties—the buyer and the seller. However, in health care, there is the buyer (the patient), the seller (the provider/doctor), and the payer (the insurance company). This makes the process more complex because in order for the buyer to receive maximum benefit and the seller to receive payment, the payer's rules must be followed. Unfortunately, every payer has different rules and guidelines and even an individual payer can have multiple different plans—each with different requirements and coverage levels. Our experienced Financial Coordinators do their best to be familiar with the insurance coverage and plans, but your assistance in obtaining as much information as possible about your plan is very helpful.

In this process, it is ___ objective and mission to be ethical in its dealings with both our patients and insurers. Therefore, we have established the following protocol for determining benefits and payment requirements for our patients.

- As soon as we are notified of a patient's intent to receive services, we will contact the patient's insurer(s) to obtain a benefit quote.
- Based on that benefit quote, we will determine the patient's financial responsibility, whether that be copayments, deductibles, or payment for the full amount if benefits do not exist for the services provided. Payment of the amount determined is due two weeks prior to the beginning of the cycle start.
- We will bill insurers for all services provided. If the insurer makes payment for services that are not consistent with the benefit quote originally received, we will contact the insurer to be certain that the benefit payment is correct. If it is correct (and the benefit quote was incorrect) we will promptly refund any patient overpayment. If the payment is not correct, we will return the payment to the insurer.

Our objective is for you to obtain every penny of benefit to which you are entitled, but we have a contractual obligation with the insurers to not accept incorrect benefit payments.

Participation with Specific Insurers

Currently, ___ is a participating provider with the following insurers:

While the provider's office may feel that these actions are excessive, it is important to do them frequently so that the message is ingrained in the minds of the employees (and, thereby, the culture of the practice), has been heard at least once (if not more) by the patient, and there is a clear understanding by all parties regarding intentions and expected behaviors (Figure 12.11).

Thinking It Through 12.4

1. What is it about conflict that makes communication difficult?
2. Describe how making the provider's intention known helps avoid ethical dilemmas at a later time.

CHAPTER REVIEW

Chapter Summary

Learning Outcomes	Key Concepts/Examples

12.1 Describe key strategies for avoiding ethical problems in medical billing and coding. Pages 378–382	• The government classifies improper conduct related to medical billing and coding in three different categories:
	  1. Waste
	  2. Abuse
	  3. Fraud
	• The degree of severity in conduct is based on the level of intent behind the action.
	• The best way to avoid allegations of improper conduct is to always engage in ethical behavior.
	• Three key strategies for ensuring consistent ethical behavior are:
	  1. Corporate ethics policy.
	  2. Specific billing/coding policies and protocols.
	  3. Excellent communication with patients.

12.2 Identify the purpose and characteristics of effective ethics policies in the health care arena. Pages 382–387	• The reasons for establishing an ethics policy are:
	  1. A values statement clarifies the desires of the organization and sets the tone for the organization.
	  2. The ethics policy provides a detailed guide to acceptable behavior.
	  3. The policy communicates the ethical principles of the company to all stakeholders.
	• For an ethics policy/code to be effective, it must:
	  1. Have a champion.
	  2. Get "buy-in" from the Board of Directors and other leaders.
	  3. Identify issues that matter to the company.
	  4. Be made widely available and be well known.
	• In practical terms, a company must:
	  1. Talk about ethics and the ethics codes continuously.
	  2. Name an ethics officer.
	  3. Celebrate and reward ethical behavior when it is demonstrated by the employees.
	  4. Model the behavior consistently at the highest levels of the organization.

12.3 Explain how billing department protocols can help effectively avoid ethical problems. Pages 387–393	• Health care providers must have specific policies and protocols to ensure ethical conduct.
	• A direct link exists between high levels of customer service and ethical conduct.
	• Key elements of billing department protocols include:
	  1. Empowering employees to resolve issues in a timely fashion.
	  2. Developing specific policies and procedures.
	  3. Establishing policies before problems occur.

12.4 Construct strategies for communicating with patients that reduce the opportunity for ethical dilemmas to occur. Pages 393–396	• Communicating with patients is a critical element in facilitating ethical conduct with patients. This can be done by:
	  1. Communicating the provider's objectives.
	  2. Telling the patient in advance what will occur if certain events transpire.
	  3. "Overcommunicating" with the patient.

Multiple Choice

Circle the letter that best completes the statement or answers the question.

1. **LO 12.1** The best way to deal with an ethical problem is to
   a. Eliminate the circumstances that create them before they occur
   b. Establish protocols that provide guidance in resolving them
   c. Refine the practice's compliance plan
   d. Instruct employees to not discuss the matter with anyone

2. **LO 12.1** On the continuum of wrongdoing, which of the following is most severe?
   a. Abuse
   b. Waste
   c. Fraud
   d. Negligence

3. **LO 12.1** Which of the following is the result of an intentional decision to mislead or misrepresent the services that were billed?
   a. Abuse
   b. Fraud
   c. Waste
   d. Negligence

4. **LO 12.2** Which of the following statements is true about values statements?
   a. Values statements can create conflict in understanding within organizations.
   b. Values statements generally contain the same key points and follow the same format.
   c. Values statements ensure that all employees think and believe the same way.
   d. Values statements help establish the ethical tone for an organization.

5. **LO 12.2** The primary audience for a health care provider's ethics policy includes all of the following *except*
   a. Customers/patients
   b. Employees
   c. Insurance companies
   d. Suppliers

6. **LO 12.2** Which of the following is *not* a tip that improves the opportunity for success in the use of an ethics policy?
   a. Name an ethics officer
   b. Have quarterly ethics training sessions
   c. Reward employees who engage in ethical behavior
   d. Have leadership continuously model ethical behavior

7. **LO 12.3** Which statement most closely matches the intent of the statement "The customer is always right"?
   a. The statement is literally correct—the customer is *always* right.
   b. The customer should have his or her concerns heard and addressed in a timely fashion.
   c. In health care, the provider should adjust its coding to maximize benefits for the patient.
   d. The customer must believe that he or she is being heard.

8. **LO 12.3** Which of the following statements is most accurate related to the changing of diagnoses?
   a. Diagnoses should never be changed.
   b. Diagnoses should be changed to make a claim payable.

   c. Diagnoses should be changed if an error in the original code selection occurred.

   d. Diagnoses should be changed only by a certified coder.

9. **LO 12.4** When conflict occurs, communication often becomes difficult because

   a. Both parties are seeking the best possible ethical outcome

   b. Emotions cause each party to focus only on their own position

   c. People become less committed to their position

   d. Both parties remove their protective barrier

10. **LO 12.4** Overcommunicating with patients is

   a. Not a good practice

   b. A good practice because it increases understanding

   c. A good practice because it is less time-consuming than other alternatives

   d. Achieved by using only one method of communication

Short Answer

Use your critical thinking skills to answer the following questions.

1. **LO 12.1** Explain why "waste" generally does not originate within the realm of medical billing.

2. **LO 12.1** Discuss the best way to avoid the allegation and occurrence of waste, abuse, and fraud.

3. **LO 12.1** Describe the ethical "trouble spots" that a plastic surgery practice may experience. Identify some trouble spots that an OB/GYN practice may encounter.

4. **LO 12.2** Discuss why the ethical complexity is high in the health care marketplace.

5. **LO 12.2** In what ways can regulations cause the occurrence of unethical behavior? Explain your answer.

6. **LO 12.2** Discuss the two schools of thought related to ethics policies. With which do you agree? Why?

7. **LO 12.3** Why is it so important that employees be empowered to solve customer service problems? Explain how their ability to solve problems can help reduce the occurrence of ethical problems.

8. **LO 12.3** What factor or factors cause employers not to entrust employees to solve problems? How can this create ethical problems?

9. **LO 12.4** Why do patients most often create ethical dilemmas? What do you believe is the best way to resolve these types of problems?

10. **LO 12.4** Can you think of other alternative communication methods, beyond those presented in the chapter, that would be effective in communicating the ethical standards of a health care provider to a patient?

Applying Your Knowledge

At the beginning of this chapter, you were introduced to Melvin, who was the administrator at Downtown Internal Medicine. Melvin was facing some very serious issues that were caused by some current issues, but which had their origination in some severe ethical problems in the past.

After reading this chapter, you have been exposed to a number of concepts regarding the best approaches to avoid the occurrence of ethical problems. If you were a consultant brought in to assist

Melvin at the time he was hired at the practice, which actions would you specifically recommend that he take to address the ethical problems at the practice? Your answer should include the following:

1. What features would be included in the practice's ethics policy?

2. What specific billing department protocols would you establish?

3. How would these policies and protocols be communicated to the affected stakeholders?

Internet Research

The Internet provides many resources that encourage people to think seriously about the issue of ethics (Figure 12.12). Some websites are academic in nature, focusing on philosophical issues surrounding ethical truths. Other websites are more practical in focus, discussing current events and specific applications for ethical principles.

Identify at least three websites that discuss codes of ethics and take the following steps:

1. Identify the website and its URL.

2. Summarize the key principles that are emphasized on each website.

3. Develop an outline for a code of ethics for a health care provider or institution, using the best elements of the three websites that you identified.

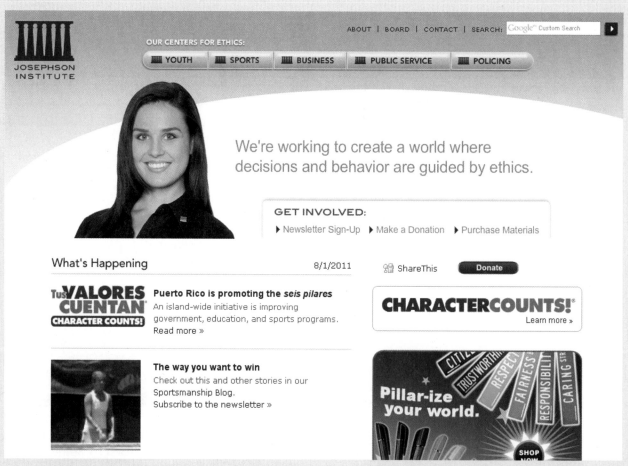

FIGURE 12.12

A significant number of websites are dedicated to the issue of ethics, including that of the Josephson Institute for Ethics (www.josephsoninstitute.org).

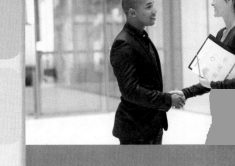

Resolving Ethical Problems When They Occur

13

Key Terms

Arbiter
Culpable
Extricate
Imminent
Intranet
Objectivity
Reciprocal

LEARNING OUTCOMES

After completing this chapter, you will be able to:

13.1 Describe the options available to individuals who are in the middle of an ethical dilemma.

13.2 Discuss methods in which individuals can resist requests to perform unethical acts, especially when the requests come from the employer.

13.3 Identify how various health care entities can use practical tips and resources for dealing with ethical problems in medical billing and coding.

13.4 Convey the value of adhering to ethical principles.

CASE STUDY

The outpatient clinic system at Southwest State University Medical School (SSUMS) was recognized nationally as a model for outstanding academic medicine. Not only was it one of the finest teaching institutions in the country for students, its multispecialty clinic system was viewed as the most well-run and financially strong academic medical system. A key component of the successful clinic operation was the billing office, which consistently exceeded all standard benchmarks for financial performance and customer satisfaction.

Aisha Irving was the director of billing services at SSUMS. She was universally liked and respected within her department. The trait that the employees liked the most was her sense of personal ethics. She treated the employees in the same manner that she wanted to be treated and she worked just as hard, if not harder, than all of the employees who reported to her. Of particular note was that she was consistent in her conduct, which served as a model for all of the employees.

Because of the multispecialty nature of the clinic system, the staff of the billing department encountered almost every imaginable ethical problem that could be faced in the field of medical billing and coding. There were no specific written protocols in place for the billing department, but Aisha's example created an environment in which the entire staff was committed to ethical conduct in relationship to their jobs. She had provided training regarding the common ethical trouble spots and discussed the legal risks to the university in engaging in abusive or fraudulent billing. In fact, when faced with an ethical problem, the staff often made decisions based on the answer to the question, "What would Aisha do?"

The medical school underwent some personnel changes at the higher administrative levels, which resulted in the hiring of a new chief financial officer (CFO), which was the person to whom Aisha reported. Aisha met frequently with the new CFO, which was expected as part of his introduction to the position. The staff noticed that Aisha often seemed upset on her return from some of these meetings, but she refused to talk about them with the staff.

When the billing office staff arrived one Friday morning, one of them remarked, "Where is Aisha?" Not seeing her was unusual, because she was usually there before everyone else arrived. As they logged into the network and retrieved their e-mails, one by one gasps went up around the department. They each received an e-mail saying that Aisha was no longer with the university because they needed to "go in a new direction." Moreover, the e-mail indicated that Arnold Porter, the new director of billing services, would be replacing Aisha on Monday. Everyone in the department was stunned because Aisha told them that things were going very well and they thought that Aisha was doing a great job in leadership.

On Monday morning, the CFO introduced Arnold Porter, the new director of billing services, to the department staff. The staff looked at each other as they learned about the background of their new boss. He had no experience in medical billing—his experience was in consulting and banking. His personality seemed completely different from Aisha's. Aisha focused on collaboration and coaching—Arnold seemed very directive and "top down" in his management style.

Problems for the department staff appeared almost immediately. A patient asked for a change in diagnosis that was completely inappropriate and demanded to speak to the director. Whereas Aisha would have unquestionably supported the staff member's position and told the patient that the change in diagnosis was inappropriate, Arnold called in the staff member and loudly criticized her within earshot of others, asking why she was not committed to customer service. He told her to make the change. When the employee began to protest, he cut her off and said, "Do you want to be in the same place as your former leader?"

Another employee who was responsible for refunds to insurance companies went to Arnold for signatures and he bellowed, "What are these for?" The employee stated, "These are refunds to insurers because the payments were made to us in error." "Did they ask for the refund?" demanded the new director. "No," replied the staff member, "but it's our policy to refund money that was paid to us in error." "Not anymore it's not!" shouted Arnold. "Insurers will get their refund checks when they ask for them. Do you have any idea of how much money we could have kept over the years if the insurer didn't notice the error?" "But it doesn't seem right," pleaded the employee. "You aren't paid to determine right and wrong," said Arnold. "Stop doing these refunds, or clean out your desk!"

1. Based on the information provided, what are some possible explanations for the personnel changes at SSUMS?

2. Have you ever been in an organization where there was a change in leadership? Was there a significant difference in leadership personality? Did this influence the direction of the organization? If so, how?

3. How would you feel if you were one of the employees in the billing department at SSUMS? How would you respond to the change in direction and apparent change in principles? What, if anything, would you do?

Introduction

An academic study of ethics can be very interesting and produce intellectually challenging discussions. This type of study is important and necessary. However, the discussion of ethics becomes most challenging and important when facing real-world dilemmas, such as those faced by the employees in the billing department at Southwest State University Medical School. Many difficult thoughts go through the minds of employees who are having their ethical systems challenged. Intense pressure can come to bear on individuals that cause them to think about doing things they would never consider doing in ordinary circumstances.

13.1 Options Available to Employees Facing Ethical Dilemmas Caused by Their Employer

Ideally, every organization would establish systems that would prevent employees from being placed in unethical positions by the organization itself. However, there are reasons why employees are placed in this position:

- The organization is not committed to ethical conduct and does not make appropriate preparations for dealing with ethical problems.
- The organization has ethics policies and procedures in place, but there are individuals (particularly those in leadership roles) within the organization who are not committed to carrying out the policies.
- The organization has ethics policies and procedures in place, but circumstances change that place extreme pressure on the organization. The commitment to adhering to the ethics policies and procedures diminishes or completely disappears.

There is no such thing as a true "organizational" ethical problem. Ultimately, all ethical problems and dilemmas are individual issues. Issues appear to become organizational in nature when people at higher levels of responsibility fail to manage their individual issues and impose the results on the rest of the organization.

An element of ethical dilemmas that is frustrating for many and leaves them feeling powerless occurs when they are not in higher levels of organizational authority and have no apparent ability to change their situation. As a result, two out of the three general options that are available to them to resolve an ethical dilemma in which they are

Those in ethical dilemmas, particularly those in lower levels of an organization, may feel that they have three options: to look the other way, to refuse to behave unethically and lose their job, or to find an acceptable alternative. Consequently, ethical dilemmas can leave workers feeling confused and powerless.

FYI

Just because an ethical dilemma occurs within an organization does not mean that the organization is unethical. There is no clear line as to the difference between ethical and unethical organizations, but the primary determining factors are (1) the frequency in which dilemmas occur, and (2) the general nature of the response to the dilemma.

involved are highly undesirable and the third option is, in large part, out of their control. The three options are to

1. Look the other way.
2. Refuse to participate.
3. Find an acceptable alternative solution.

LOOK THE OTHER WAY

There is never a circumstance when clashing with bosses or others in higher levels of administration is a desirable option. This option becomes even less favorable when unemployment levels are high and/or an employee thoroughly enjoys the job. Therefore, this is by far the easiest way to "resolve" an ethical dilemma—do not deal with it. There is certainly an element of risk that the employee will be found **culpable** if a provider is found guilty of health care fraud or abuse and the employee was actively involved in it. However, the risk of incurring the negative fallout from an employer for refusing to engage in certain unethical behavior (or reporting unethical behavior) is **imminent** and significantly higher than the possible legal risk. It is also the most passive, which, in the minds of some, is more acceptable (Figure 13.1).

The downside of looking the other way is that it can cause several adverse side effects for the employees. These include:

- *An intense emotional discomfort with the fact that they have compromised their standards.* Even though they have satisfied their employer, they have disappointed themselves.

- *Creation of a slippery slope.* Each time that an employee's ethical standards are violated, it becomes easier to violate it the next time. Developing a reputation as an unethical person does not usually happen overnight—it is often the product of a series of decisions. The first decision usually appears to be a minor ethical problem and "no big deal." The next decision, which is a more significant ethical problem, does not appear to be much more significant than the last ethical dilemma. However, if the more significant dilemma was considered in the absence of the first ethical dilemma, it would appear more unacceptable and the likelihood of choosing unethical behavior would decrease. In short, unethical choices produce more choices that are unethical.

Culpable
Deserving blame; legitimately held responsible.

Imminent
Likely to occur at any moment; happening soon.

WARNING

The most frequent response to becoming aware of an ethical problem in the workplace is to "keep your head down" and look the other way. This is often perceived as the course of least resistance.

The Scale of Risk

Risk

| Look the other way | Find an alternative | Refuse to participate |

FIGURE 13.1
Looking the other way is generally considered less risky for an employee than refusing to participate in unethical activity encouraged or required by the employer. However, this consideration of risk does not address the issues of "right" and "wrong."

Table 13.1 Ethical and Unethical Outcomes Associated with Looking the Other Way

Positive Outcome?	Ethical	Unethical
Yes	Outcome: Positive Respect: Yes	Outcome: Positive Respect: No
No	Outcome: Negative Respect: Yes	Outcome: Negative Respect: No

- *A loss of credibility and respect.* Those who ask others to do unethical things, as well as those who observe the situation/behavior, have a lower level of respect for the person if they engage in unethical behavior. John Maxwell, in his book *There's No Such Thing as Business Ethics,* tells the story of Howard Bowen, who was responsible for developing the construction of new K-Mart stores. When working on the first contract (a $40 million deal), one of the executives suggested that their group go to a strip club. Howard did not feel comfortable doing this because he thought it would be a betrayal of his wife's trust. At the risk of losing the contract (and possibly his job), he asked to be taken back to the hotel. When they arrived at the hotel, he got out of the van. Then another in their party got out of the van. Then another. Eventually, no one went out that night. Later, the executive who made the suggestion told Howard, "You have no idea how much I respect you." Howard was awarded the contract and his highly successful career got a jump start (Maxwell, 2003).

Behaving unethically does not guarantee "success," but it does guarantee a loss of credibility and respect—particularly self-respect. So even if Howard had gone out and had successfully obtained the contract, would it have been worthwhile to him? What if he had gone out and had not won the contract? He would have been disappointed on both fronts. It is not possible to behave unethically and maintain the respect of those around you, regardless of whether or not the outcome is positive. Table 13.1 shows the breakdown of outcomes in this case.

REFUSE TO PARTICIPATE

Being an employee who is placed in a position of having to refuse to participate in unethical behavior is enormously challenging. Refusing to participate puts a number of elements of the individual's life in jeopardy, and forces him or her to deal with questions such as:

- If I am fired, how will I financially support my family?
- Will I lose my home? Will I lose the respect of my spouse and friends?
- Will we have to move and will I have to uproot my children from their school?
- If I am fired, will I be able to find a job that I like as much as this one?
- Can I deal with the potential embarrassment and social stigma associated with being unemployed?
- Is it that big a deal? Is this an issue over which I should lose my job?

These serious questions have significant consequences. You cannot pretend that these issues do not matter. Therefore, this choice presents the highest level of personal risk.

> **FYI**
>
> Most financial planners recommend that people keep three to six months of salary in an "emergency savings" account, for use in unexpected circumstances such as an unplanned job loss. Knowing that this money is available relieves some of the pressure felt by an employee when placed in a difficult ethical situation.

FIND AN ACCEPTABLE ALTERNATIVE

In some cases, such as those where there is a culture that encourages unethical activity, there may appear to be only two options—either participate in (or choose to ignore) unethical behavior or seek an alternative solution. In nearly every situation there are alternatives in addition to the two primary options. Unfortunately, many do not pursue these options because

- *They may require some creative problem solving.* The mistake made by many is that they see the ethical dilemma and stop at that point—the focus becomes the dilemma. In reality, the real question is, "What are the objectives of the parties who are considering or requesting unethical behavior?" Once the objectives are understood, alternative means of achieving those objectives can be identified and pursued—means that are not unethical. Similarly, the case for avoiding risks of engaging in that behavior can be explored and a compelling case for changing course can be presented.

- *There is fear that the alternatives will be rejected.* This is a definite possibility and, depending on the circumstances, can produce a certain element of risk to the person promoting the alternatives. However, even if the proposal is completely rejected, there is less risk than a direct refusal to engage in unethical behavior.

Thinking It Through 13.1

1. Discuss the reasons that cause employees to be put in the position of behaving unethically. Which do you believe is the most frequent cause? Why?

2. What element of ethical dilemmas is most frustrating? Why?

3. When an employee looks the other way, which possible outcome do you believe is the most serious? Why?

4. Can you identify any other reasons why an employee may choose not to identify and present alternative solutions to his or her employer, who may be requesting that the employee engage in unethical behavior?

13.2 Methods That Employees Can Use When Unethical Behaviors Occur

According to the Josephson Institute of Ethics, "ethics is about how we meet the challenge of doing the right thing when that will cost us more than we want to pay." Behaving ethically is never harder than when our ethics are being challenged by the person that employs us. It is difficult because we instinctively want to trust and respect those for whom we work. There is a sense of disappointment when those we respect (or we want to respect) fall below our standards for appropriate behavior. To make matters worse, they sometimes want us to lower our standards. In addition, there is the unavoidable uncertainty and fear that occurs when the prospect of losing a valued job becomes too real.

FIGURE 13.2

Ethical dilemmas are best resolved by not allowing them to occur in the first place. There are several critical steps in preparation that will remove the pressure from employees when challenged with doing the wrong thing.

Avoid the Problem

- Create an environment that promotes ethical behavior.
- Consistently demonstrate ethical behavior at the highest levels of the organization.
- Establish policies and protocols that guide employees in ethical behavior.
- Communicate effectively with customers/patients to make them aware of how the provider will behave and what they can expect in certain circumstances.

DETERMINE HOW DILEMMAS OCCUR, EVEN AFTER PROPER PREPARATION

A major concept throughout this book is that the best way to deal with ethical dilemmas is to avoid the circumstances in which these dilemmas most frequently occur (Figure 13.2). However, it is completely unrealistic to believe that this is *always* possible. Everyone will, at some point, encounter a difficult ethical dilemma. Again, even when in the middle of a dilemma, successfully resisting and resolving the ethical dilemma requires some advance preparation before the event occurs.

Why can ethical dilemmas not be totally avoided? How can they occur even when everyone seems to make a good-faith effort to avoid behaving unethically, as demonstrated by establishing ethics policies and implementing effective procedures? There are four fundamental reasons:

1. **The situation is unique or was not previously anticipated.** Law enforcement has faced serious challenges in the last several years in dealing with Internet-based crimes such as bullying, stalking, or identity theft. The challenge was that the laws, as written, did not take into consideration the fact that such crimes could even exist. Technology moved faster than did the law. A similar situation can occur in relation to medical billing and coding ethics. Insurers may institute new coverage guidelines or the American Medical Association could create new CPT codes that allow the reporting of services that were not previously contemplated by existing policies.

2. **Leadership fails to maintain the standards of conduct required by ethics policies.** An ethics policy may be established by a strong, ethical leader who consistently demonstrates behavior consistent with his or her stated beliefs. However, change may occur in leadership that results in a new manager who does not share the same values or does not share the same level of commitment to behavior consistent with a set of values. Therefore, even though policies and protocols are in place, they are no longer followed because upper management does not support them and, in some cases, may even discourage ethical behavior. An ethical organization can become an unethical organization through simple leadership change.

3. **Employees at a level below that of leadership fail to maintain the standards of conduct required by ethics policies.** As much as

leadership is responsible for the conduct of an organization, the failure to follow ethics policies may occur at lower levels without the knowledge of upper management. Unfortunately, leadership may establish policies that unintentionally create unethical behavior. In the 1990s, the Sears Automotive Department established sales goals for mechanics of $147 per hour. The intention of the goal was to encourage mechanics to work more quickly. However, an alarming number of employees met their goal by overcharging for their services and repairing items that did not require repair. Sales goals were met, but customers were treated unethically (Bazerman & Tenbrunsel, 2011). The executives were pleased with the result—until they found out how the result was achieved.

4. **Legitimate fundamental disagreement exists about the ethics of a particular case or course of action.** In many respects, coding is an art rather than a science. There are circumstances in which it is possible to code the same service accurately in two different ways. One may be better than another, but neither is "wrong" and certainly neither is "unethical." However, an organization must have a method by which to resolve a particular case and establish a standard of practice for a given situation. It is not sufficient to let the decision for each individual case be made by different parties because it establishes a culture of inappropriate autonomy and produces nonstandard results in similar situations. This is a major step down the path of creating or maintaining an unethical organization.

RESIST REQUESTS TO ACT UNETHICALLY

It is critical to understand that formulating a strategy is essential in resolving ethical dilemmas. Dealing with dilemmas on a case-by-case basis without considering a number of factors will produce, at best, uneven results and most likely will produce unethical behavior. A number of different elements, approached from different angles, will help any person deal consistently with ethical dilemmas (Figure 13.3).

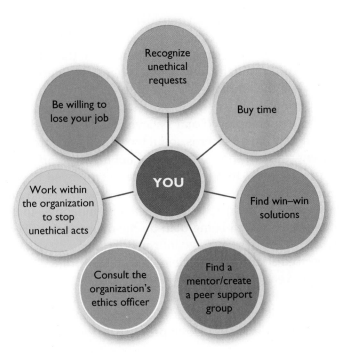

FIGURE 13.3
The wide range of options available to an individual facing an ethical challenge.

Recognize Unethical Requests and Unethical Bosses.
Sometimes it is possible to become involved in an ethical dilemma before the dilemma is even recognized. It may initially start as "This doesn't seem right" or "I don't feel comfortable with being asked to do that." However, the feeling or sense is pushed aside and loyalty to the boss, which is an admirable trait, becomes the primary focus. Analysis of the situation, including examining the responsibilities that an employee has toward all stakeholders in the process, will provide clarity as to why some situations do not seem right or are uncomfortable. Identifying the specific ethical problem is very helpful in moving toward a resolution of the problem.

Working to resolve requests for unethical behavior can begin as early as the interview process when seeking a job. The job interview process is frequently seen as a screening process that is controlled, in large part, by the employer. Usually there are more jobs than people available for a job, which seems to give the employer the upper hand. The employee is tempted to take advantage of any job opportunity presented and often does not consider ethical matters at the time of the interview. However, this is important.

Employers generally do not make a habit of stating during the interview process, "We lie, cheat, and steal—how do you feel about that?" This does not mean that potential employees are forced to walk into a job without knowing something about the ethical climate of an organization. The potential employee can ask questions about ethics policies and compliance programs. If the employer admits that the organization does not have such policies and programs, this serious red flag alerts the candidate that ethical problems may be common within the firm. If policies and programs do exist, further questions should be asked that can shed light on the ethical environment there. Asking about how the employer would respond to potential ethical scenarios that may be common for the provider lets the candidate know more about the organization. If it has not considered the problem and does not have an answer, this is a warning sign. In addition, if the employer is offended by questions of this sort, this is clear sign of potential ethical shortcomings and may be an employer that the candidate wants to avoid. On the other hand, if the employer is open and welcoming to these types of questions, it can build confidence in the relationship for both parties—the candidate knows that he or she is entering an ethical workplace while the employer knows it is getting an employee who takes ethics seriously.

Those who are unemployed may believe that they should pursue positions even if they have concerns about the ethical standards of the employer. Recent research shows that this is not a particularly good plan. A Gallup poll revealed that those who are unemployed have a lower level of well-being than those of employed people who enjoy their job. However, those who are disengaged—actively unhappy—in their jobs have a lower level of well-being than do the unemployed (Figure 13.4; Williams, 2011). This research is confirmed by a variety of other studies that produced similar results. Being forced to work within an atmosphere that actively encourages or requires unethical behavior creates employee disengagement and dissatisfaction in life. People who are looking for a new job should consider the organization's ethics a large component of their decision-making process—before they take the job.

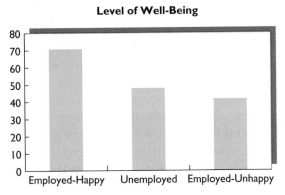

Level of Well-Being

Source: Williams, 2011.

FIGURE 13.4
People who are unemployed are happier than those who are employed, but are disengaged—actively unhappy—in their job.

Buy Time. Today's business climate is fast moving. E-mail, text messages, and remote access to systems via the Internet from nearly anywhere on earth provide a sense of immense urgency, even when the urgency is not required for a specific task. An important tool to help an employee avoid engaging in ethical behavior is to resist the urgency and delay the action to "buy time."

The purpose of buying time is not to simply delay the inevitable or passively resisting the request. The reasons that requests for unethical conduct should be delayed are:

- It provides the opportunity to gather facts about the situation.
- It allows consideration of the action on the stakeholders of the organization.
- It allows the opportunity to seek input from other people inside and outside the organization, who may have experienced a similar problem or have a solution that you have not yet considered.
- It allows you to find alternatives that achieve the objectives of all parties involved without engaging in unethical conduct.

Delaying action, even for a few hours, can provide clarity to a situation that seems irresolvable. The fact that a particular action must be performed immediately can be a sign that it is possibly an unethical action. An ethical action does not need to be done quickly for the purpose of putting it "out of sight."

WARNING

Ethics mistakes sometimes occur by making decisions too quickly. Taking some time to "cool off" and further consider the situation may help bring resolution to the issue.

Find a Mentor and a Peer Support Group. A mentor is a person who provides guidance and advice for handling situations in a variety of life circumstances, including specific career-related knowledge. When someone joins a new organization, it is important to identify, as soon as possible, which person could serve as a mentor. Ideally, the mentor will be someone who is well established and well respected within the organization and who is willing to invest time in an employee. The mentor can serve as a sounding board for given situations, can provide advice regarding how to respond to certain individuals, and, in some cases, can provide protection when conflict with a direct report (boss) is required (Mallor, Barnes, Bowers, & Langvardt, 2010).

Some medical practices are smaller and, therefore, identifying a mentor within the organization may be impossible simply because there are not enough people from which to choose a mentor. In this circumstance, the employee should look outside the organization for the guidance and support that a mentor can provide. Some possibilities

FYI

Seek out opportunities to serve as a mentor for employees as you advance throughout your career. This is one way in which you can "pay it forward" out of gratitude for what someone did for you at some point. It also helps promote and improve the general ethical environment more effectively.

include an experienced coder within a local chapter of a coder's group, an experienced colleague in a local practice manager's group, or a member in a local civic organization.

An equally important resource for obtaining advice and guidance is to identify peers inside and outside the organization who have or are encountering similar experiences in their career. They can provide significant input by offering suggestions for resolving situations and providing moral and literal support when facing difficult ethical circumstances. A peer support group does not need to be highly formal—in fact, it likely will not be formal. The important element is that it allows the person to feel supported in his or her ethical stand. Many severe ethical failures within organizations could have been avoided if a number of peer employees, even at "lower" levels, had gathered and spoken out against what was happening. These types of situations are not commonly known because a company does not usually make the news until the ethical lapses of the company grow to the point that the company implodes. Groups of employees who stand against wrongdoing are far more effective in changing the behavior of an organization than a single individual.

If a person works in a very small health care organization, a peer who shares the same values or who would be willing to provide input in assisting the resolution of an ethical dilemma may not exist. However, colleagues at other medical practices or other professional organizations can provide a certain level of support that provides encouragement to the single individual to stand up and do the right thing. Whether in a small organization or in a large organization, individuals should identify those who can provide friendship and support through their common knowledge, common experiences, and common values.

Find Win–Win Solutions. The false assumption that there is only one alternative in resolving a situation is often the cause of poor choices and ethical failings. In many circumstances, there is more than one solution. The person who desires to conduct himself or herself ethically must be willing and able to make the case for the alternative solution.

The term "win–win" sometimes leads to a false belief that it is not a positive outcome unless both parties are equally pleased (both parties get to "win"). In reality this may not always be possible, but it is frequently possible to achieve an outcome where both parties can accept the outcome. Ultimately, the objective is not an ill-defined feeling of happiness, but rather a rational resolution where all parties are treated fairly and do not compromise their ethical standards.

The win–win concept works best when the boss is willing to accept that alternatives exist and he or she truly desires to conduct business ethically. It becomes more complex and less successful if the boss does not have an equal commitment to ethical conduct. When that occurs, different approaches may be necessary.

Work Within the Organization to Stop the Unethical Actions. As it pertains to ethics and receiving support when ethical dilemmas occur, the most important part of a compliance plan is the creation of the role of ethics officer or compliance officer. The person in this position is a tremendous resource to individuals within the

Can There Be a Loser in a Win–Win Situation?

Erin, the receptionist at the physician office, answered the phone. "This is Mrs. Winsington! I can't believe you people have the nerve to claim to be a doctor's office! I spent 45 minutes in your waiting room and then the doctor saw me for barely 5 minutes. He clearly was distracted, he didn't listen to me, and he acted like he couldn't wait to get out of the room. If you send me a bill for this service, I'm going to complain to the medical board! I'm not paying for a service that wasn't worth anything." Erin assured her that she would give this information to her manager and that someone would be back in touch with her later that day.

Erin gave the information to her manager, who passed it on to the manager of the billing office, Donna. Donna knew Mrs. Winsington—she frequently complained about the service that she received. Donna wondered why she kept coming to the clinic. Following the standard procedure, Donna checked the billing system and found that Mrs. Winsington had been billed for a Level 4 E&M service (99214), with a diagnosis of malaise and fatigue (780.79) and sleep disturbance (780.50). She then pulled Mrs. Winsington's chart and found that there were two lines of illegible writing associated with the date of service in question, and nothing more. Donna did not know what happened in the exam room with Mrs. Winsington, but she knew that the documentation for that service did not support the level of service billed.

Because Mrs. Winsington was expecting an answer that same day, Donna stopped Dr. Garrigan in the hall outside an exam room. She explained the situation to the doctor and the doctor looked at the note. Dr. Garrigan said, "Oh yes, Mrs. Winsington was having trouble sleeping and so I wrote her a prescription for a sleep aid." Donna briefly explained about the patient's complaint and Dr. Garrigan said, "I'm not going to argue with her—just bill the insurance and write off the copayment—she won't owe anything. It's a win–win." Donna began to protest and Dr. Garrigan said, "Not now—I'm already running behind." She then proceeded into the next exam room.

Donna felt like she was facing a dilemma: What was she going to do with Mrs. Winsington? Should she follow the doctor's instruction?

1. Why might Donna feel that this is an ethical dilemma?

2. What could Donna have done differently in this situation to achieve a better result?

3. What should Donna do?

organization who see improper behavior. It provides them with a viable opportunity to have the issue addressed without the same degree of risk that they would incur if they were a single individual trying to stand up in opposition to a physician or other administrative officers.

Care must be exhibited when seeking help for the resolution of ethical problems. Individuals should understand several issues before they access formal programs to address ethical concerns:

- All of the facts concerning the situation must be gathered and presented before making a formal complaint. Nothing will destroy credibility more quickly than making incomplete, inaccurate, or false allegations. Just because a formal system exists to resolve ethical complaints does not mean that the employee can skip the necessary due diligence.

- While they likely will support you, do not automatically assume that your mentor and peer group will support you in your complaint against those in a position of authority. They may not share the same degree of concern that you do or they may not feel that they are in a position in which they can risk the possible fallout if they become involved in the situation. Communication with your mentor and peer group regarding this issue is important so that you know, prior to any possible conflict, what their reaction will be and what level of support you can expect.

- Attempting to work within the organization to resolve the issue does not always work. The ethics/compliance officer may be a powerless figurehead or is simply ineffective in advocating for those with ethics complaints. He or she may not agree with your assessment of the situation or may agree completely, but he or she is subsequently overruled at a higher level in the process. The existence of systems to facilitate the processing of ethics concerns does not guarantee an ethical outcome in every situation. This then requires the employee to decide whether the situation is an isolated incident, over which reasonable people can disagree, or whether it is an intolerable and corrupt environment, in which he or she cannot work.

Prepare to Lose Your Job. This is clearly a final tactic because it creates two problems:

1. You are no longer able to contribute to or influence the outcome of the ethical decision-making process within the organization. Until you leave, you may not know how much influence you actually had—it may have been more than you thought.

2. You may have obligations for a home/apartment, support of your family, and other creditors to whom you owe money, not to mention the interruption in your career path. It truly is a challenge when you decide that the situation is so intractable that you are unable to change the culture and/or you are not able to tolerate participating in the ongoing issues, because of the possible financial ramifications.

For these reasons, this should not be the first alternative pursued.

Thinking It Through 13.2

1. Explain the reasons why being asked by your employer to engage in unethical acts is such a difficult position.

2. When a situation "doesn't feel right," does it mean that something unethical is occurring? Why or why not?

3. Describe the reasons why potential employees do not actively pursue questions about ethical issues during the interview process.

13.3 Practical Tips and Resources for Dealing with Ethical Problems in Medical Billing and Coding

As discussed in Chapter 11, a compliance program is an essential element of dealing with ethical dilemmas as they occur, because it provides specific guidelines and protocols that assist in dealing with challenging ethical circumstances. The Office of Inspector General (OIG) for the Department of Health and Human Services (HHS) has created recommendations for compliance programs for a wide variety of health care entities. These entities include:

- Individual and small group physician practices.[1]
- Pharmaceutical manufacturers.
- Hospitals.
- Nursing facilities.
- Home health providers.
- Clinical laboratories.
- Ambulance providers.
- Durable medical equipment providers.
- Third-party medical billing companies.
- Medicare fee-for-service contractors (generally payers).

Although all of these vary to some degree to meet the needs of the different types of organizations, they all have seven consistent features:

1. Conducting internal monitoring and auditing.
2. Implementing compliance and practice standards.
3. Designating a compliance officer or contact.
4. Conducting appropriate training and education.
5. Responding appropriately to detected offenses and developing corrective actions.
6. Developing open lines of communication.
7. Enforcing disciplinary standards through well-publicized guidelines (OIG, HHS, 2000).

The degree and manner in which an organization implements each of these elements depends in large part on the size of the organization. It would be ridiculous for a practice with one person in the billing department to hold scheduled training sessions on ethics and compliance, whereas it would be essential for a large, multispecialty clinic system with hundreds in the billing department to do so. Communication in the large setting will be more formal than in the smaller setting, where it would be informal. An **intranet** may be a viable option for publicizing guidelines in a large and geographically diverse organization, but a simple handbook is sufficient for a single-site, single-provider practice. Whatever is implemented needs to be size appropriate and customized for the organization to obtain the maximum benefit for the program.

Intranet
A computer network with restricted access, such as an internal company network.

ESTABLISH AN EFFECTIVE PROGRAM

Regardless of how large or small an organization may be, several non-negotiable features must be present for the program to work. The size of the organization will determine what these features will look like and, particularly if it is smaller, may require some creativity to achieve the desired results.

---

[1]The definition of a "small group physician" practice is not defined by a specific number of physicians. Instead, it is named in this fashion in recognition that not all practices need, nor can afford, a full-scale compliance program (Office of Inspector General, Department of Health and Human Services [OIG, HHS], 2000).

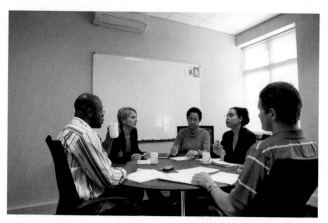

When developing an effective compliance program, the size of the organization matters. Smaller organizations may require creativity and flexibility to achieve desired results.

Meaningful, Yet Reasonable. An internal monitoring and auditing program is an essential part in ensuring ethical billing and coding practices. Unless there is some sort of self-assessment, a health care organization relies on speculation if it claims that it is billing ethically. However, care must be taken in designing and implementing this program because there are two extremes that may hamper its effectiveness:

1. The sample size is so small and the length of time between samplings is so long that the monitoring that is done is not representative of the realities of the practice's coding.

2. The sample size is so large and/or the sampling occurs so frequently that the task is so daunting that it cannot be reasonably completed. Instead of doing an exceedingly thorough review, no review occurs because there is not enough time and there are not enough resources to perform the task.

Everyone must agree at the time the program is designed on what level of monitoring is required to be *meaningful* while simultaneously being *reasonable*. In addition to considering the size of the organization, the monitoring program should be adaptable to accommodate the performance of the practice. For example, a physician whose documentation is shown to be consistently deficient may warrant more frequent or thorough monitoring than a physician whose documentation is consistently outstanding. When a physician's documentation improves and meets a certain standard, the amount of monitoring that occurs can decrease until his or her performance is proven to require more attention.

Objective. When designing a program and carrying out its ongoing performance, **objectivity** is an essential requirement. The program will not be accepted if it is believed that the original design and/or its enforcement are unfairly weighted toward one party or another. It is unrealistic to believe that the interpretation of the intent of a program will always be understood and agreed on mutually by all parties affected. Therefore, there has to be a way to obtain objective input and, in some cases, rulings regarding program interpretation.

Objectivity
Freedom from personal bias; accurate interpretation of reality.

In an extremely small practice it may seem difficult to obtain objectivity because there may not be a party within the practice who is not intimately involved in the situation. However, objectivity can always be achieved in different ways, based on the size of the organization. Some examples include:

- *Creating a coding ethics committee.* If there is disagreement in the interpretation of a policy, a coding ethics committee can be a means by which to obtain rulings or final determinations concerning how the policy is applied to a particular situation. The ethics committee could consist of a cross section of coders, physicians, and other personnel who can provide independent insight and knowledge about how a situation should be handled.

- *Establishing a protocol for coders and physicians not directly involved.* An organization may not be large enough to warrant the creation of a separate ethics committee. In such cases, an alternative is to establish a protocol by which coders and physicians who are not directly involved in the patient's care and are not directly involved in a given case are provided with the relevant facts and render an opinion regarding appropriate coding/handling of the situation.

- *Identifying an impartial coder from outside the practice.* In small practices there may not be other coders or physicians from which to obtain an opinion. An alternative is to arrange with a qualified coder and/or physician from another practice within the area to serve as an impartial **arbiter** regarding the ethics of a particular situation. This can be done without any expense if a **reciprocal** arrangement is established so that the practices provide this service for each other. This outside person does not have any bias or personal stake in the decision and, therefore, his or her decision is more likely to be correct. At the very least, the potential for allegations of bias are dramatically reduced.

Arbiter
A person with the power to make judgments or rulings.

Reciprocal
Treating each other in a similar or identical fashion.

Unquestioned Integrity in the Ethics/Compliance Officer Position. The ethics/compliance officer for a health care organization should be a person who is accountable to someone else. For example, the ethics officer of a small practice should not be the senior physician owner. Regardless of the personality and behavior of that physician, employees are not going to feel comfortable in reporting possible ethics violations involving that physician when they know that the physician can overrule any complaint they make, sweep it under the rug, or put their job in jeopardy.

The ideal ethics/compliance officer should be a person from a higher level of the practice but who is also accountable to another individual or board, to ensure that he or she does not have the exclusive power to disregard an ethics complaint unilaterally. The person should have enough authority and respect within the organization to be able to have difficult conversations with practice leaders without intimidation or concern about the status of his or her job. It may be necessary to identify an ethics officer who is not directly an employee of the practice.

Effective Disciplinary Structure. If a physician or coder is found to be engaging in unethical behavior related to billing or coding, any program is completely ineffective if the disciplinary structure

> **COMPLIANCE TIP**
>
> If you are working with a coder outside your practice, take steps to ensure that you don't violate HIPAA laws. Either execute a business associate agreement or deidentify any medical records that the coder is reviewing.

does not enforce the program or institute meaningful discipline to ensure that it does not happen in the future. The physician leadership of the practice must have complete buy-in on the disciplinary process at the time the program is established, before any possible violation is detected.

DEFINE THE UNDERLYING ASSUMPTIONS OF AN ETHICS PROGRAM

Two different policies established at two different organizations can result in two completely separate outcomes, even if the facts in question at both locations are identical. How is this possible?

The reason for the variability in outcomes can be directly linked to the values that are in place within an organization. Table 13.2 illustrates how the starting point of the policy (ethical framework) can affect the end result.

Is one method right and one method wrong? No. They are simply different. However, note the differences and note how the differences may affect the eventual outcome of their application to an ethical dilemma.

- Column 1 has more steps than column 2.
- Step 2 of the method in column 2 references consideration of consequences; the method of column 1 does not reference consequences, except perhaps as a part of step 5.
- Step 2 in column 1 draws attention back to the fundamental core values. The method in column 2 does not specifically indicate this step.
- Step 3 in column 2 encompasses steps 2, 3, and 4 from column 1. The process is more detailed in column 1.
- In column 1, after a decision is made, the results are analyzed (step 8). Such action is not indicated in column 2.

Table 13.2 Different Methods of Resolving Ethical Problems

Process Step	Column 1 Using a Framework for Ethical Decision Making	Column 2 Resolving an Ethical Dilemma
1	Identify ethical issues	Identify ethical issues
2	Clarify personal and professional values	Analyze the consequences
3	Clarify influencing factors and barriers	Analyze the actions
4	Identify guiding ethical and legal principles	Make a decision
5	Analyze alternatives	
6	Find common ground	
7	Decide and act	
8	Assess outcomes	

Sources: Column 1 data are adapted from Association of Academic Health Centers, 2003; column 2 data are adapted from Loyola Marymount University, 2009.

1. Compare and contrast the relative complexity of establishing an ethics compliance program for a very large organization and a very small organization. Which do you believe would be more difficult? Why?

2. Model compliance programs have been designed by the Office of Inspector General for the Department of Health and Human Services, as part of the Medicare program. If a health care organization does not participate with Medicare, are these programs still applicable and necessary? Why or why not?

3. What do you believe are the most significant challenges regarding the naming of an ethics/compliance officer?

13.4 The Value of Adhering to Ethical Principles

Throughout the course of this text, a case has been made for adhering to ethical principles. Significant legal risks are associated with behaving unethically. Businesses that engage in ethical behavior do better financially, not to mention the benefit that is associated with public relations for organizations that are recognized for their ethics.

However, the most important questions related to conducting yourself ethically in your career are:

- What are your values?
- How meaningful are they to you?
- Are you willing to adhere to them, even when there is temptation to do something unethical?

When reflecting back on their life, it is unlikely that anyone has thought:

- "I wish I had been less honest."
- "I should have taken more ethical shortcuts."
- "The extra money I received by cheating was really worth it."
- "The relationship I lost during a business conflict over ethics didn't mean that much."

Life is too short to live with the regret and fear that are created when we make a choice to be unethical. It should never be "okay" to violate your ethical principles—when it does, it truly is a sad occasion. By sacrificing your ethical principles during difficult times and in difficult situations, you lose the ability and the opportunity to see their real value.

In modern society, avoidance of pain and discomfort has become a primary goal. This unfortunately leads to the use of ethical shortcuts because ethical dilemmas can be painful. Those shortcuts seem the quickest way to alleviate the pain, but there is a tremendous loss of opportunity when the shortcut is chosen, in addition to creating a different set of problems.

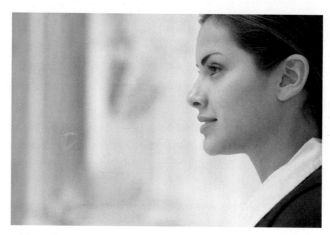

Although ethical challenges are difficult and uncomfortable, experiencing them makes an individual stronger, both as a professional and as a person.

Extricate
To remove from entanglement or complication.

If we **extricate** ourselves from all of our ethical dilemmas by taking the shortcut of unethical behavior (and avoid the hard work of doing the right thing), we miss the opportunity to develop the character and integrity that are needed to have a career and life that is fully rewarding and positively influences those around us.

It is possible to recover from a circumstance in which a person has sacrificed his or her values by behaving unethically, but it is not easy and it takes much time. The price paid for unethical behavior is withdrawn from the bank of the person's integrity, which is of great value. American financier, investor, and philanthropist Henry Kravis (1991) summarized it well when he said: "If you don't have integrity, you have nothing. You can't buy it. You can have all the money in the world, but if you are not a moral and ethical person, you really have nothing."

Thinking It Through 13.4

1. Are there other critical questions that could be asked regarding values and ethics? If so, what are they?

2. Can you think of circumstances in your life in which you were faced with an ethical struggle and chose to act unethically? Looking back, do you regret your decision? Why or why not?

CHAPTER REVIEW

Chapter Summary

Learning Outcomes	Key Concepts/Examples

13.1 Describe the options available to individuals who are in the middle of an ethical dilemma. Pages 404–407	• Employees are sometimes placed in ethical dilemmas by their employer because:
	  1. The organization is not committed to ethical conduct and does not make appropriate preparations for dealing with ethical problems.
	  2. The organization has ethics policies and procedures in place, but there are individuals within the organization who are not committed to carrying out the policies.
	  3. The organization has ethics policies and procedures in place, but circumstances change that place extreme pressure on the organization.
	• Employees generally have three options in responding to employer-generated ethical dilemmas:
	  1. Look the other way.
	  2. Refuse to deceive (and possibly lose the job).
	  3. Find an acceptable alternative.
	• There are varying levels of risk associated with each alternative.

13.2 Discuss methods in which individuals can resist requests to perform unethical acts, especially when the requests come from the employer. Pages 407–414	• It is particularly disappointing when we are asked to do unethical things by our employer, who we either respect or want to respect.
	• Even after proper preparation, ethical dilemmas can occur because:
	  1. The situation is unique or not previously anticipated.
	  2. The leadership fails to maintain the standards of conduct established by existing ethics policies.
	  3. Employees at lower levels within the organization fail to maintain the established standards of conduct.
	  4. There is legitimate fundamental disagreement concerning the appropriate course of action.
	• The key steps required to resist acting unethically are:
	  1. Recognize unethical requests and unethical bosses.
	  2. Buy time.
	  3. Find a mentor and a peer support group.
	  4. Find win–win solutions.
	  5. Work within the organization to stop the unethical actions.
	  6. Prepare to lose your job.

13.3 Identify how various health care entities can use practical tips and resources for dealing with ethical problems in medical billing and coding. Pages 414–419	• Effective ethics/compliance programs, regardless of size, must have some key features. They must:
	  1. Be meaningful, but reasonable.
	  2. Be objective.
	  3. Supply integrity/autonomy to the position of ethics officer.
	  4. Have an effective disciplinary structure.
	• An ethics program must have its fundamental assumptions defined to identify its purpose and desired results

13.4 Convey the value of adhering to ethical principles. Pages 419–420	• Although there are compelling reasons to behave ethically, the most important questions that must be asked related to ethics are:
	  1. What are your values?
	  2. How meaningful are they to you?
	  3. Are you willing to adhere to them, even when there is temptation to do something unethical?
	• Experiencing an ethical dilemma is not necessarily a bad thing. It can produce character and integrity that might not otherwise be developed.

CPT © 2011 American Medical Association. All rights reserved.

Chapter 13 | **Resolving Ethical Problems When They Occur**   **421**

End-of-Chapter Questions

Multiple Choice

Circle the letter that best completes the statement or answers the question.

1. **LO 13.1** Which of the following is *not* a reason that employees are placed by their employer in the position of behaving unethically?

    a. The organization is not committed to ethical conduct and does not prepare for ethical dilemmas.

    b. Employee-driven compliance programs are not effective.

    c. The leadership of the organization does not adhere to the existing policies.

    d. Outside circumstances put pressure on the organization to violate its ethical principles.

2. **LO 13.1** What is most frustrating for employees who are asked to engage in unethical behavior by their employer?

    a. A sense of powerlessness in changing the situation

    b. The wasted time involved in working on ethics committees

    c. The inability to find a new job

    d. The inability to realize the benefit of cooperating with the employer

3. **LO 13.1** Which of the following is *not* one of the possible side effects of looking the other way when unethical conduct is discovered?

    a. Emotional discomfort

    b. Creation of a slippery slope, encouraging more bad behavior

    c. A loss of credibility and respect

    d. Certain failure of the business

4. **LO 13.2** No matter how much preparation occurs, ethical dilemmas can never be completely avoided because

    a. Customers always ask for inappropriate actions

    b. Most people don't understand the ethical guidelines

    c. Organizational leadership sometimes fails to adhere to published guidelines

    d. There is universal agreement about what is and is not ethical

5. **LO 13.2** When applying for a job, a potential employee should be concerned if the potential employer says any of the following *except*

    a. "We don't have an ethics/compliance policy."

    b. "We haven't thought about that ethical problem before."

    c. "Why would you ask such a question?"

    d. "We are making revisions to our compliance program."

6. **LO 13.2** Which of the following is *not* a recommended option that can be used to resist unethical requests?

    a. Buy time.

    b. Circumvent the ethics officer.

    c. Be willing to lose your job.

    d. Find a win-win solution.

7. **LO 13.2** Which of the following is true regarding possible ways of resisting requests for unethical behavior?

    a. There is usually only one alternative when dealing with ethical dilemmas.

    b. A mentor and support group can be of great value.

c. There are never losers in a win–win situation.

d. Working within the organization to resolve ethical issues never works.

8. **LO 13.3** The OIG for the HHS has created recommended compliance plans for all of the following types of entities *except*

   a. Pharmaceutical manufacturers

   b. Clinical laboratories

   c. Hospitals

   d. Large physician groups and clinic systems

9. **LO 13.3** Which of the following is *not* true regarding audit and monitoring plans?

   a. They can be too comprehensive and complex.

   b. They should be the same throughout all organizations of the same size.

   c. Their samplings can be too small and inadequate.

   d. A formal plan is not necessary—assessment by consensus is adequate.

10. **LO 13.3** The ideal ethics/compliance officer is

    a. The senior physician

    b. An entry-level coder within the billing office

    c. An organizational leader who is accountable to a board of directors

    d. A senior coder within the billing office

Short Answer

Use your critical thinking skills to answer the following questions.

1. **LO 13.1** Do you agree with the statement, "There is no such thing as a true 'organizational' ethical problem"? Why or why not?

2. **LO 13.1** Why is looking the other way the easiest course of action to take when faced with unethical conduct?

3. **LO 13.1** Do you agree with the rating of risk on the scale of risk found in Figure 13.1? Why or why not?

4. **LO 13.1** Discuss the matrix in Table 13.1 related to outcomes and respect. Other than the box in the upper left corner, which scenario would you prefer to have? Why?

5. **LO 13.2** Discuss what issues should be considered when someone faces a situation that "doesn't feel right" or makes him or her feel uncomfortable?

6. **LO 13.2** What are some ways that a potential employee can learn about the ethical climate of the potential employer?

7. **LO 13.2** How do you interpret the survey results that show that people who are unemployed are happier than those who have a job but are disengaged (e.g., those who don't care about the well-being of their employer, those who don't like the environment in which they work)?

8. **LO 13.3** The OIG's recommended compliance plans do not require that every one of the seven proposed elements be included in an organization's plan if it is not appropriate for the organization (e.g., a small doctor's office). Which element(s) would be most likely to *not* be included in a small practice's compliance plan?

9. **LO 13.3** Which do you believe is the most important element in ensuring objectivity in an ethics/compliance plan?

10. **LO 13.4** What kinds of risk and fear can occur if a person engages in unethical conduct?

Applying Your Knowledge

The emotions around the lunch table in the cafeteria at SSUMC ranged from somber to furious. The employees of the billing department had experienced many changes in the past week—none of them seemed good. Their beloved leader was gone and her replacement could not be more different. Moreover, he was asking the employees to do things that were not consistent with the ethical principles with which they had all grown very accustomed. He wasn't always asking them to do anything illegal, but it did sometimes seem unethical.

"I've had it—I'm going to quit," stormed Margaret, one of the top customer service representatives.

"That's great for you," said Morris, who posted payments. "Your family has two incomes and you can make it for a while on one. I can't."

"But we can't just sit here and do nothing," said Margaret.

"Can we go talk to Morales (the new CFO)?" asked Julian, a person responsible for working unpaid insurance claims.

"That won't do any good—he replaced Aisha. He's probably behind all of these changes," muttered Elinor, the person responsible for issuing refunds.

"So, what can we do?" asked Margaret again.

1. List at least three courses of action that one or more employees in the billing department should consider. Analyze the pros and cons of each option.

2. What could Aisha have done differently prior to her departure that might have made this situation better for the remaining employees?

3. Based on the information you learned in this chapter, what do you think are the causes of the change in ethical atmosphere? Which of the tools provided do you think would be the most effective in dealing with the issues?

4. Do you believe that talking with Mr. Porter is a viable option in dealing with this situation? Why or why not? If you decide that speaking with him is best, should you meet with him individually or as a group? Why?

5. To be ethical, does every employee need to respond in the same fashion? For example, is a person who resigns in protest more ethical than a person who tries to change the environment? Why or why not?

6. If you were one of the employees in the SSUMS billing department, what would *you* do? Why?

Internet Research

The Internet provides a wide variety of resources, both academic and practical, that discuss in detail the issues associated with ethical dilemmas in the workplace (Figure 13.5). These resources are valuable because they provide both information on the topic and support to readers who are facing ethical dilemmas.

1. Find three websites that discuss ethical dilemmas in the workplace. Summarize the focus of each site and identify the strengths and weaknesses.

2. If you created a website regarding resolving ethical dilemmas, what would you include? Explain why you would include those features. Is this similar to an existing website or would this be something not currently available?

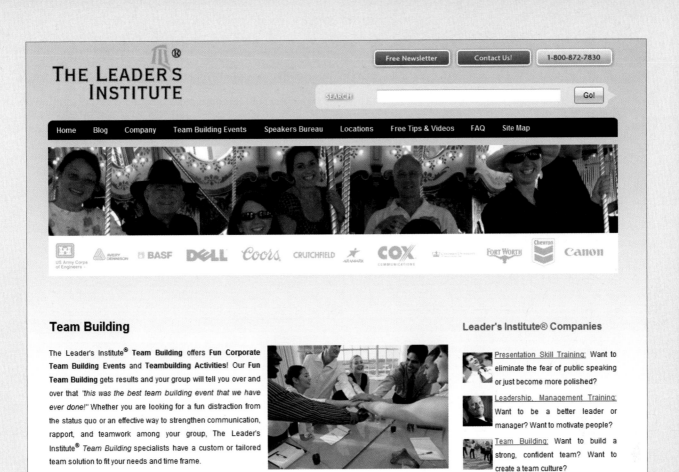

FIGURE 13.5
A variety of leadership and management websites provide resources to help people resolve conflict within the workplace.

Appendix A: AAPC Code of Ethics

Commitment to ethical professional conduct is expected of every AAPC member. The specification of a Code of Ethics enables AAPC to clarify to current and future members, and to those served by members, the nature of the ethical responsibilities held in common by its members. This document establishes principles that define the ethical behavior of AAPC members. All AAPC members are required to adhere to the Code of Ethics and the Code of Ethics will serve as the basis for processing ethical complaints initiated against AAPC members.

AAPC members shall:

- Maintain and enhance the dignity, status, integrity, competence, and standards of our profession.
- Respect the privacy of others and honor confidentiality
- Strive to achieve the highest quality, effectiveness and dignity in both the process and products of professional work.
- Advance the profession through continued professional development and education by acquiring and maintaining professional competence.
- Know and respect existing federal, state and local laws, regulations, certifications and licensing requirements applicable to professional work.
- Use only legal and ethical principles that reflect the profession's core values and report activity that is perceived to violate this Code of Ethics to the AAPC Ethics Committee.
- Accurately represent the credential(s) earned and the status of AAPC membership.
- Avoid actions and circumstances that may appear to compromise good business judgment or create a conflict between personal and professional interests.

Adherence to these standards assures public confidence in the integrity and service of medical coding, auditing, compliance and practice management professionals who are AAPC members.

Failure to adhere to these standards, as determined by AAPC's Ethics Committee, will result in the loss of credentials and membership with AAPC.

Source: Copyright © 2011 AAPC. All rights reserved.

Appendix B: AHIMA Code of Ethics

Preamble

The ethical obligations of the health information management (HIM) professional include the protection of patient privacy and confidential information; disclosure of information; development, use, and maintenance of health information systems and health records; and the quality of information. Both handwritten and computerized medical records contain many sacred stories—stories that must be protected on behalf of the individual and the aggregate community of persons served in the healthcare system. Healthcare consumers are increasingly concerned about the loss of privacy and the inability to control the dissemination of their protected information. Core health information issues include what information should be collected; how the information should be handled, who should have access to the information, and under what conditions the information should be disclosed.

Purpose of the American Health Information Management Association Code of Ethics

The HIM professional has an obligation to demonstrate actions that reflect values, ethical principles, and ethical guidelines. The American Health Information Management Association (AHIMA) Code of Ethics sets forth these values and principles to guide conduct. The code is relevant to all AHIMA members and credentialed HIM professionals and students, regardless of their professional functions, the settings in which they work, or the populations they serve.

The AHIMA Code of Ethics serves six purposes:

- Identifies core values on which the HIM mission is based.
- Summarizes broad ethical principles that reflect the profession's core values and establishes a set of ethical principles to be used to guide decision-making and actions.
- Helps HIM professionals identify relevant considerations when professional obligations conflict or ethical uncertainties arise.
- Provides ethical principles by which the general public can hold the HIM professional accountable.
- Socializes practitioners new to the field to HIM's mission, values, and ethical principles.
- Articulates a set of guidelines that the HIM professional can use to assess whether they have engaged in unethical conduct.

The Use of the Code

Violation of principles in this code does not automatically imply legal liability or violation of the law. Such determination can only be made in the context of legal and judicial proceedings. Alleged violations of the code would be subject to a peer review process. Such processes are generally separate from legal or administrative procedures and insulated from legal review or proceedings to allow the profession to counsel and discipline its own members although in some situations, violations of the code would constitute unlawful conduct subject to legal process.

A code of ethics cannot guarantee ethical behavior. Moreover, a code of ethics cannot resolve all ethical issues or disputes or capture the richness and complexity involved in striving to make responsible choices within a moral community. Rather, a code of ethics sets forth values and ethical principles, and offers ethical guidelines to which professionals aspire and by which their actions can be judged. Ethical behaviors result from a personal commitment to engage in ethical practice.

The code does not provide a set of rules that prescribe how to act in all situations. Specific applications of the code must take into account the context in which it is being considered and the possibility of conflicts among the code's values, principles, and guidelines. Ethical responsibilities flow from all human relationships, from the personal and familial to the social and professional. Further, the AHIMA Code of Ethics does not specify which values, principles, and guidelines are the most important and ought to outweigh others in instances when they conflict.

Code of Ethics 2004

Ethical Principles: The following ethical principles are based on the core values of the American Health Information Management Association and apply to all health information management professionals.

Health information management professionals:

Advocate, uphold and defend the individual's right to privacy and the doctrine of confidentiality in the use and disclosure of information.

Put service and the health and welfare of persons before self-interest and conduct themselves in the practice of the profession so as to bring honor to themselves, their peers, and to the health information management profession.

Preserve, protect, and secure personal health information in any form or medium and hold in the highest regard the contents of the records and other information of a confidential nature, taking into account the applicable statutes and regulations.

Refuse to participate in or conceal unethical practices or procedures.

Advance health information management knowledge and practice through continuing education, research, publications, and presentations.

Recruit and mentor students, peers and colleagues to develop and strengthen professional workforce.

Represent the profession accurately to the public.

Perform honorably health information management association responsibilities, either appointed or elected, and preserve the confidentiality of any privileged information made known in any official capacity.

State truthfully and accurately their credentials, professional education, and experiences.

Facilitate interdisciplinary collaboration in situations supporting health information practice.

Respect the inherent dignity and worth of every person.

How to Interpret the Code of Ethics

The following ethical principles are based on the core values of the American Health Information Management Association and apply to all health information management professionals. Guidelines included for each ethical principle are a non-inclusive list of behaviors and situations that can help to clarify the principle. They are not to be meant as a comprehensive list of all situations that can occur.

I. Advocate, uphold, and defend the individual's right to privacy and the doctrine of confidentiality in the use and disclosure of information.

Health information management professionals **shall:**

1.1 Protect all confidential information to include personal, health, financial, genetic, and outcome information.

1.2 Engage in social and political action that supports the protection of privacy and confidentiality, and be aware of the impact of the political arena on the health information system.

1.3 Protect the confidentiality of all information obtained in the course of professional service. Disclose only information that is directly relevant or necessary to achieve the purpose of disclosure.

1.4 Promote the obligation to respect privacy by respecting confidential information shared among colleagues, while responding to requests from the legal profession, the media, or other non-healthcare related individuals, during presentations or teaching and in situations that could cause harm to persons.

II. Put service and the health and welfare of persons before self-interest and conduct themselves in the practice of the profession so as to bring honor to themselves, their peers, and to the health information management profession.

Health information management professionals **shall:**

2.1 Act with integrity, behave in a trustworthy manner, elevate service to others above self-interest, and promote high standards of practice in every setting.

2.2 Be aware of the profession's mission, values, and ethical principles, and practice in a manner consistent with them by acting honestly and responsibly.

2.3 Anticipate, clarify, and avoid any conflict of interest, to all parties concerned, when dealing with consumers, consulting with competitors, or in providing services requiring potentially conflicting roles (for example, finding out information about one facility that would help a competitor).

2.4 Ensure that the working environment is consistent and encourages compliance with the AHIMA Code of Ethics, taking reasonable steps to eliminate any conditions in their organizations that violate, interfere with, or discourage compliance with the code.

2.5 Take responsibility and credit, including authorship credit, only for work they actually perform or to which they contribute.

Health information management professionals **shall not:**

2.6 Permit their private conduct to interfere with their ability to fulfill their professional responsibilities.

2.7 Take unfair advantage of any professional relationship or exploit others to further their personal, religious, political, or business interests.

III. Preserve, protect, and secure personal health information in any form or medium and hold in the highest regards the contents of the records and other information of a confidential nature obtained in the official capacity, taking into account the applicable statutes and regulations.

Health information management professionals shall:

3.1 Protect the confidentiality of patients' written and electronic records and other sensitive information.

3.2 Take precautions to ensure and maintain the confidentiality of information transmitted, transferred, or disposed of in the event of a termination, incapacitation, or death of a healthcare provider to other parties through the use of any media.

3.3 Inform recipients of the limitations and risks associated with providing services via electronic media (such as computer, telephone, fax, radio, and television).

IV. Refuse to participate in or conceal unethical practices or procedures.

Health information management professionals shall:

4.1 Act in a professional and ethical manner at all times.

4.2 Take adequate measures to discourage, prevent, expose, and correct the unethical conduct of colleagues.

4.3 Be knowledgeable about established policies and procedures for handling concerns about colleagues' unethical behavior.

4.4 Seek resolution if there is a belief that a colleague has acted unethically or if there is a belief of incompetence or impairment by discussing their concerns with the colleague when feasible and when such discussion is likely to be productive.

 4.5 Consult with a colleague when feasible and assist the colleague in taking remedial action when there is direct knowledge of a health information management colleague's incompetence or impairment.

 4.6 Health information management professionals shall not:

 4.7 Participate in, condone, or be associated with dishonesty, fraud and abuse, or deception. A non-inclusive list of examples includes:

- Allowing patterns of retrospective documentation to avoid suspension or increase reimbursement
- Assigning codes without physician documentation
- Coding when documentation does not justify the procedures that have been billed
- Coding an inappropriate level of service
- Miscoding to avoid conflict with others
- Engaging in negligent coding practices
- Hiding or ignoring review outcomes, such as performance data
- Failing to report licensure status for a physician through the appropriate channels
- Recording inaccurate data for accreditation purposes
- Hiding incomplete medical records
- Allowing inappropriate access to genetic, adoption, or behavioral health information
- Misusing sensitive information about a competitor
- Violating the privacy of individuals

V. Advance health information management knowledge and practice through continuing education, research, publications, and presentations.

Health information management professionals shall:

 5.1 Develop and enhance continually their professional expertise, knowledge, and skills (including appropriate education, research, training, consultation, and supervision).

 5.2 Base practice decisions on recognized knowledge, including empirically based knowledge relevant to health information management and health information management ethics.

 5.3 Contribute time and professional expertise to activities that promote respect for the value, integrity, and competence of the health information management profession.

 5.4 Engage in evaluation or research that ensures the anonymity or confidentiality of participants and of the data obtained from them by following guidelines developed for the participants in consultation with appropriate institutional review boards. Report evaluation and research findings accurately and take steps to correct any errors later found in published data using standard publication methods.

 5.5 Take reasonable steps to provide or arrange for continuing education and staff development, addressing current knowledge and emerging developments related to health information management practice and ethics.

 5.6 Health information management professionals shall not:

 5.7 Design or conduct evaluation or research that is in conflict with applicable federal or state laws.

 5.8 Participate in, condone, or be associated with fraud or abuse.

VI. Recruit and mentor students, peers and colleagues to develop and strengthen professional workforce.

Health information management professionals shall:

 6.1 Evaluate students' performance in a manner that is fair and respectful when functioning as educators or clinical internship supervisors.

6.2 Be responsible for setting clear, appropriate, and culturally sensitive boundaries for students.

6.3 Be a mentor for students, peers and new health information management professionals to develop and strengthen skills.

6.4 Provide directed practice opportunities for students.

Health information management professionals shall not:

6.5 Engage in any relationship with students in which there is a risk of exploitation or potential harm to the student.

VII. Accurately represent the profession to the public.

Health information management professionals shall:

7.1 Be an advocate for the profession in all settings and participate in activities that promote and explain the mission, values, and principles of the profession to the public.

VIII. Perform honorably health information management association responsibilities, either appointed or elected, and preserve the confidentiality of any privileged information made known in any official capacity.

Health information management professionals shall:

8.1 Perform responsibly all duties as assigned by the professional association.

8.2 Resign from an Association position if unable to perform the assigned responsibilities with competence.

8.3 Speak on behalf of professional health information management organizations, accurately representing the official and authorized positions of the organizations.

IX. State truthfully and accurately their credentials, professional education, and experiences.

Health information management professionals shall:

9.1 Make clear distinctions between statements made and actions engaged in as a private individual and as a representative of the health information management profession, a professional health information organization, or the health information management professional's employer.

9.2 Claim and ensure that their representations to patients, agencies, and the public of professional qualifications, credentials, education, competence, affiliations, services provided, training, certification, consultation received, supervised experience, other relevant professional experience are accurate.

9.3 Claim only those relevant professional credentials actually possessed and correct any inaccuracies occurring regarding credentials.

X. Facilitate interdisciplinary collaboration in situations supporting health information practice.

Health information management professionals shall:

10.1 Participate in and contribute to decisions that affect the well-being of patients by drawing on the perspectives, values, and experiences of those involved in decisions related to patients.

XI. Respect the inherent dignity and worth of every person.

Health information management professionals shall:

11.1 Treat each person in a respectful fashion, being mindful of individual differences and cultural and ethnic diversity.

11.2 Promote the value of self-determination for each individual.

Source: *Revised and adopted by AHIMA House of Delegates, July 1, 2004. Copyright © 2004 American Health Information Management Association. All rights reserved.*

Appendix C: AHIMA Standards of Ethical Coding

Introduction

The Standards of Ethical Coding are based on the American Health Information Management Association's (AHIMA's) Code of Ethics. Both sets of principles reflect expectations of professional conduct for coding professionals involved in diagnostic and/or procedural coding or other health record data abstraction.

A Code of Ethics sets forth professional values and ethical principles and offers ethical guidelines to which professionals aspire and by which their actions can be judged. Health information management (HIM) professionals are expected to demonstrate professional values by their actions to patients, employers, members of the healthcare team, the public, and the many stakeholders they serve. A Code of Ethics is important in helping to guide the decision-making process and can be referenced by individuals, agencies, organizations, and bodies (such as licensing and regulatory boards, insurance providers, courts of law, government agencies, and other professional groups).

The AHIMA Code of Ethics (available on the AHIMA web site) is relevant to all AHIMA members and credentialed HIM professionals and students, regardless of their professional functions, the settings in which they work, or the populations they serve. Coding is one of the core HIM functions, and due to the complex regulatory requirements affecting the health information coding process, coding professionals are frequently faced with ethical challenges. The AHIMA Standards of Ethical Coding are intended to assist coding professionals and managers in decision-making processes and actions, outline expectations for making ethical decisions in the workplace, and demonstrate coding professionals' commitment to integrity during the coding process, regardless of the purpose for which the codes are being reported. They are relevant to all coding professionals and those who manage the coding function, regardless of the healthcare setting in which they work or whether they are AHIMA members or nonmembers.

These Standards of Ethical Coding have been revised in order to reflect the current healthcare environment and modern coding practices. The previous revision was published in 1999.

Standards of Ethical Coding

Coding professionals should:

1. Apply accurate, complete, and consistent coding practices for the production of high-quality healthcare data.
2. Report all healthcare data elements (e.g., diagnosis and procedure codes, present on admission indicator, discharge status) required for external reporting purposes (e.g., reimbursement and other administrative uses, population health, quality and patient safety measurement, and research) completely and accurately, in accordance with regulatory and documentation standards and requirements and applicable official coding conventions, rules, and guidelines.
3. Assign and report only the codes and data that are clearly and consistently supported by health record documentation in accordance with applicable code set and abstraction conventions, rules, and guidelines.
4. Query provider (physician or other qualified healthcare practitioner) for clarification and additional documentation prior to code assignment when there is conflicting, incomplete, or ambiguous information in the

health record regarding a significant reportable condition or procedure or other reportable data element dependent on health record documentation (e.g., present on admission indicator).

5. Refuse to change reported codes or the narratives of codes so that meanings are misrepresented.

6. Refuse to participate in or support coding or documentation practices intended to inappropriately increase payment, qualify for insurance policy coverage, or skew data by means that do not comply with federal and state statutes, regulations and official rules and guidelines.

7. Facilitate interdisciplinary collaboration in situations supporting proper coding practices.

8. Advance coding knowledge and practice through continuing education.

9. Refuse to participate in or conceal unethical coding or abstraction practices or procedures.

10. Protect the confidentiality of the health record at all times and refuse to access protected health information not required for coding-related activities (examples of coding-related activities include completion of code assignment, other health record data abstraction, coding audits, and educational purposes).

11. Demonstrate behavior that reflects integrity, shows a commitment to ethical and legal coding practices, and fosters trust in professional activities.

Source: Revised and approved by the House of Delegates, September 2008.

How to Interpret the Standards of Ethical Coding

The following ethical principles are based on the core values of the American Health Information Management Association and the AHIMA Code of Ethics and apply to all coding professionals. Guidelines for each ethical principle include examples of behaviors and situations that can help to clarify the principle. They are not meant as a comprehensive list of all situations that can occur.

1. *Apply accurate, complete, and consistent coding practices for the production of high-quality healthcare data.*

   Coding professionals and those who manage coded data shall:

   1.1 Support selection of appropriate diagnostic, procedure and other types of health service related codes (e.g., present on admission indicator, discharge status).

   Example:

   Policies and procedures are developed and used as a framework for the work process, and education and training is provided on their use.

   1.2 Develop and comply with comprehensive internal coding policies and procedures that are consistent with official coding rules and guidelines, reimbursement regulations and policies and prohibit coding practices that misrepresent the patient's medical conditions and treatment provided or are not supported by the health record documentation.

   Example:

   Code assignment resulting in misrepresentation of facts carries significant consequences.

   1.3 Participate in the development of institutional coding policies and ensure that coding policies complement, and do not conflict with, official coding rules and guidelines.

   1.4 Foster an environment that supports honest and ethical coding practices resulting in accurate and reliable data.

Coding professionals **shall not:**

    1.5 Participate in improper preparation, alteration, or suppression of coded information.

2. *Report all healthcare data elements (e.g., diagnosis and procedure codes, present on admission indicator, discharge status) required for external reporting purposes (e.g., reimbursement and other administrative uses, population health, public data reporting, quality and patient safety measurement, research) completely and accurately, in accordance with regulatory and documentation standards and requirements and applicable official coding conventions, rules, and guidelines.*

Coding professionals **shall:**

    2.1 Adhere to the ICD coding conventions, official coding guidelines approved by the Cooperating Parties,[1] the CPT rules established by the American Medical Association, and any other official coding rules and guidelines established for use with mandated standard code sets.

    Example:

    Appropriate resource tools that assist coding professionals with proper sequencing and reporting to stay in compliance with existing reporting requirements are available and used.

    2.2 Select and sequence diagnosis and procedure codes in accordance with the definitions of required data sets for applicable healthcare settings.

    2.3 Comply with AHIMA's standards governing data reporting practices, including health record documentation and clinician query standards.

3. *Assign and report only the codes that are clearly and consistently supported by health record documentation in accordance with applicable code set conventions, rules, and guidelines.*

Coding professionals **shall:**

    3.1 Apply skills, knowledge of currently mandated coding and classification systems, and official resources to select the appropriate diagnostic and procedural codes (including applicable modifiers), and other codes representing healthcare services (including substances, equipment, supplies, or other items used in the provision of healthcare services).

    Example:

    Failure to research or confirm the appropriate code for a clinical condition not indexed in the classification, or reporting a code for the sake of convenience or to affect reporting for a desired effect on the results, is considered unethical.

4. *Query provider (physician or other qualified healthcare practitioner) for clarification and additional documentation prior to code assignment when there is conflicting, incomplete, or ambiguous information in the health record regarding a significant reportable condition or procedure or other reportable data element dependent on health record documentation (e.g., present on admission indicator).*

Coding professionals **shall:**

    4.1 Participate in the development of query policies that support documentation improvement and meet regulatory, legal, and ethical standards for coding and reporting.

    4.2 Query the provider for clarification when documentation in the health record that impacts an externally reportable data element is illegible, incomplete, unclear, inconsistent, or imprecise.

---

[1]The Cooperating Parties are the American Health Information Management Association, American Hospital Association, Centers for Medicare & Medicaid Services, and National Center for Health Statistics.

4.3 Use queries as a communication tool to improve the accuracy of code assignment and the quality of health record documentation, not to inappropriately increase reimbursement or misrepresent quality of care.

Example:

Policies regarding the circumstances when clinicians should be queried are designed to promote complete and accurate coding and complete documentation, regardless of whether reimbursement will be affected.

Coding professionals **shall not:**

4.4 Query the provider when there is no clinical information in the health record prompting the need for a query.

Example:

Query the provider regarding the presence of gram-negative pneumonia on every pneumonia case, regardless of whether there are any clinical indications of gram-negative pneumonia documented in the record.

5. *Refuse to change reported codes or the narratives of codes so that meanings are misrepresented.*

Coding professionals **shall not:**

5.1 Change the description for a diagnosis or procedure code or other reported data element so that it does not accurately reflect the official definition of that code.

Example:

The description of a code is altered in the encoding software, resulting in incorrect reporting of this code.

6. *Refuse to participate in or support coding or documentation practices intended to inappropriately increase payment, qualify for insurance policy coverage, or skew data by means that do not comply with federal and state statutes, regulations and official rules and guidelines.*

Coding professionals **shall:**

6.1 Select and sequence the codes such that the organization receives the optimal payment to which the facility is legally entitled, remembering that it is unethical and illegal to increase payment by means that contradict regulatory guidelines.

Coding professionals **shall not:**

6.2 Misrepresent the patient's clinical picture through intentional incorrect coding or omission of diagnosis or procedure codes, or the addition of diagnosis or procedure codes unsupported by health record documentation, to inappropriately increase reimbursement, justify medical necessity, improve publicly reported data, or qualify for insurance policy coverage benefits.

Examples:

A patient has a health plan that excludes reimbursement for reproductive management or contraception; so rather than report the correct code for admission for tubal ligation, it is reported as a medically necessary condition with performance of a salpingectomy. The narrative descriptions of both the diagnosis and procedures reflect an admission for tubal ligation and the procedure (tubal ligation) is displayed on the record.

A code is changed at the patient's request so that the service will be covered by the patient's insurance.

Coding professionals **shall not:**

6.3 Inappropriately exclude diagnosis or procedure codes in order to misrepresent the quality of care provided.

Examples:

Following a surgical procedure, a patient acquired an infection due to a break in sterile procedure; the appropriate code for the surgical complication is omitted from the claims submission to avoid any adverse outcome to the institution.

Quality outcomes are reported inaccurately in order to improve a healthcare organization's quality profile or pay-for-performance results.

7. *Facilitate interdisciplinary collaboration in situations supporting proper coding practices.*

   Coding professionals **shall:**

   7.1 Assist and educate physicians and other clinicians by advocating proper documentation practices, further specificity, and re-sequence or include diagnoses or procedures when needed to more accurately reflect the acuity, severity, and the occurrence of events.

   Example:

   Failure to advocate for ethical practices that seek to represent the truth in events as expressed by the associated code sets when needed is considered an intentional disregard of these standards.

8. *Advance coding knowledge and practice through continuing education.*

   Coding professionals **shall:**

   8.1 Maintain and continually enhance coding competency (e.g., through participation in educational programs, reading official coding publications such as the Coding Clinic for ICD-9-CM, and maintaining professional certifications) in order to stay abreast of changes in codes, coding guidelines, and regulatory and other requirements.

9. *Refuse to participate in or conceal unethical coding practices or procedures.*

   Coding professionals **shall:**

   9.1 Act in a professional and ethical manner at all times.

   9.2 Take adequate measures to discourage, prevent, expose, and correct the unethical conduct of colleagues.

   9.3 Be knowledgeable about established policies and procedures for handling concerns about colleagues' unethical behavior.

   9.4 Seek resolution if there is a belief that a colleague has acted unethically or if there is a belief of incompetence or impairment by discussing their concerns with the colleague when feasible and when such discussion is likely to be productive.

   9.5 Consult with a colleague when feasible and assist the colleague in taking remedial action when there is direct knowledge of a health information management colleague's incompetence or impairment.

   Coding professionals **shall not:**

   9.6 Participate in, condone, or be associated with dishonesty, fraud and abuse, or deception. A non-exhaustive list of examples includes:

   - Allowing inappropriate patterns of retrospective documentation to avoid suspension or increase reimbursement
   - Assigning codes without supporting provider (physician or other qualified healthcare practitioner) documentation
   - Coding when documentation does not justify the diagnoses and/or procedures that have been billed
   - Coding an inappropriate level of service
   - Miscoding to avoid conflict with others
   - Adding, deleting, and altering health record documentation
   - Copying and pasting another clinician's documentation without identification of the original author and date
   - Knowingly reporting incorrect present on admission indicator
   - Knowingly reporting incorrect patient discharge status code
   - Engaging in negligent coding practices

10. *Protect the confidentiality of the health record at all times and refuse to access protected health information not required for coding-related*

activities (examples of coding-related activities include completion of code assignment, other health record data abstraction, coding audits, and educational purposes).

Coding professionals **shall:**

10.1 Protect all confidential information obtained in the course of professional service, including personal, health, financial, genetic, and outcome information.

10.2 Access only that information necessary to perform their duties.

11. *Demonstrate behavior that reflects integrity, shows a commitment to ethical and legal coding practices, and fosters trust in professional activities.*

Coding professionals **shall:**

11.1 Act in an honest manner and bring honor to self, peers, and the profession.

11.2 Truthfully and accurately represent their credentials, professional education, and experience.

11.3 Demonstrate ethical principles and professional values in their actions to patients, employers, other members of the healthcare team, consumers, and other stakeholders served by the healthcare data they collect and report.

A

Absolute Nonnegotiable, unchangeable.

Abstractor A billing/coding professional (usually in a facility setting) who is responsible for identifying diagnosis codes by reviewing the medical record.

Abuse Excessively or improperly using government resources.

Accommodative approach An approach to ethics in which the individuals or businesses behave legally and ethically and do their best to balance the interests of different stakeholders, even in difficult situations.

Accounts receivable (A/R) The cumulative amount of all balances due to a provider by insurers and/or patients.

Accreditation entity An organization that gives recognition to an individual or group that meets certain standards. In addition, the organization usually offers an assurance or guarantee that the recognized person has knowledge about a given subject area.

Acute condition Condition in which the symptoms are sharp, severe, or intense in effect.

Adjudicate To settle or determine.

Administrative costs In the case of an insurance company, it is the cost of real estate, employee salaries and benefits, advertising, and so on.

Advance beneficiary notice (ABN) A document that must be signed by patients covered by Medicare, whenever they are receiving services that may not be covered by the Medicare program in circumstances when they are receiving the service more frequently than Medicare allows or they do not have a diagnosis that is required for the service to be covered.

Affirmative unethical act An active choice to engage in an unethical act.

Algorithm A computational procedure that arrives at the correct solution through a step-by-step process.

Allowed amount The amount that a payer will recognize as the reimbursable amount for a particular CPT code.

Ambulatory surgery center Ambulatory surgery centers (ASCs) are defined differently in different locations. Services provided in ASCs are usually not urgent or emergent in nature, the surgeries are not "major" in the sense they do not require long-term hospitalization, and they are often owned by nonhospital entities, such as corporations or physician groups.

Applied ethics The application of ethical principles to real-world situations.

Apprentice A person who is learning a trade, often working under the supervision of another, more experienced person.

Arbiter A person with the power to make judgments or rulings.

Aspirational Establishing an objective or goal to be achieved; something to which someone aspires.

B

Billing cycle The amount of time that passes between each billing statement sent to patients.

Billing protocol The specific pattern and guidelines for billing medical services to insurance companies.

Bundling Billing for a package of related services, instead of billing for every element provided in the course of a procedure.

Business model The rationale of how a business creates and delivers value. A plan as to how the company will conduct business.

C

Capitated A third-party reimbursement program that compensates providers on a per-patient basis—not on a production basis. Generally, insurers pay providers a fixed amount per month for each patient assigned to them, whether or not the provider supplies treatment in that month. The purpose of this methodology is to discourage providers from supplying unnecessary services and to spread some of the financial risk.

Carved out In some negotiations, services that are ordinarily included as part of the agreement are separated from the negotiated payment. A service that is designated as separately payable is considered carved out of the agreement.

Cash flow A significant measure of a company's health. It is calculated by taking cash receipts and subtracting cash payments (expenses) for a specific period. Cash flow is important to ensure that a company can meet its obligations at a given time. A company can be very successful in sales, but if collections on those sales are not efficient or effective, the company may not have enough cash on hand to pay its bills.

Chief complaint A brief summary that describes why the patient presents for treatment during that encounter.

Chronic condition A condition that is constant or habitual, but may or may not be particularly intense at any given time.

Chronological Time-based; usually presented in order from first to last.

Clean claim A claim submitted to a third-party payer that has no errors that originated in the provider office.

Codification Formalized, written organization of rules or guidelines.

Cognitive Mental processes related to memory, judgment, and reasoning. For physicians, this usually involves making diagnoses based on observation, examination, and analysis of relevant data.

Coinsurance An amount, usually a percentage of the total or allowed charge, that is due from the patient for medical care.

Collegial Communication that occurs among a group of colleagues. Generally perceived to be friendly and mutually beneficial.

Commensurate Appropriate or proportionate, fair.

Commodities Articles of trade or commerce; something useful that can be turned to commercial or other advantage.

Comorbidity (CG) A coexisting, but unrelated disease process.

Compliance program Established by health care entities to ensure that the conduct of their billing program meets both internal and governmental requirements for the performance of the billing task. Compliance programs usually consist of an audit component, by which the quality of compliance is measured and protocols for addressing compliance deficiencies are prescribed.

Complicit Cooperative in a project or process, usually with the implication that the action is inappropriate or illegal. With insurance fraud, a person could voluntarily give his or her insurance card to another person to use, or could refuse to cooperate with authorities if the card is misused by a friend or family member.

Consultation A type of evaluation and management (E/M) service provided by a physician at the request of another physician or other appropriate source to either recommend care for a specific condition or problem *or* to determine whether to accept responsibility for entire care or care of a specific condition or problem.

Continuing education unit (CEU) A measurement of educational services received. Most accreditation organizations equate one hour of classroom or lecture time with one CEU.

Conundrum A puzzling or difficult situation.

Convention Rule or method of conducting a task.

Copayment Generally a fixed dollar amount, such as $10, $20, or $50, that must be paid as part of the patient's insurance agreement each time a patient visits a provider.

Corporate integrity agreement (CIA) A program often required by the federal government when a provider or institution is found to be noncompliant in its billing/coding practices. The purpose is to facilitate monitoring of future billing and ensure corrective action on the part of the provider.

Cottage industry A small-scale, loosely organized industry.

Credential Place the person through a specified approval process. Usually, the mid-level practitioner is also listed separately in the payer's provider manual when it is individually credentialed.

Culpable Deserving blame; legitimately held responsible.

D

De facto arbiter A decision maker who was not specifically assigned the task, but became the decision maker through a chain of events or by default.

Deductible The financial responsibility of the patient that must be met prior to his or her insurer making any payments for the medical services.

Defensive approach An approach to ethics in which the individuals or businesses are ethical to the degree that they

are required to do so by law, but they take no steps beyond the minimum standards of the law to be ethical.

Deferred compensation A form of compensation in which payment is delayed until some later date. The most common types of deferred compensation are pensions, retirement plans, and stock options. The primary advantage for the employee is that taxes are deferred until the compensation is actually received.

Deontological ethics An ethical system that focuses on the action itself, regardless of the result that it produces.

Diagnosis-related group (DRG) A payment system for inpatient hospital services. Payments are issued based on the patient's diagnosis and not on the quantity of service provided to the patient.

Differential diagnoses A list of possible diagnoses, based on the symptoms present, that are gradually ruled out until the final diagnosis is determined.

Discharged A person who has been released from the practice, no longer able to be seen as a patient, usually as the result of the need for some sort of disciplinary action.

Documentation Guidelines (DG) A document created by the Centers for Medicare and Medicaid Services (CMS) to provide direction as to the documentation requirements necessary for the use of a particular evaluation and management (E/M) code. The first version was published in 1995, with a second version published in 1997.

Due diligence Satisfactory performance of a person's duties at a minimally acceptable level. Usually involves research or investigation.

Dysmenorrhea Painful menstrual periods.

E

Economies of scale The principle that products and services can be provided on a more cost-efficient basis (per unit) when produced in larger batches.

Emergent Requiring immediate action or attention to prevent permanent physical harm.

Entitlement mentality A guarantee of access to benefits by right or by law. In more common language, it is the belief that a person deserves or has a right to a benefit—most commonly paid for by a third party.

Erosion of agency The theory that people are more likely to allow their moral

positions or beliefs to "erode" when they are acting on behalf of another party (agency), such as an employer.

Essential modifier Appears within the alphabetic index of the ICD-9-CM code book. For the code to be used, the patient must have the condition described in the modifier.

Ethical challenge Ethics are the philosphical framework on which decision making is conducted or, more practically, the guiding principles uses to determine how to behave. That philosphical framework or those principles are challenged when the situation calls for a response in which the "right" or "consistent" thing may produce an uncomfortable or undesirable result.

Ethical dilemma An occasion when a person is in a point of decision concerning a conflict between his or her *values* and the *action* the person will ultimately take.

Ethical relativism An ethical theory in which the definition of *ethical* varies from circumstance to circumstance and person to person.

Ethics officer A designated person within an organization with the responsibility to ensure that the ethics policies of the organization are followed consistently.

Exemplary Worthy of imitation or commendable.

Explanation of benefits (EOB) The form provided by third-party payers to both providers and patients, informing them of the way in which a particular claim was processed.

Exploratory A surgical procedure performed to diagnose a condition or otherwise visualize the internal organs.

Extenuating Explanatory or unusual.

Extrapolation Making an assumption about an entire group based on a relatively small sample of that group.

Extricate To remove from entanglement or complication.

F

Flexible spending account (FSA) A benefit program offered by many employers that allows employees to put away money on a pretax basis to cover out-of-pocket health care expenses such as copayments, deductibles, and other non-covered medical services.

Fraud The intentional submission of a claim that has inaccurate or misleading information to obtain payment to which the person submitting the claim is not entitled.

G

Global period Many payers have established rules that all services provided in a given period of time before or after a major procedure are assumed to be associated with that procedure. Payment for the care related to that procedure is included in the reimbursement for the procedure itself and therefore related services within the global period are not separately billable or payable.

Global procedure The concept that the reimbursement for a particular procedure includes the services before and after the procedure, as well as all of the individual components required to complete the procedure.

H

Health maintenance organizations (HMOs) HMOs were developed with the intended purpose of reducing health care costs by improving the general health of the patients. This was originally accomplished by requiring that all services provided to a given patient be provided or approved by a single physician. This theoretically would ensure that one physician was supervising the patient's care and that unnecessary medical services would not be provided.

Health Insurance Portability and Accountability Act (HIPAA) Most commonly, HIPAA is considered the law that specifies privacy rules and regulations when dealing with protected health information (PHI). However, this is just one element of HIPAA. Its primary and original purpose was to allow patients to obtain health coverage without underwriting or preexisting condition limitations when a person changed jobs. Other elements of the law include security regulations, code set definitions, and the requirement of filing claims to insurance electronically.

History of present illness (HPI) A chronological description of the development of the patient's present illness from the first sign and/or symptom to the present.

I

Imminent Likely to occur at any moment; happening soon.

Implied warranty of merchantability The legal principle that a product or service must do what it is advertised to do.

Inadvertent Unintentional or caused by a lack of care.

Incident to A concept associated with the Medicare program in which employed nonphysician practitioners, such as nurse practitioners or physician assistants, are allowed to bill under the name and identification number of the employing physician. In effect, the non-physician provider is acting as an extension of the physician, providing services that are incident to other services delivered by the physician. There are very specific rules concerning the circumstances in which this billing can occur.

Individual ethics Personal standards and values that determine how people view their responsibilities to other people and groups and how they should act when their own self-interests are at stake.

Intractable Unmanageable; impossible to resolve cooperatively.

Intranet A computer network with restricted access, such as an internal company network.

Intuitive A perception of truth, without any particular reasoning process.

Iteration A procedure in which an operation is repeated, often to achieve the desired result more closely. There were several iterations of the various claim forms, with each one an improvement over the previous version.

J

Justice theory A theory that is consistent with "rights theory," but also includes an element that seeks justice by ensuring that the prospects of the least fortunate are as great as they can be.

L

Late effects Conditions that remain after the acute phase of an injury or illness is over.

Laterality The sides of the body on which a disease is located or a procedure is performed.

Lowest common denominator A mathematics term referring to least common value; the lowest common standard.

M

Macroeconomics The study of an economy at the highest level, such as that of an entire nation, a particular sector of the economy, and so forth. It does not involve the study of economics as it relates to individual people or companies.

Market share The percentage of the total number of possible enrollees insured by a given company in a given marketplace.

Meaningful Use Federal guidelines that encourage openness and improvements in health care by setting standards for electronic health record (EHR) software.

Medicaid Medicaid was created at the same time as Medicare, with a focus on caring for low-income children, their caretaker relatives, elderly and blind individuals, and individuals with disabilities. Over the years, eligibility for Medicaid coverage expanded. The addition of coverage for pregnant women and infants in 1986 was the most significant addition to the coverage.

Medical decision making The selection of the best possible course of action to treat a particular patient's condition.

Medical necessity The provision of services that are appropriate to treat the patient's condition.

Medicare Medicare was signed into law on July 30, 1965, 20 years after President Harry Truman first proposed it. Its original purpose was to ensure health insurance coverage to elderly people, and the Social Security Administration operated it. Later it was expanded to include other groups of people, such as people with disabilities and certain severe diseases. In 1977, the Health Care Financing Administration (HCFA) was created and the oversight of Medicare was shifted to this government agency.

Medicare carrier A company that contracts with the federal government to process Medicare claims from physicians and other providers in a given state or region.

Metaethics A discipline that investigates where ethical principles come from and what they mean.

Mitigate To make less severe; to minimize damage.

Modifier A two-digit numeric code indicating that a service or procedure that has been performed has been altered by some specific circumstance, but not changed in its definition or code. Modifiers also enable health care professionals to effectively respond to payment policy requirements established by other entities.

Morbidity The statistical reporting of the incidence of disease.

Mortality The statistical reporting of the incidence of death.

N

National Correct Coding Initiative (NCCI) edits A publication of guidelines that detail what codes can and cannot be billed during the same encounter. It serves, in part, as the definition of what services are bundled.

Neoplasm Abnormally fast-growing tissue. Malignant neoplasms are considered cancerous in nature.

Net revenue Often exchangeable with the term *profit,* it refers to the amount of money that remains after expenses are subtracted from income.

Nonessential modifier Appears in parentheses after the code; the patient *may* have the condition described, but is not required to have the condition for the code to be used.

Nonparticipating When no contract exists between a third-party payer and a provider.

Normative ethics An attempt to establish "normal" ethical standards for behavior, based on metaethical principles.

O

Objectivity Free of personal bias; accurate interpretation of reality.

Obsolete No longer in general use; out-of-date.

Obstructionist approach An approach to ethics in which the individuals or businesses are aware of right and wrong and the basic principles of ethics, but choose not to follow them.

Occupational ethics Standards that govern the manner in which members of a profession, trade, or craft, conduct themselves while working within the context of their industry.

Office of Inspector General (OIG) An arm of the federal government responsible for the investigation and enforcement of rules and regulations of a given governmental department (e.g., Office of Inspector General of the Department of Health and Human Services).

Operability The ability of a product to function according to its stated capabilities.

Ophthalmic Related to the eye.

Organizational ethics Standards that govern the manner in which members of a particular company or organization conduct themselves in their role as an employee of the entity.

Outlier Something that occurs outside the expected or normal range.

Outpatient surgery center Outpatient surgery centers are similar to ASCs, with the primary difference being that they are usually affiliated with hospitals and/or are located in conjunction with a hospital facility. This is not a universal rule as hospitals sometimes own ASCs and definitions may vary based on geographic location.

Overcoding Selecting an evaluation and management (E/M) code that is above the level documented in the medical record.

Overcommunicate A common principle in management theory that recommends that more communication than would normally be perceived as necessary be performed to ensure that the message reaches its intended audience with an appropriate level of effect.

Overzealousness Excessively interested or committed to a cause.

P

Paradigm A model, pattern, or way of thinking.

Participating When a contract exists between a third-party payer and a provider to supply services to the insured in exchange for a negotiated reimbursement rate.

Past, family, and/or social history (PFSH) The recording of components of the patient's past used in helping the physician diagnose and properly treat the patient.

Pay-for-performance New programs by which providers are compensated by payers based on the quality of care that they deliver, not simply the number of procedures. The quality measures are often defined by the billing codes submitted.

Payment differential Medicare pays mid-level providers 85% of the amount that physicians are paid for any given service.

Policy A course of action adopted and followed by an organization to provide guidance in future conduct.

Postoperative period The period following a surgical procedure during which any services related to that procedure are provided.

Preauthorization Similar to a referral, except that it is usually provided directly by the insurance company to the physician who desires to provide a service.

Generally, these services are either expensive diagnostic tests or surgery.

Preoperative period The period prior to a surgical procedure during which any services related to that procedure are provided.

Prepaid Historically, the consumer paid the hospital or insurer prior to requiring the service. In exchange, the hospital or insurer would provide service to the consumer when the consumer required it.

Prescriptive Giving direction or instruction.

Price controls Price controls have been implemented by the U.S. government on several occasions, including both world wars, the Korean Conflict, and by the Nixon administration between 1971 and 1973. The theory behind these controls is that it will limit and control inflation—the dramatic increase of prices. However, most economists do not agree that these are useful in controlling inflation and, in fact, they have many unintended consequences.

Principal diagnosis The condition chiefly responsible for causing the admission of the patient to the hospital.

Proactive approach An approach to ethics in which the individuals or businesses specifically go out of their way to conduct themselves in an ethical fashion.

Professional component (PC) The services delivered in conjunction with a procedure by the provider, including the performance of the procedure, the interpretation of the results, and the preparation of a report.

Proficiency Demonstrating skill; an expert.

Profit margin Total revenue less total expenses in producing that revenue. For example, if a company collected $100 in the sale of product, and it cost $98 to produce that product, the profit margin would be $2.00.

Profit maximization An ethical theory that focuses on results (profits), but requires that it occur within the constraints of the law.

Prognosis A professional opinion of the likelihood of a particular outcome.

Proprietary Privately owned and controlled.

Protocol Formal rules, guidelines, and regulations adopted by an organization to ensure specific, consistent conduct in the future.

Publicly traded A company that sells shares in the company on a public stock exchange. A private company can sell interests in the company only with the agreement of the owners of the company. The selling of shares in a company is one way to raise large sums of capital to facilitate the operation and expansion of the business.

Q

Quantified Defined; concretely measured.

R

Reciprocal Given or felt by each toward the other; treating each other in a similar or identical fashion.

Referrals A tool used by health maintenance organizations (HMOs) and health insurers, intended to ensure that the appropriate level of care is delivered. In most cases, before a patient can receive specialty care, the patient's primary care physician must approve the service via a referral. The assumption is that the primary care physician will not approve an unnecessary service.

Resource-based relative value scale (RBRVS) A reimbursement/compensation system introduced in 1992 as the method of payment for services provided to Medicare patients. Since that time, many commercial insurers have adopted this system for their physician compensation systems. Each CPT code is assigned a work value, a practice expense value, and a malpractice value. These values are multiplied by a conversion factor to determine the amount of payment for each CPT code.

Return on investment (ROI) A calculation that defines the length of time needed to recover the expenditure associated with a project and make the project financially advantageous.

Revenue The total amounts of money received by a company before any deductions, such as expenses, are made.

Revenue cycle The period of time that occurs between the initiation of service and the time that payment for service is received. For a cash transaction, the revenue cycle is virtually zero. In health care, the revenue cycle can extend from 30 to 90 days and more.

Review of systems (ROS) An inventory of body systems obtained through a series of questions seeking to identify signs and/or symptoms that the patient may be experiencing or has experienced.

Rights theory A theory that states the belief that certain human *rights* are fundamental and should be respected by all other humans.

Risk pooling The concept in which a group of people join together in anticipation of a possible undesirable event such as injury, illness, property damage, or death. Statistically, not all people will experience that adverse event during the period in which the risk is pooled. Therefore, everyone pays a relatively small amount in exchange for compensation/coverage if the adverse event happens to them. Those who do not experience the event will have paid more than they otherwise would, but they are offered "peace of mind" in knowing that they would be protected if the event occurred. Those who do experience the event obtain protection at a cost significantly less than if they had to pay the expenses associated with the event.

Rorschach test A psychological test in which participants explain what they think an inkblot looks like, used to gain insight into the participant's mindset and assumptions.

S

Secured debt Debt for which the lender has some means to require repayment, or the option to repossess the item purchased.

Sequelae Negative effects of a previous disease.

Sign Physical manifestation that can be felt, heard, measured, or observed by medical professionals.

Situational ethics A theory in which judgment can be rendered about a behavior only if the judge knows all of the relevant details associated with the situation.

Societal ethics Standards that govern how members of a society should deal with one another in matters such as fairness, justice, poverty, and the rights of the individual.

Stakeholder A person with an interest in a company or organization; usually financial, sometimes personal.

Standardized Universally used, understood, and accepted in the same fashion.

Stock options Often used by companies to compensate employees without immediate financial expense, stock options are generally given to employees as part of their compensation package. The advantage of a stock option for the company is that it costs nothing at the

time. The advantage of a stock option for the employee is that if the value of the company goes up, so does the value of the stock. Therefore, the stock option may eventually be worth much more than its cash value at the time it was issued.

Subordinate The employee who reports to a particular individual.

Superbill Charge ticket; a tool (often paper) on which the provider marks the services provided and diagnoses associated with the visit.

Supply and demand curves A fundamental component of economic theory, it is believed that as demand increases, supply decreases, resulting in higher prices. Conversely, if supply exceeds demand, then prices will fall.

Symptom Abnormal physical experience that is subjective in nature, that cannot be seen or confirmed by health care providers.

T

Technical component (TC) The technical aspects of delivering a procedure, including the purchase, maintenance, and operation of the required equipment; compensation for the staff that performs or assists in the exam; and the general overhead associated with the care delivery.

Teleological ethics An ethical system that focuses on the results of an action, as opposed to underlying principles or rules.

Time value of money The principle that the possession of money now is more valuable than the potential of receiving money in the future.

Transposition The improper interchange of two or more numbers within a sequence. For example, the ID number A123456 could be typed in as A123465. In this case, the numbers "5" and "6" are transposed.

U

Unbundling The improper practice of billing separately for every service element provided in the course of a procedure.

Undercoding Selecting an evaluation and management (E/M) code that is below the level documented in the medical record.

Unsecured debt Debt for which the lender's only recourse if the debt is unpaid is to sue the borrower in civil court.

Urgent Requiring action or attention in the very near future to prevent permanent physical harm.

Usual, customary, and reasonable (UCR) rates As a payment methodology, third-party payers made determinations about the amount they would pay for each service. The term adopted by the payers for these rates was UCR.

Value A principle that someone considers important.

Venue The scene of an action or event; a location.

Veracity Correctness or accuracy.

Verification Evidence that establishes or confirms the validity or truth of something.

Vignette Brief case study.

Virtue ethics An ethical system that is based on the idea that a person's life should be committed to the achievement of an ideal or ideals (virtues).

Wage controls Wage controls have been implemented by the U.S. government on several occasions, including both world wars, the Korean Conflict, and by the Nixon administration between 1971 and 1973. The theory behind these controls is that it will limit and control inflation—the dramatic increase of wages. However, most economists do not agree that these are useful in controlling inflation and, in fact, they have many unintended consequences.

Waste Unnecessary costs as a result of deficient management, practices, or controls.

References

Chapter 1

Braff, D. (2009, October 26). *Legitimate Work from Home Jobs at WomansDay.com*. Retrieved November 18, 2009, from *Woman's Day* website: www.womansday.com.

Centers for Medicare and Medicaid Services. (2008). *ICD-10: Clinical Modification/Procedure Coding System*. Washington, DC: Government Printing Office.

Coding. (2002). Retrieved November 19, 2009, from *The Free Dictionary* website: http://medical-dictionary.thefreedictionary.com/coding

Dunn, C. (2008). *What Is Medical Coding?* Retrieved November 19, 2009, from easyarticles.com website: www.easyarticles.com

Frequently Asked Questions. (2007). Retrieved November 30, 2009, from National Uniform Claim Committee website: www.nucc.org

Medical Insurance Coding. (2009). Retrieved April 8, 2011, from Medical Insurance Coding website: http://medicalinsurancecoding.org/

Moss, M. (2009). *What Is Medical Billing and Coding?* Retrieved November 19, 2009, from eHow: How to Do Just About Everything website: www.ehow.com

National Center for Health Statistics. (2005, April 1). *ICD-9-CM Official Guidelines for Coding and Reporting*. Retrieved November 25, 2009, from Centers for Disease Control and Prevention website: www.cdc.gov/nchs

National Uniform Claim Committee. (2009). Retrieved November 30, 2009, from National Uniform Claim Committee website: www.nucc.org

Pew Research Center's Project for Excellence in Journalism. (2006). *Principles of Journalism*. Retrieved November 20, 2009, from Journalism.org website: www.journalism.org/resources/principles

Times Reporter Who Resigned Leaves a Long Trail of Deception. (2003, May 11). Retrieved November 20, 2009, from *The New York Times* website: www.nytimes.com

Chapter 2

Barna, G. (2002, July 22). *Americans Speak: Enron, WorldCom and Others Are Result of Inadequate Moral Training by Families*. Retrieved January 6, 2011, from The Barna Group website: www.barna.org

Brown, G., & Sukys, P. (2009). *Business Law with UCC Applications*. New York: McGraw-Hill Irwin.

Ethics and Compliance Officer Association. (2006). *Program Evaluation Survey Report*. Waltham, MA: Ethics and Compliance Officer Association.

Ethisphere Magazine. (2010). 2010 World's Most Ethical Companies. Retrieved January 6, 2011, from *Ethisphere* website: http://ethisphere.com/wme2010/

Fieser, J. (2003, June 29). *Ethics*. Retrieved January 5, 2011, from Internet Encyclopedia of Ethics website: www.iep.utm.edu/ethics/

Frankel, M. (1989). Professional Codes: Why, How, and with What Impact? *Journal of Business Ethics*, 109–115.

Hill, C. W., & McShane, S. L. (2008). *Principles of Management*. New York: McGraw-Hill.

Jones, G., & George, J. (2009). *Contemporary Management*. New York: McGraw-Hill Irwin.

Mallor, J., Barnes, A. J., Bowers, T., & Langvardt, A. (2010). *Business Law: The Ethical Global, and E-Commerce Environment*. New York: McGraw-Hill Irwin.

Maxwell, J. (2003). *There's No Such Thing as "Business" Ethics*. New York: Center Street Publishing.

Chapter 3

American Medical Association. (1999, November). *CPT Assistant*. Chicago: AMA Press.

American Medical Association. (2010). *Current Procedural Terminology 2011—Professional Edition*. Chicago: AMA Press.

Gellerman, S. (1989). Why "Good" Managers Make Bad Ethical Choices. In K. R. Andrews, *Ethics in Practice: Managing the Moral Corporation* (p. 22). Cambridge, MA: Harvard Business Press.

Ghillyer, A. (2010). *Business Ethics: A Real World Approach*. New York: McGraw-Hill Irwin.

Hill, C. W., & McShane, S. L. (2008). *Principles of Management*. New York: McGraw-Hill.

Jones, G., & George, J. (2009). *Contemporary Management*. New York: McGraw-Hill Irwin.

Lewis, C. (2001). *Mere Christianity*. San Francisco: Harper.

Lewis, M. (2002, November 11). *A Dwindling Band of Brothers*. Retrieved February 10, 2011, from Forbes.com website: www.forbes.com/2002/11/11/cx_ml_1111vets.html

Maxwell, J. (2003). *There's No Such Thing as "Business" Ethics*. New York: Center Street Publishing.

Chapter 4

Achenbaum, W. A. (1988). *Social Security: Visions and Revisions: A Twentieth Century Fund Study*. Cambridge, England: Cambridge University Press.

Akin, Gump, Strauss, Hauer & Feld, LLC. (2006, December 18). Winning a False Claim Act Against the Government. *Client Alert*. Washington, DC: Author.

Card, R. F. (2005). Individual Responsibility within Organizational Contexts. *Journal of Business Ethics*, 397–405.

CMS History Quiz. (n.d.). Retrieved October 26, 2009, from Centers for Medicare and Medicaid Services website: www.cms.hhs.gov/History/Downloads/QUIZ08.pdf

Hartocollis, A. (2006, May 14). Out of Prison, Doctor Hopes to Regenerate His Lost Fame. *The New York Times*.

Hinson Neely, M. (2006, January). *Brand New World: Medical Marketing the Business Way*. Retrieved October 28, 2009, from Medical

Group Management Association website: www.mgma.com /article.aspx?print=y&id=310

Klukowski, K. (2009, October 22). *Doctors Stir, Half Asleep.* Retrieved October 28, 2009, from the *Washington Times* website: http://washingtontimes.com/news/2009/oct/23 /doctors-stir-half-asleep/

Lauersen, N. (n.d.). *Home Page.* Retrieved September 2, 2009, from the Niels H. Lauersen, MD, PhD, website: www.nielslauersenmd.org

Medicaid's Milestones. (n.d.). Retrieved October 26, 2009, from Centers for Medicare and Medicaid Services website: www.cms .hhs.gov/History/Downloads/MedicaidMilestones.pdf

Medicare Glossary. (2008, March 27). Retrieved October 28, 2009, from Medicare website: www.medicare.gov/glossary/search.asp? Language=English&SelectAlphabet=L

Merritt Hawkins & Associates. (2008). *Physician Salary, Compensation, and Practice Surveys.* Retrieved October 28, 2009, from Merritt Hawkins & Associates website: www.merritthawkins.com/pdf /2008-mha-survey-primary-care.pdf

Moore, S. (2009, September 22). Obama's Expert on Medicare Fraud. *Wall Street Journal.*

National Coalition on Health Care. (2009, September). *Health Care Facts: Costs.* Retrieved October 28, 2009, from National Coalition on Health Care website: www.nchc.org

Pharmaceutical and Health Insurance Companies Seen in Negative Light by Public, Says New Survey. (2004, July 12–19). *Insurance Advocate,* p. 34.

Preston, J. (2005, February 19). Gynecologist's Sentence Is Reduced. *The New York Times.*

Rockoff, H. (2008). *Price Controls.* Retrieved October 26, 2009, from Library of Economics and Liberty website: http://econlib.org /library/Enc/PriceControls.html

Senterfitt, B. A. (2007, February). False Claim Act Proves Difficult to Fight. *Managed Healthcare Executive,* p. 13.

Shrestha, L. (2006, August 16). *Life Expectancy in the United States.* Retrieved November 2, 2009, from CRS Report for Congress website: http://aging.senate.gov/crs/aging1.pdf

Steinhauer, J. (2000a, August 12). Fertility Doctor Loses License During Review. *New York Times,* p. B6.

Steinhauer, J. (2000b, March 7). Mistrial for Fertility Doctor Accused of Insurance Fraud. *The New York Times,* p. B7.

Steinhauer, J. (2001, January 10). Doctor Convicted of Insurance Fraud in Fertility Procedures. *The New York Times,* p. B1.

Chapter 5

American College of Rheumatology. (2010). *Legislative Action Center—Elimination of Consultation Codes.* Retrieved October 19, 2010, from American College of Rheumatology website: www .rheumatology.org/advocacy/consultation.asp

American Medical Association. (2009). *Current Procedural Terminology (CPT 2010).* Chicago: AMA Press.

American Medical Association. (2010). *Current Professional Terminology (CPT 2011),* 4th ed. Chicago: AMA Press.

Centers for Medicare and Medicaid Services. (n.d.). Retrieved September 21, 2010, from www.cms.hhs.gov

Centers for Medicare and Medicaid Services. (1999, March 4). *1995 Documentation Guidelines for Evaluation and Management Services.*

Retrieved September 21, 2010, from Centers for Medicare and Medicaid Services, Medicare Learning Network website: www .cms.gov/MLNProducts/Downloads/1995dg.pdf

Centers for Medicare and Medicaid Services. (2010a, September 3). *Medicare Learning Network.* Retrieved September 28, 2010, from Centers for Medicare and Medicaid Services website: www.cms .gov/MLNEdWebGuide/25_EMDOC.asp

Centers for Medicare and Medicaid Services. (2010b, September 3). *1997 Documentation Guidelines for Evaluation and Management Services.* Retrieved September 28, 2010, from Centers for Medicare and Medicaid Services website: www.cms.gov/MLNEdWebGuide /25_EMDOC.asp

Cohen, F. (2002). *Projection of Financial Impact of E/M Coding Variances on Family Physicians.* Clearwater, FL: Frank D. Cohen.

Grogan, J. (2011, June 15). *Compensation Greater for Specialty-Care Physicians, Says MGMA.* Retrieved June 27, 2011 from MDNews.com website: www.mdnews.com/news/2011_06 /compensation-greater-for-specialty-care-physicians

Office of Inspector General. (2005, November). *Office of Inspector General Reports.* Retrieved October 18, 2010, from Office of Inspector General, U.S. Department of Health and Human Services website: http://oig.hhs.gov/oei/reports/oei-07-03-00470.pdf

Chapter 6

American College of Emergency Physicians. (2008). *NCCI-CCI FAQs.* Retrieved November 15, 2010, from American College of Emergency Physicians website: www.acep.org/PrintFriendly.aspx?id=48111

American Medical Association. (2009, May). *CPT Category III Codes: The First Ten Years.* Retrieved November 23, 2010, from American Medical Association website: www.ama-assn.org /ama1/pub/upload/mm/362/cat3-codes-first-10-yrs.pdf

American Medical Association. (2010a). *Applying for CPT Codes.* Retrieved November 23, 2010, from American Medical Association website: www.ama-assn.org/ama/pub/physician-resources /solutions-managing-your-practice/coding-billing-insurance/cpt /applying-cpt-codes.shtml

American Medical Association. (2010b). *Current Procedural Terminology (CPT),* 4th ed. Chicago: AMA Press.

Andrews, S. (2009, May). Modifier 59: Five Tips for Effective Use. *Practical Dermatology,* p. 23.

Centers for Medicare and Medicaid Services. (2006, January 1). *Medicare Learning Network.* Retrieved November 15, 2010, from MLN Matters website: www.cms.gov/MLNMattersArticles /downloads/SE0545.pdf

Centers for Medicare and Medicaid Services. (2010). *Medically Unlikely Edits—National Correct Coding.* Retrieved November 15, 2010, from Centers for Medicare and Medicaid Services website: www.cms.gov/NationalCorrectCodInitEd/08_MUE.asp

Harvard Pilgram Health Care. (2009, November). *Unlisted and Unspecified Procedure Codes.* Retrieved November 23, 2010, from Harvard Pilgram Health Care website: https://www.harvardpilgrim .org/pls/portal/docs/page/providers/manuals/payment%20 policies/H-6%20unlisted_unspec%20codes_111509.pdf.

Noridian Administrative Services. (2009). *Modifier 52 and 53 Reimbursement Clarification.* Retrieved November 22, 2010, from Noridian Medicare website: https://www.noridianmedicare .com/provider/updates/docs/Modifier_52_53_Reimburse_ Clarification.pdf%3f

Pharmacist Services Technical Advisory Coalition. (2005, July 7). *Professional Service Billing Codes Approved for Pharmacists.* Alexandria, VA.

Physician Advocacy Institute. (2010). *Welcome to HMO Settlements.* Retrieved November 24, 2010, from HMO Settlements website: www.hmosettlements.com

Witt, M. (2005, January). 4 CPT Gems for 2005. *OBG Management,* 36–41.

WPS Insurance Corporation. (2007, October 10). *Modifier 53 Fact Sheet.* Retrieved November 22, 2010, from WPS Medicare website: www.wpsmedicare.com

Chapter 7

American Congress of Obstetricians and Gynecology. (2010). *The Essential Guide to Coding in Obstetrics and Gynecology.* Washington, DC: Author.

American Medical Association. (1999). *Report of the Council on Medical Service.* Chicago: AMA.

Brittain, A., & Mueller, M. (2010, December 12). N.J. Doctor Supplied Steroids to Hundreds of Law Enforcement Officers, Firefighters. *Newark Star-Ledger,* pp. 1, 7–8.

Buck, C. (2010). *ICD-9-CM Volumes 1 & 2 for Physicians, Professional Edition.* St. Louis, MO: Elsevier Saunders.

Centers for Disease Control and Prevention. (2010, August 9). *Classification of Diseases, Functioning, and Disability.* Retrieved December 15, 2010, from Centers for Disease Control and Prevention website: www.cdc.gov/nchs/icd/icd9cm_addenda_guidelines .htm

Centers for Medicare and Medicaid Services. (2008). *FY 2009 OIG Work Plan.* Washington, DC: Government Printing Office.

Centers for Medicare and Medicaid Services. (2009). *ICD-9-CM Official Guidelines for Coding and Reporting.* Washington, DC: Government Printing Office.

Centers for Medicare and Medicaid Services. (2010a, November 30). *Diagnosis and Procedure Codes: Abbreviated and Full Code Titles.* Retrieved December 15, 2010, from Centers for Medicare and Medicaid Services website: www.cms.gov/ICD9ProviderDiagnosticCodes /06_codes.asp

Centers for Medicare and Medicaid Services. (2010b, January 20). *Glossary.* Retrieved December 7, 2010, from The Official US Government Site for Medicare: www.medicare.gov/glossary/m.html.

Centers for Medicare and Medicaid Services. (2010c, July 20). *Process for Requesting New/Revised ICD-9-CM Procedure Codes.* Retrieved December 2, 2010, from Centers for Medicare and Medicaid Services website: www.cms.gov/ICD9ProviderDiagnosticCodes /02_newrevisedcodes.asp.

Cinquino, S. (2010). Medical Necessity: Is It Reasonable and Necessary? *Coding and Compliance Focus News,* 3–4.

Fraud Prevention. (2010, June 12). *Top 10 Largest False Claims Act Cases.* Retrieved December 11, 2010, from Fraud Prevention website: http://fraudusa.us/1768/top-10-largest-false-claims-act-cases-top-10-largest-fraud-cases-whistleblowers-receive-over-50-million-each/

Mattise, J. (2010, November 26). *Vero Beach Couple Agrees to Settlement in Medicare Claim Case, Denies Fraud Allegations.* Retrieved December 8, 2010, from *Orlando Sentinel* website: www .orlandosentinel.com.

Medical-Billing-Coding.org. (2006, March 24). Retrieved December 11, 2010, from Articles: www.medical-billing-coding.org /NewsArticleDetail1159.htm.

Office of Compliance, Privacy & Internal Audit. (2010). *How to Use the ICD-9 Book.* Retrieved December 3, 2010, from NYU Langone Medical Center website: http://compliance.med .nyu.edu/departments/faculty-group-practice-compliance /physician-office-training/how-use-icd-9-book.

Sindelar, T. (2002). *The "Medical Necessity Requirement" in Medicaid.* Boston: Disability Law Center.

Chapter 8

American Academy of Family Practice. (2011). *ICD-10 Codes for Signs and Symptoms.* Retrieved May 9, 2011, from American Academy of Family Practice website: www.aafp.org/online/etc /medialib/aafp_org/documents/prac_mgt/codingresources /signssymptoms.Par.0001.File.dat/ICD10SignsSymptoms.pdf.

American Medical Association. (2010, June 2). *The Differences Between ICD-9 and ICD-10.* Retrieved May 6, 2011, from American Medical Association website: www.ama-assn.org/ama1/pub /upload/mm/399/icd10-icd9-differences-fact-sheet.pdf.

Barta, A., McNeill, G., Meli, P., Wall, K., & Zeisset, A. (2008, May). *ICD-10-CM Primer.* Retrieved May 6, 2011, from American Health Information Management Association website: http: //library.ahima.org/xpedio/groups/public/documents/ahima /bok1_038084.hcsp?dDocName=bok1_038084.

Conn, J. (2008, August 22). *ICD-10 Estimated to Cost Vendors, Providers Billions.* Retrieved May 6, 2011, from ModernHealthcare .com website: www.modernhealthcare.com/article/20080822 /REG/738760.

Grider, D. (2010). *Preparing for ICD-10-CM: Make the Transition Manageable.* Chicago: AMA Press.

National Committee on Vital and Health Statistics. (2003). *Attachment II: Hearings on ICD-10-CM and ICD-10-PCS Timeline.* Washington, DC: Government Publishing Office.

Chapter 9

American Credit Counseling Service, Inc. (2010, September 23). *Payment Priorities.* Retrieved March 14, 2011, from American Credit Counseling Service website: www.accs.org/PaymentPrior .html

American Medical Association. (2010a). *Current Procedural Terminology,* 4th ed. Chicago: AMA Press.

American Medical Association. (2010b, June 14). *New AMA Health Insurer Report Card Finds Need for More Accuracy.* Retrieved March 12, 2011, from *AMA News* website: www.ama-assn.org /ama/pub/news/news/2010-report-card.shtml

American Medical Association. (2011). *Heal the Claim Process.* Retrieved March 12, 2011, from American Medical Association website: www.ama-assn.org/ama/pub/physician-resources /solutions-managing-your-practice/coding-billing-insurance /heal-claims-process/htc-toolkit.shtml

Centers for Medicare and Medicaid Services. (2011, March 8). *PFS Relative Value Files.* Retrieved March 11, 2011, from Centers for Medicare and Medicaid Services website: www.cms.gov /PhysicianFeeSched/PFSRVF

Chapter 10

American Academy of Professional Coders. (2009, March 9). *AAPC Membership Reaches 75,000*. Retrieved April 12, 2011, from American Academy of Professional Coders website: http://news .aapc.com/index.php/2009/03/aapc-membership-reaches-75000/

American Academy of Professional Coders. (2010, December 15). *2010 Medical Coding Salary Survey*. Retrieved April 22, 2011, from American Academy of Professional Coders website: http://news .aapc.com/index.php/2010/12/2010-salary-survey/

American Academy of Professional Coders. (2011a). *AAPC Code of Ethics*. Retrieved April 23, 2011, from American Academy of Professional Coders website: www.aapc.com/AboutUs/code-of-ethics.aspx

American Academy of Professional Coders. (2011b). *About AAPC*. Retrieved April 12, 2011, from American Academy of Professional Coders website: www.aapc.com/AboutUs/

American Academy of Professional Coders. (2011c). *Certified Interventional Radiology Cardiovascular Coder*. Retrieved April 14, 2011, from American Academy of Professional Coders website: www .aapc.com/certification/circc.aspx

American Academy of Professional Coders. (2011d). *Certified Professional Coder*. Retrieved April 14, 2011, from American Academy of Professional Coders website: www.aapc.com/certification/cpc.aspx

American Academy of Professional Coders. (2011e). *Certified Professional Coder—Hospital*. Retrieved April 14, 2011, from American Academy of Professional Coders website: www.aapc .com/certification/cpc-h.aspx

American Academy of Professional Coders. (2011f). *Certified Professional Coder-Payer*. Retrieved April 14, 2011, from American Academy of Professional Coders website: www.aapc.com /certification/cpc-p.aspx

American Academy of Professional Coders. (2011g). *Specialty Medical Coding Certification*. Retrieved April 14, 2011, from American Academy of Professional Coders website: www.aapc .com/certification/specialty-credentials.aspx

American Health Information Management Association. (2005, August). *Employers Value Credentials in Healthcare*. Retrieved April 21, 2011, from American Health Information Management Association website: www.ahima.org/downloads/pdfs/certification /EmployeeValuesurvey.pdf

American Health Information Management Association. (2011a). *AHIMA Facts*. Retrieved April 20, 2011, from American Health Information Management Association website: www.ahima.org /about/facts.aspx

American Health Information Management Association. (2011b). *AHIMA History*. Retrieved April 20, 2011, from American Health Information Management Association website: www.ahima.org /about/history.aspx

American Health Information Management Association. (2011c). *Committees*. Retrieved April 21, 2011, from American Health Information Management Association website: www.ahima.org /about/committeecharts.aspx

American Health Information Management Association. (2011d). *Component State Association*. Retrieved April 21, 2011, from American Health Information Management Association website: www.ahima.org/about/csa.aspx

American Health Information Management Association. (2011e). *House of Delegates*. Retrieved April 21, 2011, from American Health Information Management Association website: www.ahima.org /about/hod.aspx

American Health Information Management Association Foundation. (2011). *Research and Education in HIM*. Retrieved April 21, 2011, from AHIMA Foundation website: www.ahimafoundation .org/Default.aspx

American Health Information Management Association House of Delegates. (2008, September). *American Health Information Management Association Standards of Ethical Coding*. Retrieved April 23, 2011, from American Health Information Management Association website: http://library.ahima.org/xpedio/groups/public /documents/ahima/bok2_001166.hcsp?dDocName=bok2_001166

Commission on Certification for Health Informatics and Information Management. (2011, January 1). *Candidate Guide*. Retrieved April 20, 2011, from Commission for Certification for Health Informatics and Information Management website: www.ahima .org/downloads/pdfs/certification/Candidate_Guide.pdf

Chapter 11

American Congress of Obstetricians and Gynecologists. (2011). CPT-4 and ICD-9 Coding Workshop 2011. *ACOG Coding Workshop*, p. 88. Washington, DC: Author.

American Medical Association. (2011). *Current Procedural Terminology 2011*. Chicago: AMA Press.

Centers for Medicare and Medicaid Services. (2011, April 18). *EHR Incentive Program Timeline*. Retrieved April 29, 2011, from Centers for Medicare and Medicaid Services website: https://www.cms .gov/ehrincentiveprograms/

Grider, D., Linker, R., Thurston, S., & Levinson, M. S. (2009, April 3). *The Problem with EHRs and Coding*. Retrieved April 27, 2011, from Modern Medicine website: www.modernmedicine.com /modernmedicine/article/articleDetail.jsp?id=590411

Hsiao, C.-H. P., Hing, E., Socey, T., & Cai, B. (2010, December 8). *Electronic Medical Record/Electronic Health Record Systems of Office-Based Physicians: United States, 2009 and Preliminary 2010 State Estimates*. Retrieved April 29, 2011, from Centers for Disease Control and Prevention website: www.cdc.gov/nchs/data/hestat /emr_ehr_09/emr_ehr_09.htm#figures

Kaiser Health Care. (2010, March). *U.S. Health Care Costs*. Retrieved May 2, 2011, from Kaiser Health Care website: www.kaiseredu.org/Issue-Modules/US-Health-Care-Costs /Background-Brief.aspx

U.S. Department of Justice. (2011, March 9). *Statement of Acting Deputy Assistant Attorney General Greg Andres of the Criminal Division Before the Senate Committee on Homeland Security and Governmental Affairs*. Retrieved May 1, 2011, from Justice News website: www.justice.gov/criminal/pr/testimony/2011 /crm-testimony-110309.html

Woodcock, E. (2010). *Understanding the "Meaningful Use" Regulations*. Tampa, FL: Sage Software Healthcare.

Chapter 12

Ghillyer, A. (2010). *Business Ethics: A Real World Approach*. New York: McGraw-Hill Irwin.

Google. (2009, April 8). *Code of Conduct*. Retrieved March 18, 2011, from Google Investor Relations website: http://investor.google .com/corporate/code-of-conduct.html

Institute of Business Ethics. (2011). *Making Codes of Ethics Effective.* Retrieved March 18, 2011, from Institute of Business Ethics website: www.ibe.org.uk/index.asp?upid=76&msid=11

Kansas Department on Aging. (2010). *Definition and Examples of Fraud and Abuse.* Retrieved March 18, 2011, from Senior Health Insurance Counseling for Kansas website: www.aging.state.ks.us /SHICK/Fraud_Abuse/Examples.htm

Mallor, J., Barnes, A. J., Bowers, T., & Langvardt, A. (2010). *Business Law: The Ethical, Global, and E-Commerce Environment.* New York: McGraw-Hill Irwin.

Merck, Inc. (2010). *Code of Conduct.* Retrieved March 18, 2011, from Merck, Inc. website: www.merck.com/about/code_of_conduct.pdf

Ministry Health Care, Inc. (2010). *Mission and Values Statement.* Retrieved March 18, 2011, from Ministry Health Care website: http: //ministryhealth.org/Careers/home/MissionandValuesStatement .nws

Office of Inspector General. (2009). *Avoiding Medicare and Medicaid Fraud and Abuse: A Roadmap for New Physicians.* Retrieved March 17, 2011, from U.S. Department of Health and Human Services Office of Inspector General website: http://oig.hhs.gov/fraud /PhysicianEducation/

Van de Water, P. (1995, July 31). *Fraud, Waste, and Abuse in Medicare.* Retrieved March 18, 2011, from Congressional Budget Office website: www.cbo.gov/doc.cfm?index=5497&type=0

Zaibak, O. (2010, October 13). *20 Customer Service Statistics for 2011.* Retrieved March 25, 2011, from Customer 1 website: www .customer1.com/blog/customer-service-statistics

Chapter 13

Association of Academic Health Centers. (2003). *A Framework for Resolving Ethical Dilemmas in Healthcare.* Retrieved April 5, 2011, from Partnerships for Training, George Washington University Medical Center website: http://learn.gwumc.edu/hscidist /LearningObjects/EthicalDecisionMaking/

Bazerman, M., & Tenbrunsel, A. (2011, April). *Ethical Breakdowns.* Retrieved April 4, 2011, from *Harvard Business Review* website: http://hbr.org/2011/04/ethical-breakdowns/ar/1

Kravis, H. (1991, February 12). Avatar of American Finance.

Loyola Marymount University. (2009). *Resolving an Ethical Dilemma.* Retrieved April 5, 2011, from Loyola Marymount University, Center for Ethics and Business website: www.lmu .edu/Page27945.aspx

Mallor, J., Barnes, A. J., Bowers, T., & Langvardt, A. (2010). *Business Law: The Ethical, Global, and E-Commerce Environment.* New York: McGraw-Hill Irwin.

Maxwell, J. (2003). *There's No Such Thing as Business Ethics.* New York: Center Street.

Office of Inspector General, U.S. Department of Health and Human Services. (2000). OIG Compliance Program for Individual and Small Group Physician Practices. *Federal Register,* 59434–59452.

Williams, R. (2011, April 2). *A Bad Job May Be Worse for Your Wellbeing Than Being Jobless.* Retrieved April 4, 2011, from *Psychology Today* website: www.psychologytoday.com/blog/wired-success /201104/bad-job-may-be-worse-your-wellbeing-being-jobless

Credits

Photo Credits

Chapter 1: **Page 1, 15:** © Ingram Publishing/RF

Chapter 2: **Page 30:** ©Anderson Ross/Blend Images LLC/RF; **35:** © Randy Faris/Corbis/RF

Chapter 3: **Page 70:** © John Feingersh Photography Inc./Blend Images/Getty Images/RF; **84:** © Dream Pictures/Blend Images LLC/RF

Chapter 4: **Page 100:** © Ingram Publishing/RF

Chapter 5: **Page 133:** © Jose Luis Pelaez Inc/Blend Images LLC/RF

Chapter 6: **Page 174:** © Comstock Images/Jupiter Images/RF; **205:** © Image Source/Getty Images/RF

Chapter 7: **Page 221:** © Blend Images/Getty Images/RF; **228, 235:** © Image Source/Veer/RF

Chapter 8: **Page 259:** © Polka Dot Images/Jupiter Images/RF; **264:** © Image Source/Veer/RF

Chapter 9: **Page 283:** © DreamPictures/Pam Ostrow/Blend Images LLC/RF

Chapter 10: **Page 321:** © Plush Studios/Bill Reitzel/Blend Images LLC/RF; **339:** © Image Source/Getty Images/RF

Chapter 11: **Page 348:** © Comstock/Jupiter Images/RF; **357:** © Purestock/Getty Images/RF

Chapter 12: **Page 376:** © Abel Mitja Varela/Getty Images/RF

Chapter 13: **Page 401:** © David Lees/Getty Images/RF; **404:** © David Wasserman/Getty Images/RF; **416:** © Alistar Berg/Getty Images/RF; **420:** © Dave and Les Jacobs/Blend Images LLC/RF

Text and Illustrations

Chapter 1: **Page 11,** Fig. 1.5: American Medical Association. All Rights Reserved.; **12,** Fig. 1.6: American Medical Association. All Rights Reserved.; **14,** Fig. 1.7: American Medical Association. All Rights Reserved.; **16,** Fig. 1.8: American Medical Association. All Rights Reserved.; **18,** Fig. 1.9: American Medical Association. All Rights Reserved.; **19,** Fig. 1.10: American Medical Association. All Rights Reserved.; **20,** Fig. 1.11: American Medical Association. All Rights Reserved.; **21,** Fig. 1.12: American Medical Association. All Rights Reserved.

Chapter 2: **Page 44,** Fig. 2.8: From Ethisphere Magazine, 2010 "2010 World's Most Ethical Companies," http://ethisphere .com/wme2010/. Reprinted with permission.; **49,** Fig. 2.13: From Charles W.L. Hill, Principles of Management 1E. Copyright © 2008. Reprinted with permission of The McGraw-Hill Companies, Inc.; **57,** Fig. 2.18: From Gareth Jones and Jennifer George, Contemporary Management 6E, p. 136. Copyright © 2009. Reprinted with permission of The McGraw-Hill Companies, Inc.

Chapter 8: **Page 268,** Table 8.2: American Medical Association. All Rights Reserved.

Chapter 9: **Page 312,** Fig. 9.17: American Medical Association. All Rights Reserved.; **313,** Fig. 9.19: American Medical Association. All Rights Reserved.

Chapter 11: **Page 364,** Fig. 11.9: From Lauren Alloy, et al., Abnormal Psychology: Current Perspectives 8E. Copyright © 1999. Reprinted with permission of The McGraw-Hill Companies, Inc.; **374,** Fig. 11.12, Reprinted courtesy of eCareSoft, Inc.

Chapter 12: **Page 385,** Fig. 12.7: Reprinted courtesy of Ministry Health Care.; **396,** Fig. 12.11: Reprinted with permission of the Josephson Institute.

Chapter 13: **Page 425,** Fig. 13.5: Reprinted with permission of The Leaders Institute.

Appendix A: AAPC Code of Ethics: Reprinted with permission of AAPC.

Appendix B: AHIMA Code of Ethics: Reprinted with permission of AHIMA.

Appendix C: AHIMA Standards of Ethical Coding: Reprinted with permission of AHIMA.

Index

Metaethics, 33–34, 44
Milgram, Stanley, 125–126
Ministry Health Care System
    (Wisconsin), values statement
    from, 383
Misstating severity of a condition, 247
Mitigation of potential damages, 76
Modern rights theory, 39
Modifiers
  -22, 203–205
  -24, 198–199
  -25, 162–163
  -26, 199–201
  -52, 201–202
  -53, 202–203
  -59, 196–198
  essential, 226
  ethical procedural coding and,
    195–205
  nonessential, 226
Morbidity, 9
Mortality, 9
Multiple diagnosis coding for single
    condition, 234–235
Multiple procedure bundling and
    unbundling, 190–191
Mutually exclusive edits, 194–195

N

Name-calling in health care financing
    debate, 123–124
National Center for Health Statistics
    (NCHS), as cooperating party for
    ICD-9-CM, 224
National Coalition on Health Care, 114
National Correct Coding Initiative
    (NCCI) edits, 192, 324
National Health Insurer Report Card,
    American Medical Association
    introduction of, 311–312
National Provider Identifier (NPI), 11
National Uniform Billing Committee
    (NUBC), 13
National Uniform Claim Committee, 12
New patients
  classification of, 164–165
  CPT requirements to be met or
    exceeded for office or outpatient
    visits, 139
  Medicare Documentation Guideline
    requirements to be met or
    exceeded
    for office or outpatient visits, 140
    for the past, family, and/or social
      history component of office or
      outpatient visits, 146
    for review of systems component
      of office or outpatient visits, 144
  proper coding and, 303–304
1995 Examination Guidelines, 150–152
1997 Examination Guidelines, 152–155
1997 Medicare Documentation
    Guidelines, 157
Nonessential modifiers, 226
Non-participating status, 16

Nonpayment, patient, 303
Normative ethics, 34, 44
Norms, ethical, 36–42
"Not elsewhere classifiable (NEC)" in
    Tabular List, 230
"Not otherwise specified (NOS)" in
    Tabular List, 230

O

Obama, Barack, on physician
    performance of unnecessary
    surgeries, 107
Objectivity, 416–417
Obsolete codes, 7
Obstructionist approach to ethics,
    57–58
Occupational ethics, 50–51
Office visit codes, 136
Open-access health maintenance
    organizations (HMOs), 105
Ophthalmic manifestations, 9
Organizational culture, unethical, 81
Organizational ethics, 51
Organizations, working within, to
    stop unethical actions, 412–414
Outliers, 179
Out-of-network benefits, 105
Outpatient surgery centers, use of
    CPT codes by, 7
Overcoding, 137, 363

P

Parent-child codes, 189–190
Participating status, 16
Participation, refusal of, 406
Past, family, and/or social history
    (PFSH) in E/M services, 146–150
Past history, 146–147
Patient nonpayment, 303
Patient Protection and Affordable
    Care Act (PPACA) (2010),
    367–369
  mandatory compliance programs
    and, 366–370
Patients. See also Established patients;
    New patients
  activities in facility or clinic,
    301–305
  appropriately classifying new and
    established, 164–165
  billing of, for balances due, 294–295
  in coding, 14–16, 112–113
  communication with, 381
  constructing strategies
    communicating with, in avoiding
      ethical problems, 393–396
  encounter at facility or clinic,
    289–290
  ethical challenges driven by, 241
  ethical considerations related to,
    301–303
  ethical issues in registering, 295–301
  expectations of, 112–113
  identity of, 296–297
  insurance coverage of, 297–299

overcommunication with, 395–396
  record management and, 351
  role of, in medical coding, 112–113
Patient statements, ethical issues in,
    313–316
Payers. See also Third-party payers
  patient's insurance coverage and,
    298–299
Pay-for-performance, 264
Payment expectations, 300–301
Peer support group, finding, 411–412
Performance goals, unrealistic, 81–82
Personal business
  conflict between business ethics
    and, 49
  difference between business ethics
    and, 48–49
Personal discipline, developing, 87–88
Personal ethics, 44
  development of standards in, 44–45
  employees with poor, 81
  practical, 46–47
  roots of, 46
Personal integrity, 46–47
Physician offices, use of CPT codes by, 7
Physicians
  choice of diagnosis code, 249
  problem of supply, 102–103
Place of service (POS), 19
  improper reporting of, 20–21
  reimbursement and, 21
Pleasure, effect on ethical decision
    making, 78
Policies
  creating specific, 391–392
  defined, 391
  establishing, before problems occur,
    392–393
Postoperative period in surgical and
    procedural services, 181–185
Postoperative services, proper coding
    and, 305
Power, effect on ethical decision
    making, 78–79
Preauthorization, specialists approval
    of, 105
Preferred provider organizations
    (PPOs), 105
Preoperative services, 177–181
  proper coding and, 305
Prepaid health plans
  hospitals development of, 103
  origin of, 103
Pressure, effect on ethical decision
    making, 77–78
Price controls, 103
Pride, effect on ethical decision
    making, 79
Primary care physicians, approval of
    specialty care, 105
Principal diagnosis, 231
Priorities
  aligning, with values, 88
  effect on ethical decision making,
    79–80

Technical services, differences between professional services and, 124
Technology adoption, history of, in health care, 351–353
Teleological ethics, 40–42
Theft, identity, 296–297
A Theory of Justice (Rawls), 39
There's No Such Thing as Business Ethics (Maxwell), 47, 73, 405–406
Third-party payers, 108
  as ethical challenge of ICD-10-CM, 274–276
  ethical issues in relation to, 308–313
  filing of claims with, 292–293
  intervention of, in payment process, 287
  level of reimbursement for, 116
  in medical coding, 118–120
  in payment process, 287–288
  provider's role in obtaining payment from, 308–311
  in revenue cycle, 311–313
Time
  buying, 411
  ethical dilemmas associated with in code selection, 159
Time value of money, 309
Treatment, distinguishing between diagnosis and, in insurance policies, 391*n*
Truth, simple, 46

U

UB-82, 13
UB-92, 13
Unbundling, 186–195
Undercoding, 137
Unethical behaviors. *See also* Ethical behavior
  allegations of, 380–381
  methods employees can use against unethical behaviors, 407–414
  reasons for continuation of, 82–85
  root and influences of personal, 75–76
  roots of, in business, 80–82
  working within organization to stop, 412–414
Unethical organizational culture, 81
Unintentional unethical acts, 272
Unlisted codes
  ethical choices regarding procedure methods and, 205–214
  purpose and use of, 208–210
Unsecured debt, 314
Unspecified diagnoses, 266
Urgent services, 179–180
"Use additional code" in Tabular List, 227–228
Usual, customary and reasonable (UCR) rates, 103–104
Utilitarianism, 40–41
  traditional, 41

V

Values, 46
  aligning priorities with, 88
  importance of, 75
  instrumental, 46
  intrinsic, 46
Values state, 382–383
V codes, 23, 24
Veil of ignorance, 39*n*
Venues, 11
Virtue ethics, 37–38

W

Wage controls, 103
Waste
  defined, 378
  examples of, 379–380
Weaknesses, knowing, 88
Win-win solutions, finding, 412
Wisdom, 37
"With" in Tabular List, 229
Work Group for Electronic Data Interchange (WEDI), 13
World Health Organization (WHO), 9
  ninth revision of the International Classification of Diseases (ICD-9), 222–223
Wrongdoing, admitting, 88